CANCER CARE FOR ADOLESCENTS AND YOUNG ADULTS

Books of Interest

Cancer and the Adolescent (Second Edition)
Edited by Tim Eden, Ronald Barr, Archie Bleyer and Myrna Whiteson
9780727918109

Cancer in Children and Young People
Faith Gibson and Louise Soanes
9780470058671

Cancer Nursing (Second Edition)
Edited by Jessica Corner and Christopher Bailey
9781405122535

Evidence-Based Palliative Care
Huda Huijer Abu-Saad
9780632058181

CANCER CARE FOR ADOLESCENTS AND YOUNG ADULTS

Editors

Dr Daniel Kelly
Reader in Cancer and Palliative Care
School of Health and Social Science,
Middlesex University,
London

Dr Faith Gibson
Senior Lecturer in Children's Cancer Nursing Research,
UCL Institute of Child Health
and Great Ormond Street Hospital for Children NHS Trust,
London

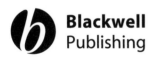

Blackwell
Publishing

Blackwell Publishing editorial offices:
Blackwell Publishing Ltd, 9600 Garsington Road, Oxford OX4 2DQ, UK
  Tel: +44 (0)1865 776868
Blackwell Publishing Inc., 350 Main Street, Malden, MA 02148–5020, USA
  Tel: +1 781 388 8250
Blackwell Publishing Asia Pty Ltd, 550 Swanston Street, Carlton, Victoria 3053, Australia
  Tel: +61 (0)3 8359 1011

First published 2008 by Blackwell Publishing Ltd

ISBN: 9781405130943

Library of Congress Cataloging-in-Publication Data
Cancer care for adolescents and young adults / editors, Daniel Kelly, Faith Gibson.
    p. ; cm.
  Includes bibliographical references and index.
  ISBN-13: 978-1-4051-3094-3 (pbk. : alk. paper)
  ISBN-10: 1-4051-3094-6 (pbk. : alk. paper)   1. Cancer in adolescence.   2. Cancer in
adolescence—Patients—Care.   I. Kelly, Daniel, 1959–   II. Gibson, Faith, 1960–
  [DNLM: 1. Neoplasms—psychology.   2. Adolescent.   3. Quality of Life. QZ
275 C2148 2008]

RC281.C4C347 2008
616.99′400835—dc22
2007027069

A catalogue record for this title is available from the British Library

Set in 10/12.5pt Palatino by Graphicraft Limited, Hong Kong
Printed and bound in Singapore by Utopia Press Pte Ltd

The publisher's policy is to use permanent paper from mills that operate a sustainable forestry
policy, and which has been manufactured from pulp processed using acid-free and elementary
chlorine-free practices. Furthermore, the publisher ensures that the text paper and cover board
used have met acceptable environmental accreditation standards.

For further information on Blackwell Publishing, visit our website:
www.blackwellpublishing.com/nursing

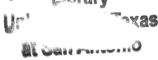

Contents

Contributors

Julia Arbuckle, social worker, Children's Rights Office, Edinburgh, UK.

Maggie Bissett, nurse consultant in palliative care, Camden and Islington Primary Care Trust/University College London Hospitals, London, UK.

Professor Tim Eden, Teenage Cancer Trust Chair of Paediatric Oncology and honorary consultant paediatric haematologist and oncologist, Christie Hospital NHS Trust and Central Manchester and Manchester Children's University Hospitals Trust, Manchester, UK.

Debra Eshelman, certified paediatric nurse practitioner, Children's Medical Centre Dallas, Centre for Cancer and Blood Disorders, Dallas, Texas, USA.

Dr Lorna Fern, research development coordinator, National Cancer Research Institute Teenagers and Young Adult Clinical Studies Development Group, University College London Hospitals NHS Trust, London, UK.

Alison Finch, ward sister, Haemato-Oncology Unit, University College London Hospitals NHS Trust, London, UK.

Dr Faith Gibson, senior lecturer in children's cancer nursing research, UCL Institute of Child Health/Great Ormond Street Hospital NHS Trust, London, UK.

Dr Anne Grinyer, senior lecturer in health research, Institute for Health Research, Lancaster University, UK.

J. Neale Harvey, divisional nurse director, Rare Cancers Division The Royal Marsden Hospital NHS Foundation Trust, London, UK.

Sue Hutton, clinical services manager, Palliative Care Department, Camden Primary Care Trust/University College London Hospitals, London, UK.

Dr Daniel Kelly, reader in cancer and palliative care, School of Health and Social Science, Middlesex University, London, UK.

Dr Nelia Langeveld, research nurse, Academic Medical Centre, Department of Paediatric Oncology, University of Amsterdam, The Netherlands.

Dr Gill Levitt, consultant in oncology and late effects, Great Ormond Street Hospital for Sick Children NHS Trust, London, UK.

Susie Pearce, formerly clinical nurse specialist (practice development and research), University College London Hospitals NHS Trust, now independent consultant in Health and Wellbeing, London, UK.

Dr Jeremy Whelan, consultant medical oncologist, University College Hospital NHS Trust, London, UK.

Dr Roberta Woodgate, associate professor, Helen Glass Centre, University of Manitoba, Winnipeg, Canada.

Young people

Kelly Denver, Leicester, UK.

Rebecca Lofts, East Sussex, UK.

Dr Alan Pitcairn, Linlithgow, UK.

Foreword

One of the most remarkable medical stories of the last 40 years has been the success in improving survival for children with cancer and leukaemia from little expectation to 75–80% cure rates. There has until recently been lack of focus on teenagers and young adults (TYA), who have been described as 'The Forgotten Tribe'. Yet the UK incidence figures show a progressive rise from 10.1 per 100,000 population for 12–14 year olds to 14.4 for those aged 15–19 years and 22.6 for 20–24 year olds, and these cancers account for 11% of deaths in this age range. The first challenge has been to define the incidence figures and what type of tumours occur in this age range. The patterns seen provide clues to causation which require more in depth investigation.

Care issues have focused on the challenges which face young people, their families and their professional carers. It is a common perception that young people are slow or poor at accessing all health care, but especially do delay in seeking help for worrying signs or symptoms. Furthermore that they are non compliant or non adherent with treatment and they are reported to be reluctant to enter into clinical trials. Evidence is accumulating that for some young people there are issues well spelt out in this book relating to health care access and of risk taking with their health. However much diagnostic delay, low clinical trial entry rates and lack of adherence can be laid fairly and squarely at the door of the professions, with doctors not recognising or trivialising symptoms/signs, not listening to, misinterpreting or communicating badly with their young patients and deciding a young person does not know his or her own will and choice is denied. Repeatedly in studies young people say that far too often professionals talk to their parents but not to them, ignoring the fact that most often they can give very valid consent. All of these issues are well covered in excellent chapters especially the challenges facing us all as we transit from childhood to adult life.

We will not achieve the goals of optimising care, curing adolescent cancer and ensuring good quality of life after treatment if we don't listen to our patients and recognise the need for excellence in supportive care, the challenges of treatment and provide support to rebuild the future. Accessing the voice of young people is a critical component of that and most welcome from my perspective in this book are the very insightful experiences from the young people. Rebecca Lofts describes no medical delays but nevertheless the far from straight forward pathway to diagnosis, the frightening nature of so many investigations and not knowing 'what is going on'. This is especially hard when you have been previously healthy, and fit and you know nothing about hospitals and doctors. Kelly Denver shares her thoughts on treatment, and when you may as a patient seem to be coping admirably but inside are suffering. We often mistake stoicism for there being no problems. What she describes could be resolved by common sense explanation and better observation and understanding of the patient's pathway. She does emphasise the importance of the place of care. This message is clearly evident from Anne Grinyer's research. Finally Alan Pitcairn relates life after treatment and trying to re-enter normal life. It is not easy. Despite having not faced too many crises or recurrence he still has felt that he has lost three years of his life which is difficult to get back. For that sort of limbo, professionals must find a way to help.

The topics of the chapters are well chosen and beautifully written by quite clearly dedicated and experienced professionals. The challenges before us are highlighted by the young people. It is an excellent book. It is a 'must' for all professionals who wish to work with young people who have acquired cancer, but also an essential read for health care workers who might be sceptical about the needs of young people to have dedicated services. Many patients and families themselves would find the book very helpful. The voice of young people and their advocates does appear at last starting to be heard and this book makes an invaluable contribution to that exercise.

Professor Tim Eden

Introduction

Daniel Kelly and Faith Gibson

Improving our understanding of the impact of a cancer diagnosis during adolescence and young adulthood is the aim of this book. Colleagues with experience of caring for young people with cancer have generously agreed to share their considerable knowledge and experience. We felt that such a book was needed as the debate continues about the inequalities facing different groups of cancer patients – including those in the earliest years of adulthood. More emphasis is being placed on this age group, such as the need for improved cure rates that can match the improvements already achieved in childhood cancer.

Three young people with personal experience of having survived cancer have added their voices to the book. The final chapter also includes the views of parents, young people, and colleagues. These strategies reflect our goal of making the book as inclusive and relevant to those who may wish to use it, namely health professionals from a range of disciplines, parents, teachers, and young people themselves.

The book is divided into three sections. The first is broadly concerned with 'life before cancer' and its impact on the young person and their family and friends. The second section focuses on the treatment phase and the importance of appropriate supportive care strategies, as well as the challenges facing professionals caring for this unique population. The final section is concerned with 'life beyond cancer', whether the outcome is recovery or appropriate end of life care.

Throughout the book there is an emphasis on the unique nature of this age group and the extra burdens they will face when diagnosed with cancer. A recurring message is the importance placed on the 'cognitive tasks' associated with this phase of the human life course, such as individual identity formation, as well as rebellion, separation from parents, close identification with peer groups, and allegiance to the cultural symbols of difference such as fashion and music. For young adults who have experienced cancer there are additional challenges associated with establishing a career, sustaining intimate relationships, and achieving other life goals.

Most of us can probably recall aspects of our own adolescence and the impact that memorable events played in shaping our present values, lifestyle, and personalities. It is a time of immense awareness of the developing sense of self – both in a physical and emotional sense – but also of increasing awareness of the wider world and the excitement of becoming an independent individual within it. It has been said that the human species is unique in having such a long lead in to adulthood via childhood and adolescence, although it has also been claimed that adolescence is now changing, with girls, in particular, maturing earlier. Despite this, it remains a phase of human existence characterised by intense physical growth and emotional and social development. Striving to separate or rebel against parental/authority figures is balanced by the need to be accepted by members of one's peer group. Image matters. Usually the process allows a transition into early adulthood with personal values and preferences intact – and with the experiences of education, employment, and relationships leading to a degree of social responsibility in early adulthood. The time between 12 and 24 years of age is uniquely challenging: these years are certainly emotionally charged (as any parents will tell you!), yet they are also full of excitement, possibility, and wonder.

However, this life phase is increasingly been presented as 'problematic', with rebellious behaviours leading to young people being seen as disruptive and, occasionally, even dangerous or threatening. Recent gang murders in some urban centres in the UK exemplify the threat associated with some young people, who not only seek to challenge authority symbols in everyday contexts, but also in more tragically violent ways. Those seeking to restore order struggle to confront the adolescent's desire to flout the rules (by carrying illegal drugs or knives) without alienating them entirely. There may be parallels in clinical situations where authority figures are also challenged by adolescents, while simultaneously being expected to provide help and emotional support in times of crisis. It is challenging and skilled work.

The phrase 'youth is wasted on the young' reflects the yearnings of an older generation for what is usually a carefree time before the demands of adulthood. Antagonism may be directed towards those able to enjoy the freedom associated with life without the constraints of responsibility and adulthood. Since the 1950s adolescence has become more than a chronological phase of the human life course. Teenagers have gradually secured a place in the consciousness of Western culture, provoking feelings of envy, fear, ridicule, and bewilderment by members of adult society. Music, fashion, and 'antisocial' behaviours are usually the tools used for challenging the *status quo* and, to varying degrees, they usually succeed.

Each generation reacts as the taboos are challenged and rules are bent and then broken by the young. If adolescence and young adulthood are marked by acts of separation and rebellion, then the sudden introduction of cancer into the frame is particularly traumatic – bringing in its wake more sombre concerns of hospitals, sickness, dependence, and even the threat of death. Cancer has few positive associations, especially in adolescence. For those seeking to be 'one of the crowd' cancer singles them out as different, even special, but certainly destined for a unique adolescence. It is the nature of this difference that we explore in these pages.

The fact that cancer occurs in these age groups is a reality. However, little attention has been paid to the nature of the services needed to help young people and those closest to them in coping with cancer. The aim of this book is to add to the process of debate and understanding by drawing on the experience of colleagues who have cared for adolescents and young adults with cancer. We are grateful to them all for their contributions, and trust that their wisdom will serve young people well. For professionals, there is much still to think about. A case has to be made to secure the resources and the evidence needed to enhance the care of young people with cancer further. We hope this book contributes to this process, as well as providing guidance for those involved in the challenging but immensely rewarding work of caring for adolescents and young adults with cancer.

A Young Person's Experience 1
Life Before Treatment

Rebecca Lofts

I had always been a relatively healthy child, and my parents had no reason to be concerned about my health during my childhood. I was very active and was involved a great deal with sports at school. In fact, just 5 days prior to my diagnosis I had taken part in the high jump and 800 m at my local county games, which is why I still find it hard to comprehend I had such a large 'aggressive' tumour growing inside my spine.

When you tell people you have had cancer as a teenager the first thing they ask is how I found out that I had cancer. At the time I thought I felt well and did not notice my health slowly deteriorating. In retrospect, I was more lethargic than usual, my appetite had slowly decreased, and I had steadily been losing weight. I was always very slim, but at my time of diagnosis, when I was 14 years old, I was 168 cm tall and weighed only 44 kg. We had put this down to the sports I had taken up.

My initial onset of symptoms happened quickly, over 3–4 days. It started with feeling weak and my legs became shaky and unsteady. On my way into a class at school my legs suddenly gave way and I fell to the floor and could not move my legs. They felt heavy and I had a strange sensation, similar to that of pins and needles. My tutor thought I was just playing around and ordered me to stand up – despite my telling her I could not move my legs. During the next 20 minutes my legs came back to life, but during the day they continued to give way randomly.

That night as I lay in bed the pins and needles feeling returned, this time accompanied by a sharp pain running down my legs. My legs became restless and spasmed uncontrollably. The pain was excruciating and continued to get worse – shooting from my back to my legs. I was literally crawling up the walls with pain. The only thing that relieved it was moving around, which was hard work as my legs were so weak.

During the next day the pain and peculiar tingly feeling subsided, although the weakness and giving way remained. I got ready for bed and, as I lay down, I felt a huge pressure on my lower back and the pain began again. My mother wanted to take me to hospital but I insisted that I would be fine. I spent another night in agony and without any sleep. My mother called the telephone advice service NHS Direct for advice and to ask whether an ambulance should be called. They told her that my symptoms did not match any known illness and that I was probably having problems at school and wanted time off! However, my mother knew that this was not the case.

The next morning, when I felt strong enough, we went to my general practitioner (GP), by which time I could no longer feel areas of my legs at all. I was also extremely weak. My GP did a pin test on my legs and sent me straight to the accident and emergency unit of our local hospital with a letter requesting an immediate magnetic resonance imaging (MRI) scan.

The MRI scan was extremely difficult, as I could not lie still: lying on my back was the main cause of pain and made my legs go into spasm. At this point I had not even started to think about what could be wrong. All I could think about was the pain. As the table of the MRI machine moved down I noticed only one technician in the control room. The next time I looked there were at least five doctors in there: some were looking at the MRI computer screen while others were staring at me with blank expressions. I will never forget that moment, as that was when I realised something was seriously wrong.

After a long wait on a trolley in the corridor of the accident and emergency department the doctors returned and asked to see my mother. They began to explain that something abnormal had been found on the scan. My mother asked if they would explain what they had found to both of us, rather then her alone, as she knew that was what I would have wanted. It was explained to us that there was a 'shadow' on the scan: it was inside the vertebrae of my lumbar spine L3, L4, and L5. It was putting pressure on my spinal cord and this was what was causing all the numbness and pain. For the next 3 weeks I was in a state of shock. I was taken straight to a London hospital by ambulance. The seriousness of the situation was reaffirmed by the fact there was not even enough time for us to go home and pack our bags for the stay.

When I arrived at the hospital, where two different registrars saw me, I was given morphine, but this provided little relief from the pain. I spent another night awake in agony. The next morning I had further pin tests, reflex tests, and numerous other examinations. I was then taken for another MRI scan, but I could not keep my legs still and had to be sedated so that a clear image of my spine could be obtained. When I came round my mother and the doctors were there waiting and they explained what had been found. This was the first time the word 'tumour' was used. It seems silly but I had not even thought what they had meant by 'a shadow' on the first scan. I had just gone along with events around me and did not feel I had time to think or question what was happening. I was told that they were unable to say what kind of tumour it was until they operated and examined it more closely.

I met my surgeon a short while later and he explained the procedure to me – including the possible risks. However, I knew in my heart that I did not really have a choice. At this point I was not really scared. I just wanted the pain to stop and did not give the operation a second thought – it was just something that had to be done.

I had to wait until the following day before the operation, so I asked if I could have access to a laptop. I decided I wanted to know as much as I could about this illness and what was causing so much pain. This helped me to understand my body and made me feel more at ease about the situation. It was as though taking the mystery away from 'my enemy' made it easier to fight and I was determined to win!

I went in to the operation without any fear at all. It was a very strange situation to be in. I was more worried about how everyone was going to cope without me for 11 hours! All I can remember was feeling hopeful and excited by the prospect that, when I awoke, I would not be in pain any more.

The week or so after the operation was a blur. I was on so many painkillers that I did not function normally for some time. I remember being unable to move my legs and lying flat on my back for a number of days. Things slowly became clearer and, after being in intensive care for nearly 2 weeks, I was moved into a side room. By this point I had not even thought about whether I had cancer. This may sound very naive, but I am not even sure it had even been mentioned by that time. I was simply in too much pain. When you are in such a state of shock I think you tend to choose to hear what you want to hear – and no one wants to hear the word cancer.

As the nights passed I had more time to think and began to accept what was happening and the possibility that I could actually have cancer. I had asked on several occasions if my biopsy results were back: however, one night I could not sleep so I asked for the registrar on call, who came and spoke to me. My mother and I sat on my bed and, as the registrar began to sit down, I said 'It's cancer, isn't it?' She took my hand and said that they could not be certain, but that it did look that way. They would know more, however, when the results came through. That was the first time since I had become ill that I cried, and also the last time for over a year, until I finished my treatment. It was not because I felt scared or angry, but because I felt an enormous sense of relief! I felt that I now knew what I was dealing with and that I could start forming 'a game plan', as it were. That night I had the most peaceful night's sleep in over 3 weeks. I felt at peace with my body.

Over the next week I saw a physiotherapist, who began to help me get back on my feet. My legs were still very weak, but each day I managed to walk a little further. The results came through and it was explained to me that I had a Ewing's sarcoma. Of course I got straight back on the Internet to find out what I was dealing with. I had the different kinds of treatment open to me explained and I agreed that I wanted to go ahead. I was referred to a specialist cancer hospital in London, but before that all began I was given 2 weeks' respite.

Everyone at the hospitals where I was diagnosed and treated was amazing. I owe my life to them all. I cannot fault my care during the time of diagnosis, and my surgeon was an exceptional man. I have do doubt that, without the quick actions of both himself and my GP, I would not be here today. My GP knew instantly that he was dealing with something serious and he took the correct action. He was calm and reassuring and was involved throughout my diagnosis, making sure that the best care was taken of me. He continues to be a pillar of support for me.

Chapter 1

Cancer in Adolescence: Incidence and Policy Issues

Jeremy Whelan and Lorna Fern

Introduction

There is a growing acknowledgement that teenagers with cancer are caught between two worlds: the world of childhood that they are outgrowing and adulthood, a world for which they are preparing and aspire to, but one which they have not yet reached. Nowhere is this contrast more apparent than when they come into contact with healthcare services. The special needs of young people with cancer have attracted increasing attention, particularly over the past 10 years in the UK. More focused epidemiological data and a growing body of evidence relating to the differing outcomes of treatment, which frequently affect young people adversely, have assisted this debate. Health policy initiatives in the UK are now beginning to reflect this new information. Here we describe the epidemiology of cancer occurring in teenagers and young adults (TYAs) and outline relevant developments in health policy.

Incidence of cancer in young people

Cancer arising in TYAs is a rare occurrence, accounting for less than 2% of all cancers in the USA and less than 1% in Europe (Birch *et al.*, 2003; Bleyer *et al.*, 2006). Nevertheless, within the UK cancer accounts for 11% of deaths within this cohort, making cancer the second most frequent cause of death in young people aged 15–24 years, preceded only by accidental death. Despite this, research into cancer within this group remains scarce. Consequently, the risk factors, aetiology, and, indeed, the optimal treatments for many tumours remain poorly defined. However, what is clear from analysis of both European and American data is that cancer arising in 15–24 year olds represents a heterogeneous group of malignancies with a unique distribution of tumour types that is replicated in no other age group. When this is combined with the psychosocial and emotional needs of TYAs, delivering high-quality cancer care is exceptionally challenging.

The International Classification of Diseases system and its derivative for childhood cancer describe tumours by the primary anatomical site (Percy *et al.*, 2002). This is routinely used for describing and classifying adult tumours, but is being recognised as insufficient for grouping tumours within TYAs usefully. In light of this, Birch *et al.* (2002) proposed an alternative classification based on the morphology for patients aged 15–24 years that more accurately describes a tumour type. When applying this coding system to TYA cancers, the unique spectrum of malignancies occurring in this age group becomes apparent.

Types of cancer affecting TYAs

Tumours found frequently in childhood, particularly those derived from embryonic tissues, become less common in the TYA cohort. Similarly, common epithelial tumours arising in adulthood are not as prevalent in the TYA age group, but do first become apparent at very low frequencies in this age group. As such, TYA tumours can be classified as belonging to one of three categories. The first two are those that typically arise in children and represent the tail end of these tumours, i.e. 'late paediatric' and those typically arising in adults, which can be viewed as 'early onset adult' cancers. The third group is comprised of true 'TYA cancers', demonstrating a peak incidence between 13 and 24 years of age (Birch, 2006). True TYA tumours include nodular sclerosis Hodgkin's lymphoma, osteosarcoma, Ewing's sarcoma, certain soft tissue sarcomas such as alveolar soft part sarcoma, and gonadal germ cell tumours encompassing testicular, ovarian, and intracranial germ cell tumours (Birch *et al.*, 2003; Bleyer *et al.*, 2006; Stiller *et al.*, 2006a). Examples of solid tumours occurring in TYAs are shown in Table 1.1. Tumours of the central nervous system (CNS) occur across all these age ranges, although there is a change in subtype. Leukaemias also occur across all age ranges but the frequency declines with advancing age: for patients between 13 and 14 years 22% of cancers will be leukaemias, whereas this falls to just 7.7% of cancers in patients between 20 and 24 years (Birch, 2005).

Whilst 60% of tumours arising in TYAs are early onset adult tumours, the distribution of tumour types is markedly different from that found in adults. Carcinomas of the lung, breast, colon, rectum, and bladder, which account for 50% of all cancers, are rare in the TYA cohort, accounting for only 2% of malignancies

Table 1.1   Spectrum of solid tumour subtypes occurring in TYAs

TYA tumour	Example
'Late paediatric' (predominately embryonal)	Wilms' tumour, rhabdomysarcoma, and neuroblastoma
'True TYA tumours'	Ewing's sarcoma, osteosarcoma, germ cell, some rare soft tissue sarcomas (alveolar soft-part sarcoma), and Hodgkin's lymphoma
'Early onset' carcinomas	Melanoma, thyroid, and nasopharyngeal

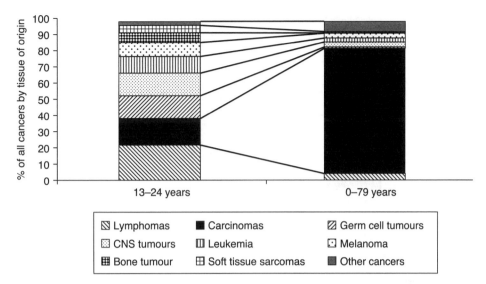

Fig. 1.1 The tumour distribution in TYAs is unique and is not replicated in any other age group (J. M. Birch, unpublished data, reproduced with the authors' permission)

in patients aged between 15 and 24 years (Birch *et al.*, 2003; Birch, 2005; Bleyer *et al.*, 2006; Stiller *et al.*, 2006b).

The tumour distributions arising in TYAs are unique compared with those found in any other age group: Fig. 1.1 illustrates the striking difference between tumours arising in all ages (0–79 years) compared to those arising between the ages of 13 and 24 years (J. M. Birch, unpublished data). The distributions of tumour types found in TYAs are different from those found in both adult and paediatric cancers; furthermore, the frequency of tumour types within the TYA cohort also changes with increasing age, so that the distribution of a tumour type found at the lowest age (13–14 years) does not resemble the tumour distribution in older patients (20–24 years). This is illustrated in Fig. 1.2 using data from cancers in young people aged 13–24 years in England between 1979–2000 (Birch, 2005). As discussed previously, approximately 22.6% of cancers diagnosed in the 13–24 years age group are leukaemias, but this represents just 7.7% of tumours in the 20–24 years cohort: the most frequently diagnosed tumours in this group are lymphomas, which account for 24% of tumours, followed by carcinomas, which represent 21.1% of cancers.

Adolescent cancer incidence in England

The cancer incidence in children is well described, both nationally and internationally. Despite an increased incidence of cancer in TYAs compared to children, large-scale data on cancer incidence and survival in adolescents have been less often described.

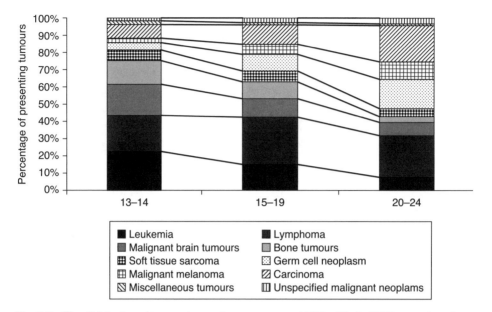

Fig. 1.2 The distribution of tumour types changes amongst TYAs (Birch, 2005, reproduced with the author's permission)

Birch *et al.* (2002, 2003) applied a morphology-based classification to a cohort of young people diagnosed with cancer between 1979 and 1997 using cancer registration data from the UK Office of National Statistics. This classification grouped the various malignancies into ten main groups with several subdivisions. The largest diagnostic group was lymphomas, accounting for 25.5% of the total incidence (the age-standardised incidence in 1979–1997 was 46.7 per million years at risk) including Hodgkin's disease (18.5%) and non-Hodgkin's lymphoma (7.0%). This group was followed by carcinomas (17.1% with age-standardised risk (ASR) 30.5), germ cell tumours (13.8% with ASR 24.5), leukaemia (10.7% with ASR 20.2), CNS tumours (8.9% with ASR 16.5), melanomas (8.4% with ASR 15.0), bone tumours (5.7% with ASR 10.8), and soft tissue sarcomas (5.4% with ASR 9.9).

The overall incidence rates for 12–24 year olds, 15–19 year olds, and 20–24 year olds between 1979 and 1997 were 101, 144, and 226 per million person years, respectively (Birch *et al.*, 2003). These reports also showed an increased incidence over the 20-year study period in all cancers. The cancers accounting for this increase included acute myeloid leukaemia, non-Hodgkin's lymphoma, certain CNS tumours, and, in particular, melanomas, gonadal germ cell tumours, and thyroid cancer.

Adolescent cancer incidence in Europe

Stiller *et al.* (2006a) recently reported the largest review of cancer incidence in adolescents across Europe. This large-scale analysis was carried out using the

Automated Childhood Cancer Information System (ACCIS). The ACCIS is an initiative between European cancer registries that aims to collect and analyse data on the cancer incidence in children and adolescents in Europe (Steliarova-Foucher *et al.*, 2004). The database contains data from 78 population-based cancer registries that cover approximately 50% of the population aged 0–14 years and about 25% of the population aged 15–19 years living in the 35 participating countries. It covers 1.3 billion person years, giving rise to over 160 000 cases of childhood and adolescent cancer being diagnosed during the period 1968–2001 (Sankila *et al.*, 2006). The geographical regions of Europe were grouped according to socio-economic characteristics and data availability. For the purpose of this analysis, Northern Europe was grouped to include Denmark, Finland, Iceland, and Norway, Southern Europe was grouped to include Italy, Malta, Slovenia, Spain, and Turkey, Eastern Europe was grouped to include Belarus, Estonia, Hungary, Slovakia, and parts of Germany, and Western Europe was grouped to include France, Germany, the Netherlands, and Switzerland, while the British Isles included Ireland (national) and the UK. For more geographical details included in this analysis the reader is referred to the paper by Stiller *et al.* (2006a).

Data on 15 399 adolescents (15–19 years) diagnosed with cancer during 1978 and 1997 were reported. The incidence cancer in the 15–19-year-old cohort across Europe was uniformly greater than that in children. The total incidence of cancer in this group was 186 per million, which compares to 138.5 per million from a similar analysis carried out using the ACCIS on children less than 15 years old (Stiller *et al.*, 2006a,b). The rates of cancer in 15–19 year olds within Europe were less than those reported in the USA: using 1975–2000 US SEER data the incidence of invasive cancer was reported to be 203 per million for 15–19 year olds, while the incidence in children was similar to that reported in Europe at 147.3 per million (Bleyer *et al.*, 2006). The disparity, in the incidence rates in patients of 15–19 years between the USA and Europe is likely to be due to differences in the completeness of TYA cancer registration, in that the current European analysis only covers 25% of the population aged 15–19 years in the 35 participating countries in the ACCIS.

Geographical variation is apparent across Europe, with the incidence ranging from 169 per million in the east to 210 per million in the north (Stiller *et al.*, 2006a). This fluctuation may not be attributed to true differences in incidence and may be a result of different registration policies, for example some registries including non-malignant CNS tumours. Further, during this analysis large areas of Europe were not covered and so the adolescent figures are less accurate than those reported for children. As such, the actual incidence of cancer in adolescents in Europe is likely to be higher. Further studies of geographical variation may provide some clues to the aetiology of cancer in this age group.

Incidence data for young adults, say 20–24 years, were missing from this large-scale analysis, further highlighting the lack of recognition in cancer within this cohort. However, other studies of data from the UK and USA suggest that the incidence in the 20–24 years groups is almost double that in children. Figure 1.3 shows the increasing incidence across age groups in the USA and England.

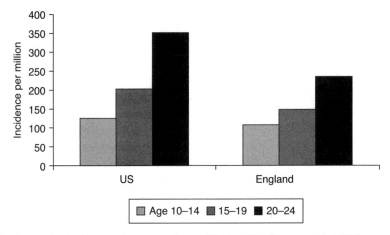

Fig. 1.3   Increasing incidence of cancer with age (Birch, 2005; Bleyer *et al.*, 2006).

Birch (2005) reported that, between 1979 and 2000 in England, the incidence of cancer in children aged between 13 and 14 years was 107 per million: this rose to 235 per million for those aged 20–24 years. Similarly, in the USA cancer in those aged 10–14 years was 125 per million and steadily increased to reach 352 per million in people aged 20–24 years (Birch, 2005; Bleyer *et al.*, 2006). These data would support further efforts to persuade healthcare providers, researchers, the pharmaceutical industry, and policy makers to extend their focus beyond children's cancer.

The distribution of tumours arising in adolescents is similar between the USA and Europe. Throughout Europe the most frequently diagnosed cancer amongst patients aged 15–19 years are lymphomas, which account for 24.6% of diagnoses, which is similar to the USA where lymphomas account for 26% of all invasive cancers occurring between the ages of 15 and 29 years (O'Leary *et al.*, 2006; Stiller *et al.*, 2006a).

Changes in incidence in Europe

Supporting the report from Birch (2005) on English data, there is now evidence that the incidence of cancer in teenagers elsewhere in Europe and the USA is increasing. In the analysis by Stiller *et al.* (2006a) the overall rate of cancer in the 15–19 years age group increased by 2% per year during 1978–1997. While the focus of research and development remains with paediatric and adult oncology, the increase in the incidence of childhood cancer across Europe during 1978–1997 was found to be less than that of the TYA cohort at 1.1% per year (Kaatsch *et al.*, 2006). Melanomas, Hodgkin's lymphoma, and testicular cancer have demonstrated the greatest annual increases at 4.1%, 3.5%, and 2.5%, respectively (Stiller *et al.*, 2006a). Inadequacies in TYA cancer registration have been proposed, so it is possible that the actual increase is higher. Recent analysis carried out in the north of England demonstrated that, between 1968 and 1972, the rate of cancer in the 15–24 years age group increased from 161 per million to 202 per million in 1993–1997 (Pearce *et al.*, 2005). Within this study significant increases were observed in bone tumours, testicular tumours, and malignant melanomas, although it also appears that the incidence rate for some of these cancers such as Hodgkin's disease, Ewing's sarcoma, melanomas, and carcinomas may now be stabilising in the north of England, similar to data produced in the USA (Bleyer *et al.*, 2006). The highest increased incidence was observed for testicular cancers, in keeping with most industrialised nations, suggesting an environmental role in transformation (Huyghe *et al.*, 2003).

Gender differences

There are gender-specific differences apparent in TYA tumours. Throughout Europe, the incidence of cancer in TYA males was 1.2 times that among females between 1978 and 1997 (Stiller *et al.*, 2006a). There exists an unequal sex distribution in acute lymphoblastic leukaemia (ALL), non-Hodgkin's lymphoma (NHL), bone tumours, and brain tumours, which are all more common in males, while carcinoma of the thyroid and melanomas are more common in females (Birch, 2005).

Changes in the male:female ratio with age implies developmental changes in the body to be casually related to the development of these cancers. Evidence for this is suggested by a reversal in the ratio of Ewing's sarcoma and osteosarcoma. The male:female ratio of both osteosarcoma and Ewing's sarcoma demonstrates an excess in females aged 13–14 years; this changes to an excess in males aged 20–24 years (Birch, 2005). This change in the male:female ratio with time mirrors the lag of onset of puberty/maturation in males compared to females and suggests that developmental changes occurring during puberty may be associated with the development of these tumours.

Outcomes of treatment

The majority of TYAs will present with tumours for which curative therapy has been demonstrated. Hodgkin's disease has a favourable outcome: the 5-year survival within Europe has recently been reported to be 89%. A moderate survival for NHL of 64% was also recently reported. However, patients presenting with other haematological malignancies, such as ALL and acute myeloid leukaemia (AML), had poorer survival rates at 50% and 35%, respectively (Stiller *et al.*, 2006a). The prognosis is also poor for patients with bone cancers, with the lowest survival in all tumour types across Europe occurring in those patients with Ewing's sarcoma, at just 31%. The 5-year survival for osteosarcoma was a modest 52% (Stiller *et al.*, 2006a).

Overall, the 5-year survival for Europe between 1978 and 1997 was 73%. Survival was highest in the north at 78% and lowest in Eastern Europe at 57% (Stiller *et al.*,

Table 1.2 Five-year survival of adolescents and children across Europe

	Five-year survival (%)	
	0–14 years	15–19 years
Leukaemia	73	44
Lymphoma	84	81
CNS	64	70
Bone	61	48
Soft tissue	65	67
Germ cell and gonadal	84	87

Sankila *et al.* (2006) and Stiller *et al.* (2006a).

2006a). The overall 5-year survival was reported to be similar to that in children at 72% (Sankila *et al.*, 2006). However, further breakdown of these data reveals that survival in adolescents is not comparable to children, as adolescents have significantly lower rates of survival for certain tumour types, as shown in Table 1.2.

When compared to US SEER data, the 5-year survival in Europe was similar, a notable exception being Ewing's sarcoma, with survival being 31% across Europe, but approximately 60% within the USA (Bleyer *et al.*, 2006; Stiller *et al.*, 2006a). The advances observed in the survival of some paediatric tumours hinges on inclusion in clinical trials, and there is evidence from the USA and UK to suggest that TYAs are significantly under-represented in clinical trials (Bleyer *et al.*, 2005).

Delivery of care

Children under the age of 16 years diagnosed with cancer are routinely treated in a specialised paediatric unit by a team of professionals dedicated to the care of children with cancer, a result of specialised paediatric oncology training. This specialised treatment, care, and support has been associated with improvements in cure rates from less than 30% to ~75% over the past 40 years (De Angelo, 2005). The application of rigid age boundaries between adult and paediatric cancer services, protocol designation, and institute referral may be disadvantageous for TYAs.

Despite the incidence of malignancy in the 15–24 years age group being almost twice that in children, the needs of TYAs remain under-recognised and, in comparison to paediatrics, financial investment into care and research within this age group has been considerably less. This may be linked to the failure of improvements in survival in this cohort to mirror those of their child or adult counterparts. Furthermore, the emotional and psychological needs of TYAs have been given little consideration in the application of cancer treatments for this age group. The Teenage Cancer Trust (www.teenagecancertrust.org), a charitable organization that creates wards specifically tailored towards the needs of TYAs, has highlighted the psychosocial needs of TYAs and importance of environment in the UK. As yet there is no evidence that care in such units is associated with better survival.

Influence of protocols

The outcomes for paediatric ALL have improved considerably: children with B-cell ALL can be expected to achieve complete remission at a rate approaching 98% and the 5-year estimated event-free survival is between 63% and 78% (Gaynon *et al.*, 2000; Gustafsson *et al.*, 2000; Pui *et al.*, 2000). The biology of ALL changes with age and this is reflected in response to therapy and, ultimately, survival. In comparison, adults with ALL have a 5-year survival rate of 30–39% (Gokbuget *et al.*, 2000; Thomas *et al.*, 2004). The event-free survival also decreases with age. The event-free survival for patients with pre-B ALL aged 1–5 years is around 80% however, this reaches approximately 40% for patients of 15–18 years. The event-free survival for adults with pre-B ALL is similarly around 40%, while for patients with T-cell ALL the event-free survival is 60% independent of age (Reiter, 1994; Gokbuget *et al.*, 2000; Schrappe *et al.*, 2000; Thomas *et al.*, 2004). The decrease in event-free survival with age is, in part, related to an increase in the frequency of adverse karyotypes including the presence of the Philadelphia chromosome and a decrease in abnormalities associated with better prognosis, such as hyper-diploidy and molecular markers such as tel/AML. In addition, elderly patients with ALL are likely to present with co-morbid conditions and are unable to tolerate intense chemotherapy, particularly L-asparaginase and high-dose metho-trexate (Boissel *et al.*, 2003).

Whether an adolescent with ALL is treated on an adult protocol in an adult ward or on a paediatric protocol in a paediatric ward will, in many countries, depend on the referring physician. However, there is an increasing body of evidence to suggest that TYAs have better outcomes when treated on paediatric protocols for some tumour types. Comparative analysis of ALL patients treated on the paediatric FRench Acute Lymphoblastic Leukaemia Group-93 trial (FRALLE-93), compared to the adult Leucémies Aiguës Lymphoblastiques de l'Adulte-94 trial (LALA-94), showed that, at a median of 3.5 years follow-up, although the complete remission rates were similar at 94% for the adult protocol and 83% for the paediatric, the overall survival was found to be 78% versus 45% in favour of the paediatric protocol (Boissel *et al.*, 2003). Within this study the median age of patients on the paediatric protocol was 2 years older than those on the adult protocol, but otherwise the patients were well matched for sex, immunophenotype, and cytogenetic profiling. Similar results have been reported from other groups and are summarised in Table 1.3.

Thus, TYAs with ALL treated on paediatric protocols appear to have more favourable outcomes. The reasons for this are not wholly understood, but are likely to be multiple and inter-related involving the effect of patient, physician, protocol, and, potentially, carer influence. Biology, drug doses, compliance, and supportive care are all key influences. It can be anticipated that similar data for other TYA cancers will emerge.

Table 1.3 Comparison of adolescent ALL patients treated with paediatric or adult protocols

Protocol	Number of patients	Age (years)	Complete remission (%)	Overall survival (%)	Event-free survival
FRALLE 93	77	15–20	94	78	67 (5 years)
LALA 94	100	15–20	83	45	41 (5 years)
CCG 1850*	196	16–21	96	–	64 (6 years)
CALBG*	103	16–21	93	–	38 (6 years)
DCOG ALL6-0*	47	15–18	98	–	69 (5 years)
HOVON ALL 5, 18*	44	15–18	91	–	34 (5 years)

Boissel *et al*, (2003), Stock *et al*, (2002), Debont *et al*, (2004).
* Paediatric protocols: CCG, Children's Cancer Group; CALBG, Cancer and Leukaemia Group B; DCOG, Dutch Childhood Oncology Group; HOVON, Hemato-Oncologie voor Volwassenen Nederland.

Long-term issues

A greater understanding of the molecular and biochemical changes which drive malignant growth together with advances in drug development have resulted in long-term survival for many cancer patients who would have previously succumbed to their disease. While the triggers for malignant transformation in TYAs are not fully elucidated, those with diseases such as NHL and Hodgkin's disease still benefit from current treatment strategies and the long-term survival for these patients is real. However, this success story is somewhat marred by the appearance of the long-term effects of curative therapy. Early menopause, cardiac failure, and secondary neoplasms have all been documented. The British Childhood Cancer Survivor Study is tracking the survival rates and long-term effects for all children diagnosed with cancer since the 1950s (Taylor *et al.*, 2004). Longitudinal studies into the long-term effects of cancer therapy in TYAs are awaited to demonstrate the full extent of long-term consequences.

National health policy in the UK

The most easily defined starting point for the current UK national cancer strategy was the publication of *A Policy Framework for Commissioning Cancer Services: a Report by the Expert Advisory Group on Cancer to the Chief Medical Officers of England and Wales* by the Department of Health (1995). The so-called Calman–Hine Report, named after the then chief medical officers, provided a blueprint for the ordered disposition of cancer care between hospitals providing a full range of cancer services ('cancer centres') working in conjunction with smaller hospitals responsible for less complex cancer treatments in common cancers ('cancer units'). The report emphasised that there should be uniform access to high-quality cancer care for all. The services that would be present in most cancer centres were stated to include 'paediatric *and adolescent* cancer services' (authors' emphasis). Further, in a short separate section of the report ('4.4 Children and Adolescents with Cancer') clear direction for future development is given:

> 4.4.2 Purchasers should look for opportunities for developing the treatment of adolescents with cancer. They present special medical and psychological problems and require specialised care in the Cancer Centre. The development of Centres for the care of adolescents with cancer is less complete and refurbishment, or in some instances new building, may be necessary (Department of Health, 1995, p. 14).

These statements represented a limited consensus of professional views rather than the summary of evidence from research studies. Indeed at the time of publication of the Calman–Hine Report very little research had been published on the 'special . . . problems' of cancer in teenagers. This remains true a decade later, but progress has certainly been made in expanding support for this consensus view.

Development of specialist services

There appears to be two main drivers for change to services for young people. The first is the specific social and psychological differences associated with adolescence which, when interacting with a cancer diagnosis, create a dynamic between teenager, family, and professionals that is unique to this age group. This has been the main force for change in the UK. An alternative focus is apparent elsewhere, for example in the USA, where inequalities of access to care and poorer health outcomes, including survival, have dominated the debate. Neither of these two streams is exclusive of the other. Indeed, there is far more that is complementary, and any perceived differences are more a matter of balance and approach.

In the UK, separate inpatient units have been at the centre of the growth of dedicated services for the treatment of teenagers with cancer. Exclusively the consequence of locally driven initiatives fuelled by set-up funding for capital costs from the Teenage Cancer Trust, there has been a steady increase in the number of such units since the first opened at the Middlesex Hospital in London in 1990. There are now eight units with others planned. They provide a focus around which specialist multi-disciplinary teams have grown. The development of expertise by a range of professional groups, but particularly doctors, nurses, and social workers, has provided a platform from which pressure to extend service improvement beyond these specialist units has been exerted. Interestingly, an equally important force lobbying for more widespread change has been the community of young people themselves. A loose community has grown up from those treated in the specialist units, facilitated by such events as the Teenage Cancer Trust's Find Your Sense of Tumour conferences. Particular regard has been paid in the messages delivered by young people themselves about how they wish to be cared for.

Young people and the national cancer policy

The National Cancer Plan of 2000 set out the first comprehensive national cancer programme for England (Department of Health, 2000). It had four aims:

1. To save more lives.
2. To ensure people with cancer get the right professional support and care as well as the best treatments.
3. To tackle the inequalities in health that mean unskilled workers are twice as likely to die from cancer as professionals.
4. To build for the future through investment in the cancer workforce, through strong research and through preparation for the genetics revolution, so that the National Health Service never falls behind in cancer care again.

Key means of delivering these objectives have now been introduced, including the following:

1. The establishment of local cancer networks: geographical areas serving a population of around 1 million in which the delivery of cancer services is coordinated from community through to tertiary care. Each network has a cancer centre in conjunction with related cancer units. Comprehensive services for all common cancers are provided within the network. Highly specialised services, including those for children and young people with cancer, are present in some but not all networks.
2. Comprehensive, evidence-based descriptions of appropriate care for individual tumour types and services. This 'improving outcomes guidance' was pr duced under the aegis of the National Institute for Health and Clinical Excellence. The documents provide the template against which funders of services can set standards and review the quality and completeness of provision.
3. The National Cancer Research Institute and network aims to provide a co-ordinated network for clinical research. National committees for each tumour type and for generic topics such as palliative care are charged with developing portfolios of clinical research. At a local level, a research network to support the conduct of clinical trials mirrors each cancer network. This led to an improvement in accrual to cancer trials that had more than doubled by 2005/2006 to 14.0% of new incident cases (National Cancer Research Network, 2006). In 2005, a new National Cancer Research Institute group was set up to improve the recruitment of TYAs to clinical trials and to improve knowledge of other aspects of care.

Within this framework the needs of TYAs with cancer have been specifically recognised. The service outline *Improving Outcomes in Children and Young People with Cancer, The Manual. Guidance on Cancer Services* was published in August 2005 (National Institute for Health and Clinical Excellence, 2005). It includes a range of recommendations to strengthen the well-established network of services for children with cancer delivered by the Childhood Cancer and Leukaemia Group (formerly the United Kingdom Children's Cancer Study Group). Critically it recognises that the needs of teenagers should be defined and provided as a distinct group from children and older adults.

Selected recommendations directly relevant to young people are as follows:

1. The identification of principal treatment centres for each cancer type for both children and for young people, with associated referral pathways, including to centres outside the network of residence when necessary.
2. All care for children and young people under 19 years must be provided in age appropriate facilities. Young people of 19 years and older should also have unhindered access to age appropriate facilities and support when needed. All children and young people must have access to tumour-specific or treatment-specific clinical expertise as required.
3. Centres providing care for TYAs should ensure that the skills and experience represented in multidisciplinary team meetings are appropriate to their age-related needs. Members should be familiar with the communication issues specific to working with TYAs and their families, and appropriate training and support should be available.
4. Clinical nurse specialist posts, to address the care and support needs of young people with cancer, should be developed, and appropriate training provided.
5. Partnerships between age-appropriate facilities, such as teenage wards/units and tumour-specific services, which may be primarily located within an adult setting, are required.

Up to 90% of children with cancer will be treated in one of 20 specialist centres in the UK. Each of these centres aims to offer a comprehensive multidisciplinary service for at least the majority of tumour types occurring in young children. Many of the recommendations described above are already in place or are established aspirations.

The prevalence of expertise for young people, as mandated above, is far lower. The recommendation for treatment within 'age-appropriate facilities' also represents a significant challenge. As previously stated, there are currently only a handful of Teenage Cancer Trust units in place. The definition of such facilities remains vague, reflecting the limited research undertaken in this field. Finally, further work is required to persuade clinicians of the wider benefits that patients may experience by treatment within dedicated services.

The proportion of teenagers treated in such centres varies according to such factors as region, age, and diagnosis. A study using regional cancer registry data of patients with a new cancer diagnosis aged between 10 and 24 years in south east England investigated referral patterns to specialist care by recording the place of first chemotherapy. When the group was divided into three cohorts (10–14 years, 15–19 years, and 20–24 years) referral rates to specialist care fell from 87% to 32%.

Current level of implementation

Since the publication of the guidance, work is under way to implement its recommendations. This is particularly complex and challenging. The range of agencies with direct interest in these developments is considerable, from charities through to local authorities. The latter have simultaneously been charged under the 'Every Child Matters' agenda laid out in the Children's Act 2004 with facilitating inter-agency working to meet the five goals of being healthy, staying safe, enjoying and achieving, making a positive contribution, and achieving economic wellbeing.

The Department of Health has brought together all stakeholders on an advisory board to oversee implementation. The process will be led through specialist commissioning services, who will take responsibility for the designation of services, and hence funding, after review against a series of standards or measures derived from the guidance itself. This is very much in line with the peer review process which UK cancer centres have undergone since 2000 to ensure quality control and equality of care for common cancers. It is expected that designation of centres to provide TYA services will take place in 2007–2008.

Summary

New epidemiological data from the UK, Europe, and the USA have clearly identified the unique spectrum of cancer arising in those aged 12–24 years. Although still only a small proportion of the overall population cancer burden, cancer in this age cohort is two to three times more common than in younger children and is increasing in evidence. These and other data have also identified poorer outcomes for TYAs, both from treatment and from the experience of care. In the UK, a number of specific initiatives are being undertaken to improve the care of young people with cancer as part of the national cancer strategy. For example, the National Cancer Research Institute Teenage and Young Adult Clinical Studies Development Group was established in December 2005 and is making progress in addressing some of the issues raised by the previously mentioned National Institute for Health and Clinical Excellence (2005) guidance for children and young adults with cancer (www.ncrn.org.uk). Within this group, research proposals are under way to investigate cancer registration for TYAs, health services research, late effects and survivorship, and benchmarking TYA clinical trial activity and availability for TYAs.

Much of the successes observed in the paediatric setting are the result of large-scale, multi-centre clinical trials from which chemotherapy regimens can be optimised, combined modality treatments can be tested, and best supportive care examined. The success of these trials hinges on the accrual of patients. Historically, the recruitment of TYAs to trials has been poor: this has been demonstrated in the USA and Australia. More recently, data emerging from the UK have suggested that the accrual of patients aged 20–24 years with solid tumours is only 2.7%, compared to a national accrual rate of 14% (National Cancer Research Network, 2006; J. Whelan and L. Fern, unpublished data). The lack of progress in survival rates for TYAs, compared to paediatric and adult oncology patients, may in part be related to lack of clinical trial availability and accrual.

It would appear that the progress currently been witnessed in the UK is beginning to be replicated internationally, particularly in the USA, Australia, and France. This should in turn be translated into universal recognition of the unique needs of TYAs and lead to more widespread improvements in treatment, service provision, and, ultimately, survival.

References

Birch, J. M. (2005) Patterns of incidence of cancer in teenagers and young adults: implications for aetiology. In: *Cancer and the Adolescent*, 2nd edn (eds T. O. B. Eden, R. D. Barr, A. Bleyer, & M. Whiteson), pp. 13–31. Blackwell Publishing Ltd, Oxford.

Birch, J. M. (2006) Why do teenagers get cancer? *Fourth International Conference on Teenage and Young Adult Cancer Medicine*, Royal College of Physicians, London, Teenage Cancer Trust.

Birch, J. M., Alston, R. D., Kelsey, A. M. *et al.* (2002) Classification and incidence of cancers in adolescents and young adults in England 1979–1997. *British Journal of Cancer*, **87**(11), 1267–1274.

Birch, J. M., Alston, R. D., Quinn, M. *et al.* (2003) Incidence of malignant disease by morphological type, in young persons aged 12–24 years in England, 1979–1997. *European Journal of Cancer*, **39**(18), 2622–2631.

Bleyer, A., Montello, M., Budd, T. *et al.* (2005) National survival trends of young adults with sarcoma: lack of progress is associated with lack of clinical trial participation. *Cancer*, **103**(9), 1891–1897.

Bleyer, A., Viny, A., & Barr, R. (2006) Cancer in 15–29 year-olds by primary site (SEER Site Recode), U. S. SEER, 1975–2000. In: *Cancer Epidemiology in Older Adolescents and Young Adults 15 to 29 Years of Age, Including SEER Incidence and Survival: 1975–2000* (eds A. Bleyer, M. O'Leary, R. Barr, & L. A. G. Ries), pp. 1–14. National Cancer Institute, Bethesda, MD.

Boissel, N., Auclerc, M. F., Lheritier, V. *et al.* (2003). Should adolescents with acute lymphoblastic leukemia be treated as old children or young adults? Comparison of the French FRALLE-93 and LALA-94 trials. *Journal of Clinical Oncology*, **21**(5), 774–780.

De Angelo, D. J. (2005) The treatment of adolescents and young adults with acute lymphoblastic leukemia. *American Society of Hematology Education Program Book*, **2005**, 123–130.

De Bont, J. M., van der Holt, B., Dekker, A. W., Van der Does, A., Senneveld, P., Pietus, R. Significant difference in outcome for adolescents with ALL treated on pediatric versus adult ALL protocols in the Netherlands. *LeuKaemia* 2004; **18**: 2032–53.

Department of Health (1995) *A Policy Framework for Commissioning Cancer Services: a Report by the Expert Advisory Group on Cancer to the Chief Medical Officers of England and Wales* (the Calman–Hine Report). Department of Health and Welsh Office.

Department of Health (2000) *The NHS Cancer Plan: a Plan for Investment, a Plan for Reform*, Department of Health, The Stationery Office, London.

Gaynon, P. S., Trigg, M. E., Heerema, N. A. *et al.* (2000) Children's Cancer Group trials in childhood acute lymphoblastic leukemia: 1983–1995. *Leukemia*, **14**(12), 2223–2233.

Gokbuget, N., Hoelzer, D., Arnold, R. *et al.* (2000) Treatment of adult ALL according to protocols of the German Multicenter Study Group for Adult ALL (GMALL). *Hematology/ Oncology Clinics of North America*, **14**(6), 1307–1325, ix.

Gustafsson, G., Schmiegelow, K., Forestier, E. *et al.* (2000) Improving outcome through two decades in childhood ALL in the Nordic countries: the impact of high-dose methotrexate in the reduction of CNS irradiation. Nordic Society of Pediatric Haematology and Oncology (NOPHO). *Leukemia*, **14**(12), 2267–2275.

Huyghe, E., Matsuda, T., & Thonneau, P. (2003) Increasing incidence of testicular cancer worldwide: a review. *Journal of Urology*, **170**(1), 5–11.

Kaatsch, P., Steliarova-Foucher, E., Crocetti, E. *et al.* (2006) Time trends of cancer incidence in European children (1978–1997): report from the Automated Childhood Cancer Information System project. *European Journal of Cancer*, **42**(13), 1961–1971.

National Cancer Research Network (2006) *National Cancer Research Network, Annual Report, 2005/06*. National Cancer Research Network Coordinating Centre, Leeds.

National Institute for Health and Clinical Excellence (2005) *Improving Outcomes in Children and Young People with Cancer, the Manual. Guidance on Cancer Services*, National Institute for Health and Clinical Excellence, London.

O'Leary, M., Sheaffer, J., Keller, F., Xiao-Ou, S., & Cheson, B. (2006) Lymphomas and reticuloendothelial neoplasms. In: *Cancer Epidemiology in Older Adolescents and Young Adults 15 to 29 Years of Age, Including SEER Incidence and Survival: 1975–2000* (eds A. Bleyer, M. O'Leary, R. Barr, & L. A. G. Ries), pp. 25–39. National Cancer Institute, Bethesda, MD.

Pearce, M. S., Parker, L., Windebank, K. P. *et al.* (2005) Cancer in adolescents and young adults aged 15–24 years: a report from the north of England young person's malignant disease registry, UK. *Pediatric Blood Cancer*, **45**(5), 687–693.

Percy, C., van Holten, V., & Muir, C. (1990) *International Classification of Diseases for Oncology (ICD-0)*, 2nd edn. World Health Organization, Geneva.

Pui, C. H., Boyett, J. M., Rivera, G. K. *et al.* (2000) Long-term results of total therapy studies 11, 12 and 13A for childhood acute lymphoblastic leukemia at St Jude Children's Research Hospital. *Leukemia*, **14**(12), 2286–2294.

Reiter, A. (1994) Therapy of B-cell acute lymphoblastic leukaemia in childhood: the BFM experience. *Baillieres Clinical Haematology*, **7**(2), 321–337.

Sankila, R., Martos Jimenez, M. C., Miljus, D. *et al.* (2006) Geographical comparison of cancer survival in European children (1988–1997): report from the Automated Childhood Cancer Information System project. *European Journal of Cancer*, **42**(13), 1972–1980.

Schrappe, M., Camitta, B., Pui, C. H. *et al.* (2000) Long-term results of large prospective trials in childhood acute lymphoblastic leukemia. *Leukemia*, **14**(12), 2193–2194.

Steliarova-Foucher, E., Stiller, C., Kaatsch, P. *et al.* (2004) Geographical patterns and time trends of cancer incidence and survival among children and adolescents in Europe since the 1970s (the ACCIS project): an epidemiological study. *Lancet*, **364**(9451), 2097–2105.

Stiller, C. A., Desandes, E., Danon, S. E. *et al.* (2006a) Cancer incidence and survival in European adolescents (1978–1997). Report from the Automated Childhood Cancer Information System project. *European Journal of Cancer*, **42**(13), 2006–2018.

Stiller, C. A., Marcos-Gragera, R., Ardanaz, E. *et al.* (2006b) Geographical patterns of childhood cancer incidence in Europe, 1988–1997. Report from the Automated Childhood Cancer Information System project. *European Journal of Cancer*, **42**(13), 1952–1960.

Stock, W., Sather, H., Dodge, R. K., Bloomfield, C. D., Larson, A. and Nachman, J. Outcome of adolescents and young, adults with ALL: a comparison of Childrens Cancer Group (CCG) and Cancer and LeuKaemia Group B (CALGB) regimens. *Blood*, 2000, **96**: 467a.

Taylor, A., Hawkins, M., Griffiths, A. *et al.* (2004) Long-term follow-up of survivors of childhood cancer in the UK. *Pediatric Blood & Cancer*, **42**(2), 161–168.

Thomas, D. A., Faderl, S. Cortes, J. *et al.* (2004) Treatment of Philadelphia chromosome-positive acute lymphocytic leukemia with hyper-CVAD and imatinib mesylate. *Blood*, **103**(12), 4396–4407.

Chapter 2
The Physical and Emotional Impact of Cancer in Adolescents and Young Adults

Daniel Kelly

Introduction

A message that recurs throughout this book is that there are unique challenges associated with a cancer diagnosis during adolescence and young adulthood. Even writing about this issue is not straightforward, as reaching agreement about the population in question is problematic. For example, when we talk about 'adolescents' and 'young adults' what age groups should we include? When does adolescence begin and childhood end? When do we reach 'adulthood', and what is the impact of a diagnosis of a life-threatening illness, such as cancer, during a phase of the human life course characterised by so much physical and emotional change?

In relation to these age groups the more generic term 'TYAS' (teenagers and young adults with cancer) is now emerging in the UK. This reflects its use at the present time in health and lobbying circles (see www.tyac.org.uk for example). Whilst abbreviations may risk appearing impersonal, they can also be helpful in terms of consistency. The term TYAS is intended to be inclusive of all those age groups who will find relevance in this book. Thus, there may be issues of relevance for those who were diagnosed as children, survive cancer, and enter their teenage years with this unique experience behind them. However, most of the clinical and support issues will be most relevant to those diagnosed with cancer during their teenage years. However, 'young adulthood' also raises difficulties in terms of agreed definitions. It is usual for clinicians to agree on an upper age range (usually placed in the mid- to late twenties) in order to maintain focus on the particular challenges of young people facing cancer. In the previous chapter, for instance, the upper age range for young adults was set at 24 years. However, this remains a cut-off point that, inevitably, will exclude the needs associated with those in their mid- to late twenties. This situation indicates that, despite the somewhat arbitrary (but also necessary) age limits applied by professionals, each phase of the human life course is far from fixed.

One of the benefits of examining the concept of age-appropriate care is that it helps to highlight how the support needs of cancer patients may differ (or indeed converge) across the different phases of life. The first task in defining what we mean by age-appropriate care is to examine the impact of a cancer diagnosis in the age groups concerned – in this case teenagers and young adults (TYAs). In particular this chapter explores the physical and emotional challenges faced by these age groups.

A unique time of life

The previous chapter outlined recent trends in the incidence of cancer in the TYA age group and emphasised the need for accurate cancer registration data, as well as more clinical trials of therapeutic interventions in order to promote an evidence-based approach to cancer treatment and supportive care. This may be considered an 'etic' (or wide-angled) view of cancer care for these groups. This chapter adopts a more 'emic' (or individual) focus to examine the physical and emotional impact of cancer in relation to everyday life. Some of the issues raised will also re-emerge in subsequent chapters as their relevance is examined further in relation to the topic addressed by each author. This is intentional, as the nature of adolescence can be seen to evoke consistent concerns for clinicians, families, and researchers interested in improving the cancer experience.

If we accept that the term TYA applies to 12–24 year olds it is clear that this will include a wide range levels of physical and emotional maturity, as well as life experience. Age is a limited variable when defining complex human needs – perhaps never more so than when a condition such as cancer is involved. Remaining aware of the importance of age-appropriate care, however, will help ensure that individual issues remain paramount. Adolescence applies to an age group that, whilst sharing some common features, is also disparate in terms of physical, emotional, and social maturity. For example the rate at which physical maturity is reached does not follow a fixed pattern, a message that will recur throughout this book. That said, we do rely on predetermined age ranges to help direct finite cancer resources. This is a point worth underlining, as it emphasises the importance of individual approaches to assessment and care in the clinical context to counterbalance the broad-stroke approach of the care needs associated with specific age groups. If resources are flexible enough then services can be directed to where they are needed, a point that we return to in the final chapter.

A period of transition and change

Whilst adolescence may be presented as a single span of development on the way to adulthood, some have divided it into three further substages (Hamburg, 1998; Klopfenstein, 1999). The first begins with early adolescence, which may extend from around the age of 10–14 years and is concerned with a shift in attachment from parents to peers. Middle adolescence, put at around 15–17 years, may be focused more on consolidation of self-image, developing a sense of achievement and power, experimentation, logical thought, and an increased ability for abstract reasoning. Late adolescence may extend to ~20 years and is characterised by awareness of others and oneself and an appreciation of meaningful relationships. Hamburg (1998) described the normal emotions involved in adolescence as involving mild, fluctuating moods, but without persistent or significant behavioural disorders. Thus, the gradual shift in adolescence is towards an increasing sense of separation from parents, autonomy in an emotional and social sense, emerging sexual identity, concern for others in the world, and a focus on a future with ambitions and opportunities. When seen in this way it is clear why cancer is so disruptive to each of these 'tasks'. The emotional discord that accompanies a cancer diagnosis is likely to be displayed through behaviours representative of each substage – and despite its limitations this construction of adolescence may help professionals appreciate some of the reactions witnessed in young people in their practice.

It is also important to consider the social and cultural determinants of adolescence, as they also shape how members of this age group behave and are perceived. It is from such shared perceptions that our understanding about the support needs of adolescents and young adults with cancer will also emerge. Anyone new to adolescent oncology is likely to be struck by the intensity of their reactions to the courage and resolve of young people confronting cancer. The accounts of the three young people in this book emphasise the shock experienced both by themselves and by those close to them. A diagnosis of cancer is always likely to evoke fear, uncertainty, and disruption in equal measures. In young people there is the additional impact of cancer on a body that is already in a state of development and almost constant change. A unique feature of cancer at this time, therefore, is that it is experienced alongside intense physical growth, emotional turmoil, and the various developmental tasks described above. Jacobs (1990), in writing about adolescence from a psychotherapeutic perspective, described this time as

> A time of awkwardness, of disproportions, of frightening sexual maturation, of pimples, and of new and untried feelings. Nothing is set. Nothing is solid. Everything is in flux and change. The aim with early adolescence is to get past it and then, not to look back. In contrast, late adolescence is idealised, especially as future experiences include disappointments and frustrations (p. 109).

This statement may resonate with those of us recalling our own adolescence – and the difficulties experienced whilst being on the threshold of adulthood. Once again this points to the additional impact of a life-threatening illness, such as cancer, at this time. For those seeking to offer help, therefore, this chapter aims to explore the significance of cancer at this time in terms of its physical and emotional impact.

A life interrupted

For those unfamiliar with cancer in this age group it is normal to experience a sense of intense injustice when it occurs. There is something almost unnatural about the situation of cancer occurring in young people, which distorts every-thing that seemed secure in the person's (and their family's) world. It is the nature of this distortion that needs to be understood and, if possible, made more bearable by the support services available.

For those who have gained experience of caring for young people with cancer, however, there is also a risk that familiarity may eventually dull their initial responses to suffering and be replaced with unintended complacency or the adoption of 'inappropriate' defence mechanisms. Susie Pearce explores this issue further in Chapter 4 when discussing the role of staff support within adolescent cancer care. Awareness of our own reactions to a young person's cancer is, there-fore, an important starting point in terms of how we approach the needs of those involved.

At this stage it is important to emphasise that, as well as this sense of unfairness, there is the 'jarring or anger' that often occurs when cancer is diagnosed in the adolescent or young adult age group. Many will have experienced repeated visits to their family doctor with symptoms that did not seem indicative of such a ser-ious outcome. The sense of threat that is experienced when cancer is mentioned interrupts and distorts the central purpose of this life stage – to grow and develop an individual identity in order to take one's place in the world as an independent adult. Cancer, normally associated with adults or the elderly, will be both un-familiar and an unwelcome constraint in those striving for an independent role in the wider world, as they have been socialised to do. Suddenly the sense of one's life stretching far ahead disappears and independence is compromised – starting with the most basic tasks of daily life. This increased dependence is further com-pounded by the demands and side effects of treatment. Supportive care assumes a particular meaning in this context and is explored in more depth subsequently by Neale Hanvey and Alison Finch in Chapter 5.

Confronting a diagnosis of cancer

In a study of a specialist adolescent cancer unit (Kelly *et al.*, 2004; D. Kelly, A. Mulhall, and S. Pearce, unpublished report) a number of hurdles seemed to pre-sent when cancer was first diagnosed. Not least was the recurring importance of others' attitudes towards the disease. According to all of the adolescents we inter-viewed the word 'cancer' was considered powerful, but was used only rarely in their presence. As one 16-year-old male patient said

> I mean you know what everyone else has got and you know it has the same name. There's not that much talk about, you know, cancer itself. Cancer, the word, is very rarely actually used apart from 'the tumour has shrunk' or some-thing like that . . . the word cancer, they don't actually say it.

This may have been a reflection of the fact that the common conditions on the unit (sarcomas, lymphomas, and leukaemias) did not actually require the use of the word itself. However, it may also support the assertions of Sontag (1991), who argued that the word cancer has come to symbolise a slow and painful death, rather than a potentially curable disease. This image still seems relevant today – few diseases are associated with so much dread, and many conditions with a far worse prognosis are accepted with less fear and dismay (Barraclough, 1999). There is also evidence that older people may cope better with a cancer diagnosis. For instance, Ramfelt *et al.* (2002) found that older people diagnosed with a cancer spoke of feeling grateful for the lives they had led and all they had enjoyed. This points once again to the 'jarring' that may be experienced following a cancer diagnosis in young people and the emotional sequelae that may be expected as a result. Research by Drew (2003) provides insight into the way that young men and women diagnosed with cancer spoke about the experience in a way suggesting that a long-term or conventional sense of security about life was replaced by unpredictability. Importantly, however, this did not prevent some from developing ideas about 'imagined futures' and making plans for them. An example from one of Drew's (2003) participants exemplifies this:

> George: I don't have a problem thinking about the future and developing ideas where I'd like to be. I would say that my cancer experience gave me an awareness that plans can change, so that's what I've got – I've got these great ideas of where I long to be – if I'm somewhere else, okay, I'm there, you know. (If) I don't have my Mustang (or other plans don't quite come to fruition), or something changes – I'm prepared to just go with it.

Each of the personal accounts by young people in this book also emphasises the way that cancer interrupts lives, and the importance of being able to rely on key individuals or routines to provide encouragement and emotional support from the point of diagnosis onwards. The disruption that cancer brings is especially challenging for adolescents, who may have been involved in the process of separating from parental figures and who suddenly have to accept being dependent on adults again as a result of cancer treatment. For cancer professionals this should be an important consideration, as they also occupy roles of authority for these young people whose lives are suddenly held in a state of suspended animation. Briggs (2002) helped to capture the nature of the challenge at such times:

> Developing identity means separating from others, becoming an individual and gaining a sense of self and other . . . The adolescent has to distinguish between self and others through formulating answers to the questions 'Who am I and who am I like? And also who am I not?' The search for identity takes place in a psychosocial matrix, forced upon the adolescent by the impact of puberty from within and the social contexts, demands and rituals from the outside (p. 12).

This suggests that it is important to understand the psychosocial matrices of everyday life (including the nature of healthcare settings) that young people encounter when they are confronting cancer. It is also important to appreciate the centrality of the new identity they will assume as 'a cancer patient'.

The 'problem' of adolescence

In Western society the transition from childhood to adulthood is marked by a series of cultural rituals such as testing the boundaries of authority and experimenting with identity and relationships. Adolescence is also considered a time of 'unfinishedness' when the individual may not yet be an adult, but is no longer a child and is engaged in establishing an identity in relation to their peer group and the wider world (Lupton and Tulloch, 1998). The nature of developmental milestones or 'tasks' is central to understanding the care and support needs of adolescents facing a cancer diagnosis (Neville, 2000). Furthermore, the complexity of the challenges facing adolescents with cancer should perhaps be sufficient to have prompted questions about the adequacy of the services available. However, there is actually a notable lack of research available to help guide adolescent cancer policy, certainly in the UK (Kelly *et al.*, 2002). This means that services have often grown out of accepted practice rather than evidence-based assessments of need (Kelly and Hooker, 2007). The culture of adolescent cancer care in this country at present, however, also demonstrates a growing consensus that needs may not be being met and that current practice should be questioned. The lack of reliable evidence for this assertion, however, is compounded by the changing image of adolescence in society.

At the time of writing there have been a number of high profile cases in London involving young people engaged in crimes that have included the use of guns, knives, or other types of gang-related violence. This has raised the profile of youth in the media and has contributed to a process of problematising of adolescence:

> If you believe everything you read about them, British children [*sic*] are in deep trouble. They are either victims, being given a terrible time by parents, other adults, school or other children; or they are – perm any three from the following – ignorant, fat drunk, promiscuous, drugged, violent, bullying, foul-mouthed, knife-wielding, illiterate and hooded. Some manage to get into both categories. Few stories and studies emphasise the normality of most children and the lives they lead: or that most are relatively happy and, on the whole, satisfied (Berlins, 2007, p. 12).

This situation appears to emerge primarily from the inner cities, where the impact of social exclusion and poverty may exacerbate behaviours that suggest a need for young people to establish an identity and to gain the approval and respect of peers (which may translate into gang-like behaviours). Chapter 9, on end of life care, provides an example of one young person who, throughout the latter stages of his illness, continued to identify closely with the street culture of his youth. It is clear that adolescents in this particular situation are viewed as increasingly problematic, or even as individuals to be feared, as Berlins (2007) also argued:

> My objection to the constant portrayal of children as problems has another dimension. The public has been persuaded to look at them in the same way. We approach a group of teenagers, even unhooded, and cross to the other side of

the street; we see a fat boy and immediately think of the more powerful word obese, and the statistics of obesity; we no longer think of the giggling girl in the pub as a bit tipsy – she is bingeing (p. 12).

The 'reality' of adolescence

Alongside these societal issues are the individual, everyday experiences of young people who, consistent with their developmental tasks, may display impulsive behaviours mirroring their own dynamic emotional state. Thus, behaviours that test the boundaries of authority may be followed by the need for reassurance and support. The demands of a cancer diagnosis, therefore, introduces a combination of stressors that previously would have been unimaginable – such as repeated admissions to hospital, coping with radical surgery or chemotherapy, risking infertility, coming to terms with the uncertainty about the outcome of treatments, and facing the reality of death (as well as the demise of other young people in the same situation). Faced with cancer it is unsurprising that some young people seem unable to comprehend the full extent of what is involved and choose to withdraw. In these cases adaptation may have to occur more gradually, with professionals making themselves available to offer support as the new reality is confronted.

Biological research studies into the function of the adolescent brain also suggest that more effort is needed to perform relatively simple experiment tasks – such as ignoring a light in the corner of the eye whilst looking straight ahead. Researchers at the University of Pittsburgh recently demonstrated that, although adolescents can perform the above task just as well as adults, they require much more 'brain power' to do so (Luna *et al.*, 2001). A range of frontal lobe regions appears to be activated just to ignore the light. Thus, an adolescent may appear like an adult, but their brain is still maturing and may need longer to process information and tasks. The researchers suggested that this may also help explain erratic moods or behaviours or inappropriate responses to risk taking. During adolescence layers of myelin are laid down in the brain that allow different areas to connect and so eventually be 'online' as an adult. It is also known that the grey matter thickens in childhood and then thins in waves from the posterior to anterior brain regions by early adulthood. This process is associated with the onset of mature thinking – it is also known to happen quicker in females, which may explain why they mature more rapidly in this respect (Powell, 2006). In view of these biological explanations for emotional lability and unpredictable behaviour it is important to consider how best to support adolescents who face the additional trauma of cancer.

The culture of care

Adolescence, as a recognised developmental stage between childhood and adulthood, is said to have emerged only after the industrial revolution in the UK. It is now an important phase in the organisation of the human life course and society (Leonard *et al.*, 1996). Adolescence can be defined in various ways such as specific age ranges and the parameters of physical growth, stage of development, or extent of social responsibility. As mentioned earlier, the exact age range included in this term actually varies widely in the literature. Lewis (1996) suggested that it may encompass individuals within the age range of 14–22 years, but that this can stretch by several years in either direction.

Importantly, however, within the psychosocial literature adolescence is presented as a 'difficult time'. This perception compounds our expectations of adolescents – and also the expectations that they may have of themselves. For instance, Maguire (1996) suggested there are particular hurdles for the adolescent to overcome as a result of a cancer diagnosis. These will include uncertainty, searching for meaning, the experience of social stigma, and actual or perceived isolation. In addition, he suggests adverse effects of treatment (such as the loss of a body part or body function), threats to personal development (such as the ability to separate from parents whilst maintaining a healthy dependence), and the challenge of developing realistic goals, as well as peer relationships, as important challenges facing this patient group. Each presents complex challenges in its own right. When occurring together, however, the multiple demands facing adolescents with cancer can be seen to be substantial – even in situations where there is little apparent psychological distress.

The nature of the care setting is important, and there are several determinants of what may be considered beneficial features for the care of teenagers with cancer: expertise in the disease, access to the necessary treatment, and specialised staff experienced in both oncology and the care of this age group probably have the most significant effect.

The context of care

In our work unfavourable comparisons are frequently made by parents with their experiences in other healthcare institutions. Paediatric, adult, or mixed adolescent wards were considered by all those we spoke to be inappropriate for the care of teenagers. Children's wards were too noisy and busy, whereas adult wards could not always make the family feel welcome. A general adolescent ward was considered less likely to engender the same degree of mutual support from being with other young people with cancer – it was also described as 'too lively'. Patients also appreciated being with their own age group. As one young man of 14 years of age said:

> My local hospital . . . I had to go there during the first two times of chemo, I had to go there because I had an infection and I was put in a side room because they didn't want me to be near anyone, but that was OK because I had my TV. But the third time I had to go they put me on an adult ward and I felt as though I was out of place because they were all middle aged and when my friends

came in I felt I was getting disapproving looks because I was talking to someone and they wanted to sleep.

A body of psychological literature already exists in the field of childhood cancer (e.g. Novakovic *et al.*, 1996). It is only relatively recently, however, that there has there been a noticeable development in literature reviews or empirical studies in relation to adolescent cancer (e.g. Hinds and Martin, 1988; Ritchie, 1992; Whyte and Smith, 1997a,b; Drew, 2003; Hedstrom *et al.*, 2003). Interestingly, many psychological studies in this area have focused on parents' perceptions in an attempt to understand the cancer experience in this age group (Eiser, 1996; Maguire, 1996).

Similarly, it is also evident that little attention has been paid to whether or to what extent specialist adolescent cancer units are more effective than other settings of care for this patient group. A small number of specialist adolescent units are currently established in the UK with financial priming being provided by charities such as the Teenage Cancer Trust (www.teenagecancertrust.org). Such developments stem from a belief that it is inappropriate to continue to offer care to adolescents in existing child or adult oncology settings. The availability of specialised care settings, whilst having the primary aim of improving standards of treatment, care, and support, also provide opportunities for examining the culture of cancer care for TYAs.

The term culture in this context is used to denote the shared meanings, experiences, and perspectives that develop around a particular event or place. The culture of adolescent cancer care, therefore, can derive from personal experiences as well as more objective sources (such as the cancer statistics presented in the previous chapter). Each combines to tell us something about the nature of the cancer experience. Similarly, we can learn about the culture of cancer care by asking young people themselves or talking to their parents or the professionals caring for them. Whilst this might derive from research studies such as those describing the functioning of one specialist adolescent cancer unit (Kelly *et al.*, 2004; D. Kelly, A. Mulhall, and S. Pearce, unpublished report), others may provide insight by exploring adolescence more generally or examining the impact of cancer on life situations (Hokkanen *et al.*, 2004), communication about cancer in consultations (Young *et al.*, 2003), the impact of cancer on their psychological state (Neville, 1996), or family relationships (Birenbaum, 1995). Together with the sharing of clinical expertise, this range of work can help us appreciate the main concerns for this group. A better understanding of the culture of TYA cancer care is also important in allowing us to understand the experience across the diagnosis–treatment–aftercare trajectory.

One of the most important concerns for people looking at the culture of care is the emotional and physical impact of cancer. It is with these issues that the remainder of this chapter is concerned. Insights from my own work, as well as others, will be used to highlight the suggestion that the essential culture of TYA cancer care may help explain the nature of the experience and the challenges confronting those diagnosed at this stage in life.

The importance of coping

Much of the research on adolescent cancer within the nursing literature has explored coping. Some studies have focused particularly on strategies for coping around the time of diagnosis (Neville, 1996; Allen, 1997). Others have investigated coping throughout the illness trajectory (Hinds and Martin, 1988). These studies have suggested that adolescents, both at the beginning and throughout their cancer experience, use a range of coping processes such as adaptive denial, which focuses on normality and a strong belief that everything will work out in the end (Neville, 1996). Following a large interview-based study, Hinds and Martin (1988) suggested four stages in the coping process: cognitive discomfort, distraction, cognitive comfort, and personal competence. Adolescents used all of these to maintain a sense of hopefulness and to cope with their cancer. More recently, Hinds *et al.* (2000) studied the effect of a three-part educational intervention for facilitating coping evaluated through psychological and clinical outcomes. In our work it was clear that some did not always want to discuss their situation openly (Kelly *et al.*, 2004). Some chose not to tell other people what was wrong or did not use the word cancer themselves, suggesting that this was a strategy for helping them cope. As one young person said:

> I don't tell everybody, just some people and then I don't want to talk about it. I don't like people saying cancer all the time. Some people say it all the time and I don't like that.

Another reiterated the importance of friendship as a coping mechanism:

> I've got a best friend I tell everything to, everyone else, I'm like, I'm fine don't worry, it's just too much to tell everybody. Best they think everything's going well.

As Cooper (1998) described, young people in this situation can be expected to experience feelings such as grief, anger, guilt, and fear. However, most can also be expected to develop effective coping mechanisms through the setting of life goals and socialising with peers. Those who demonstrate situational, transient, emotional lability (perhaps as a response to normal adolescent tasks of identity formation – or in response to treatment or disease events) – can usually be managed by the support obtained from the multi-professional team. However, more severe symptoms, such as depression, sleep disorders, dysfunctional relationships, or self-harming, may require specialist psychiatric assessment and treatment.

There is also some evidence that describes the demands that arise at key milestones of the cancer experience – such as the completion of treatment (Weekes and Kagan, 1994) or the experiences of long-term survivors (Hollen and Hobbie, 1993). Other work has focused on support and information as important components of coping. These include descriptions of support groups (Heiney *et al.*, 1990) and the examination of supportive variables (Nichols, 1995). The importance of information giving for this population is frequently highlighted. Tools have also been developed and published to help healthcare professionals elicit the information and health needs of adolescents with cancer (Hooker, 1997; Whyte and Smith, 1997a,b).

Emotional support

Although there is some evidence base for the emotional care of adolescents with cancer, our understanding needs to be developed further. Empirical research studies are few in number and may be limited by employing small sample sizes, having the characteristics of pilot studies, or reducing a complex experience (which we are yet to understand fully) into predetermined psychological variables (such as measurements of anxiety or depression) that serve professional interest more than the everyday care experience.

For instance, young people may feel more guilt at times about their cancer than other emotions, especially when they witness the worry being caused to parents, siblings, or friends. Some may also assume that something they have done has caused the cancer. Other emotions may be expected in parents who may witness the suffering of other young people or families as they did in our study (Kelly *et al.*, 2004) as the following extract shows:

> It was terrible, if you had said to me a couple of months ago that I would cope with something like this I would have said no way but you do.

After some time, however, the cancer seemed to have become ingrained as an everyday part of their life: 'we don't give our old life a second chance . . . we just accept this is our way of life.'

Witnessing teenagers coming back with secondary cancers or seeing them die was described as a particularly difficult feature of being a parent on this unit: 'seeing mums not taking their children home . . . emphasized the fact that you can never know what is round the corner.'

The recurrence of cancer or the death of other patients was also mentioned as particularly difficult experiences for the staff. As one nurse said:

> The downside is they can't be protected when someone comes back with a relapse, somebody dies on the ward . . . they come in feeling well and you look around and everyone is suffering, you want to run out.

There was also a desire for those who had been treated to reciprocate in some way, as if there is a debt to be paid. A mother summarised this sentiment: 'we want to give something back for what you have got out of it . . . say thank you for what they have done'.

Reciprocating might include raising money for the unit or talking with and trying to help those families in a similar situation. There was also a belief that, over the course of time, the experience of having cancer engendered an ambition in many patients to do something special with their lives.

The period of time towards the end of treatment was mentioned as highly significant by several parents. Interestingly, it was other parents who played an important role in helping them prepare emotionally for this event. For example, they discussed with each other the challenges now facing them in the outside world. As one mother said, 'adjusting to normal life . . . it will be a big gap in our lives when it is finished . . . a nice gap but a gap . . . it has been our life and then it won't be.'

For staff, too, the changes brought about by time seemed to become most acute around the end of treatment. Some spoke of the fear that was engendered at the end of treatment when patients were discharged and professionals would no longer be on hand to determine the significance of physical symptoms. One senior nurse said that:

> Some patients . . . they don't look as happy as maybe you'd expect them to, they almost look quite fearful but you know that it's because we're going to give them their last chemotherapy. They are going to walk out the door and then we will leave them to get on with it.

Although patients were followed up in the outpatient clinic, staff recognised that moving on from the security of the unit was perhaps the hardest part in terms of separation. According to one professional, 'physically they might be well again, but mentally they are nowhere near even going back to school or college.'

On a more day-to-day level, there existed a tension between the desire to return to normality and the need for others to appreciate the nature of the experience they had encountered. A member of the rehabilitation team said:

> They cling on to the fact that they are just the normal self they were . . . Is that still me? . . . They still want to be me yet at the same time it does make them different and it does make them special.

Despite these and other insights, there is a limited body of published research which has examined the emotional experiences and needs of parents or health-care professionals in relation to adolescent cancer rehabilitation – a situation mirrored in the adult literature (Doyle and Kelly, 2006).

Support needs of young people

Researchers such as Ball *et al.* (1996) have explored the impact that the constant threat of death has on the culture of childhood cancer care. Studies have also described parents' experiences of caring for a terminally ill adolescent (Hayout and Krulik, 1999). The classic ethnographic study by Blubond-Langner (1980) into the culture of a paediatric haematology unit should also be noted as particularly influential in describing the way that loss was a pervasive feature of the children's experience. However, making available formal models of psychological support to manage these issues may be less important than creating a generally supportive atmosphere. When we asked young people about this aspect of their care they emphasised informal support as being valuable. An example from one young man of 18 years illustrates this point:

> I think they (the nurses) really understand the whole impact, the whole family thing, and you are mates. Down there (names other hospital) they are just the

nurses that sort you out and send you home, that's it, once you're finished there off you go – a conveyer belt-type system. So yeah, this place is much better.

In the majority of interviews this informal type of support was preferred to formal therapy, which was not viewed as particularly helpful:

I've been to the counselling group a couple of times, but I'm quite open. I can talk about my illness. I'm alright, but it's there if you want it.

The emotional and support needs of adolescents within the hospital setting have been highlighted since the 1950s (Stuart-Clark, 1953). Although there has clearly been a focus on the development of appropriate children's services in the UK since the publication of a report by Platt (1959), there has been little evidence of policy developments specifically aimed at the care of adolescents. Short reports and guidelines include those from the National Association for the Welfare of Children in Hospital (1990) and the Royal College of Nursing (1994). However, Viner and Keane (1998) suggested that the Department of Health's (1991) report *Welfare of Children and Young People in Hospital* was the first to look seriously at issues such as the commissioning of adolescent healthcare services in the UK.

This report stressed the impact that hospital admission can have on the normal emotional and physical challenges experienced by adolescents, and highlighted the need to provide acceptable facilities with appropriately trained staff. In their review of the evidence concerning the development of adolescent services, Viner and Keane (1998) found that the rate of commissioning healthcare facilities for adolescents in the UK was low, and they went on to argue for the establishment and operation of more generic adolescent inpatient units. All of this work serves to emphasise the importance of an appropriate culture of care for these age groups of patients.

Although this is an important and relevant argument, the particular needs of teenagers requiring treatment for cancer raises the question of whether they could be cared for equally well in generic adolescent units. Within the framework for the development of cancer services launched by the Expert Advisory Group for Cancer Services (Department of Health, 1995) it was recommended that adolescent services should become a feature of most cancer centres. Apart from the establishment of a small number of specialist teenage cancer units in recent years in this country, adolescents have been and often still are cared for by disease or age group specialists on adult or paediatric cancer units.

Gibson (1997) argued that service planning in the future must consider the appropriateness of any particular setting, as well as other factors such as the expertise available and the adoption of a model of care that considers the adolescent's developmental needs. She also emphasised the importance of listening to the views of those teenagers and families living with cancer to determine the most appropriate setting for their care, a topic we returns to in Chapter 10.

Although individuals associated with more established adolescent cancer units, such as the one set up at the Middlesex Hospital in London in 1990, have argued the benefits and advantages of such units for some time (Souhami *et al.,*

1996), as yet, however, no formal evaluation has taken place. The ethnographic study that was undertaken in a London unit emphasised that the care setting itself allowed young people to feel that they were all 'in the same boat' and were being cared for in a place where the effects of cancer were appreciated and managed appropriately (D. Kelly, A. Mulhall, and S. Pearce, unpublished report).

The importance of the body in adolescent cancer

The focus on body image during adolescence, compounded by the changes brought about by puberty, mean that physical appearance has great significance in relation to cancer. Comparisons with peers, increasing sexual interest, and risks of appearing 'different' are considered normal stressors for adolescents (Eccles *et al.*, 1993). For those young people whose bodies are altered as a result of cancer occurring at the same time as the development of abstract thinking (such as perceived negative opinions of others) there is a real risk of negative body image and social isolation (Pendley *et al.*, 1997). Striking anatomical changes occur during puberty, including the growth of breasts and pubic hair, menstruation in girls, and growth of the penis and nocturnal emissions in boys. Both sexes also experience increased body odour, acne, changes in height and weight, and feelings of attraction to others. Thus, the adolescent body is already in a state of change. Relationships with peers are an important way of making sense of these changes by comparing what happens and when. Later, when young people move away to college or university, they will also form powerful relationships with peers that will be a memorable aspect of these formative years.

Physical manifestations of cancer such as amputation, hair loss, weight gain or loss, skin changes, and the insertion of infusion devices serve as signs that the young person is essentially different from their peers. Interestingly, those in the cancer unit study (Kelly *et al.*, 2004; Mulhall *et al.*, 2004) mentioned that these changes eventually became normal – and were actually seen as 'badges of belonging' after some time – in fact, some of the mothers were pleased when their children eventually lost their hair, as they were no longer different from the others.

This example demonstrates how complex body image issues are in relation to cancers in young people. Surprisingly, there is not a strong empirical base of evidence to draw upon – although some older research has suggested that self-perceptions of unattractiveness and negative ratings of actual appearance have been positively correlated with negative peer relations, decreased contact with peers, less school attainment, and low self-esteem (Rauste-Von Wright, 1989). Adolescents and young adults with cancer do risk becoming isolated from friends who they think cannot relate to their new life with cancer. Friends may feel uncomfortable about talking about the cancer all the time, whilst the young person themselves may feel apprehensive about forming new friendships (Chesler *et al.*, 1992). The risk of social isolation is increased due to repeat admissions to hospital or as a result of physical symptoms that are difficult to hide such as fatigue or weight gain (Zebrack, 2006).

A recurring theme in previous work (D. Kelly, A. Mulhall, and S. Pearce, unpublished report) was the seemingly innocent nature of the initial physical symptoms of cancer. This confirms the importance of the body from the outset. As one 18-year-old woman said:

> I was experiencing back pain in January and went to my GP several times about it and he eventually sent me for an X-ray of my back which revealed a tumour. They weren't sure if it was malignant or not so they operated on it and it turned out that it was.

Recurrence of disease and the body in adolescent cancer

Four of the patients who took part in the same study had since experienced a recurrence of their cancer. They were now receiving further treatment, and two had advanced disease that was threatening their lives. The experience of recurrence was recounted in one conversation with a young man who had to undergo yet another round of aggressive treatment:

> I was at the outpatients and they did an X-ray and they just said, by the way, your cancer might be back so I had treatment straight away basically . . . it was in my knee, I didn't take it that serious and I thought they would just cure it and they said something like 30% it might come back. I think I was just unlucky when it came back. There is not a lot of people like me.

Discussions of how cancer had affected the body, especially in situations involving recurrence and advanced disease, were particularly poignant. One young woman, who died a few months later, recounted being told and then shown that the cancer had returned:

> The last time I saw it was ages ago. When I saw the CT [computerised tomography] scan and they were just like little clouds, bits and bobs everywhere . . . it was quite a shock actually . . . when I saw it, it was a bit of a 'Gosh, it's bigger than I thought.'

This was despite a number of radical treatments which had already been carried out:

> 'I had a whole lot of chemo, had an operation to remove the tumour and they took a bit of bone out of my leg – fibula? They put that in the hole where the tumour was . . . more chemo but found it didn't work so I had radiotherapy but still the tumour was growing in my arm and had also spread to my lungs.'

The emphasis placed on the impact on the body underlined further the importance of appreciating this aspect of young people's cancer experience. Despite the ways they coped with the situation their child was in, there were also emotional costs for parents who had to witness the demands of repeated and sometimes unsuccessful treatments. One mother told us how 'there are days when you feel like chucking it in.' Another admitted that 'you have to be strong for them but underneath you are just breaking . . . it's your child, it's hard.'

Particularly traumatic experiences for two of the mothers were described as 'mini-death' situations. One involved seeing their child being anaesthetised prior to a clinical procedure: 'you watch them die for a moment.'

For another it was when her child was 'lost', meaning that they did not move or speak to them for 3 days.

Body work in cancer care

The importance of the body in adolescent oncology clearly offers the opportunity for further research. This is particularly true in terms of how young people experience and cope with events such as amputations or other types of radical surgery, intensive chemotherapy, or radiotherapy, as well as the side effects such as fatigue, infections, vomiting, and nausea. Some researchers have also provided interesting insights into activities that nurses may most often be involved in, such as 'basic care' involving normally private activities such as washing, dressing, feeding, and going to the toilet. In adolescence having such activities witnessed by others can be intensely traumatic, and many will have experienced attempts of young people to preserve their privacy at all costs. One piece of work that could be examined further in relation to adolescent cancer care is the nature of body work that professionals engage in – and the helpful or unhelpful techniques that might be used for learning more about the more private aspects of cancer care in young people. For example, the techniques employed to minimise the embarrassment or threat from such encounters have been examined in studies with adults. Lawler's (1991) work entitled *Behind the Screens. Nursing: Somology and the Problem of the Body*, for instance, was concerned with:

> Aspects of corporeal and embodied existence which have been privatised and designated as dirty work in social life and which therefore have been largely ignored in academia (p. 4).

She described how intimate procedures (such as washing or toileting) are managed in medical settings to minimise the embarrassment for those involved. In many instances parents (usually mothers) will play a key role in this aspect of care. However, this may not always be possible or advisable if the family members are not coping well with the effects of treatment or disease. There is a need to examine this neglected aspect of care to appreciate its impact and to ensure that we are sharing the necessary skills involved through education and training programmes. This is especially important if these aspects of care are being delegated to healthcare assistants or nursing aides.

Dealing with the body during cancer also arises during routine procedures, such as those employed for the purposes of diagnosis, and the manner in which they are carried out can have a significant impact on the overall cancer experience. The tone adopted during such procedures is normally neutral and emphasises its legitimacy for locating a tumour that would otherwise remained unseen in the body. To be diagnosed, therefore, cancer must be accessed via the external body using biopsies, computerised axial tomography scans, biopsies, blood tests, or more invasive techniques, including surgery. These will probably be amongst the most significant moments in a young person's cancer experience as they herald entry into another social world, the kingdom of the sick (Sontag, 1991). This should help to emphasise their importance: however, there is more to be done to appreciate their impact from an empirical perspective in relation to adolescents and young adults.

Procedures such as biopsies and scans, literally, open the internal body to external scrutiny. In research into embodiment and pregnancy, Schmied and Lupton (2001) cited the work of Schilder (1970), who suggested the existence of significant perceptual differences between the external and internal body. For instance, the changing nature of the pregnant body and the relationship that women gradually develop with the growing foetus is described as akin to 'having another within oneself'.

This may resonate with young people learning that they have a cancer growing inside their body; albeit that a more sinister entity is involved:

> The inner contents of the body tend to be understood as an undifferentiated mass, amorphous and indistinguishable, and awareness of the inner organs mainly comes with dysfunction (Schmeid and Lupton, 2001, p. 35).

Once again it should be remembered that the body is already the focus of considerable attention, especially in adolescents, who are vulnerable to feeling different – discovering the presence of cancer, therefore, may have a powerful negative impact on an already fragile body image and supports the need for awareness of the sensitivity surrounding this issue.

Some of the patients with more advanced disease in our study spoke of embarking on other treatment options to achieve cure and would routinely talk about the different areas of their bodies that were now involved due to the metastatic nature of cancer:

> I had some more chemo but found it didn't work, so I had radiotherapy but still the tumour was growing in my arm and it spread to my lungs. So I decided after much thought to have an amputation and, um, I'm here now to start new high intense chemo which, hopefully, will sort out my lungs.

Parents seemed to make sense of cancer in these young people's bodies in different ways. For example, some chose to focus on the prognoses attached to different cancers or use what they saw happening to other young people's bodies as a form of preparation. As one mother said in response to another child's relapse, 'knowing these things may come along . . . children dying on the ward . . . a part looming for all of us.'

Importantly, however, another mother commented that they would rather witness and be part of such suffering than be elsewhere and miss the benefits that the unit brought: '. . . the intimacy and security'.

In contrast, a parent whose son had been diagnosed only recently did not wish to become too involved with other parents. It simply felt 'too frightening . . . if something goes wrong'. This suggests that the threat of death as a result of cancer is never far away.

Awareness of this outcome has implications for care during advanced stages of cancer (Kelly and Edwards, 2005) – a topic that is also explored further in Chapter 9, on palliation and end of life care. For those who have received care on specialist units there is also the issue of a transition to adult services to be considered. Leaving familiar surroundings will raise new concerns and worries, and a poorly planned transition may present adverse effects in terms of physical, social, and emotional well-being. In the UK, the need for appropriately planned transitions is now being examined, although, once again, there is a need for a stronger evidence base in relation to the particular needs of young people with cancer (Department of Health, 2006).

Looking forward

Young people with cancer present us with unique challenges in terms of providing appropriate treatment, care, and support. This chapter has emphasised the nature of adolescence itself and the importance of considering its social, emotional, and physical dimensions in order to appreciate the extra demands associated with cancer. Much remains to be understood in order to articulate fully the challenges of caring for these age groups. It is important also to build on what is already known in order to expand our knowledge base of the needs of those in 'young adulthood' phase of life – a group about whom even less is known.

This chapter has also emphasised that the emotional and physical aspects of adolescence that compound the risks of isolation and uncertainty that young people may face when diagnosed with cancer. Appreciating that the setting of care is an important supportive variable, as our research has suggested, has also allowed the voices of young people and their parents to be heard in describing what cancer meant to them and how they can be helped to cope. The experience of parents is picked up on once again in the next chapter, where further insights are offered.

The final point I would make here is that theorists who have examined the embodied impact of cancer (albeit primarily with older adults) routinely emphasise the isolating effect of the diagnosis. For example, according to Schilling (1993), 'cancer leaves people alone with their bodies' (p. 167). This suggests that isolation in a physical, emotional, or existential sense may all too often be a reality for those facing the threat of cancer at such a young age.

If isolation and suffering is compounded in adolescents diagnosed with cancer, we have a responsibility for continuing to examine its impact on this unique population. Offering support in what is a truly challenging situation requires patients, parents, families, and professionals to have the opportunity to tell their stories and develop services that are appropriate (Mulhall *et al.*, 2001). This will go some way to help ensure that the most effective form of care is available to young people, wherever cancer treatment is offered.

References

Allen, R. (1997) Adolescent cancer and the family. *Journal of Cancer Nursing*, **1**(2), 86–92.

Ball, S., Bignold, S., & Cribb, A. (1996) Death and the disease: inside the culture of childhood cancer. In: *Contemporary Issues in the Sociology of Death, Dying and Disposal* (eds G. Howeth & P. Jupp), pp. 151–164, Macmillan Press Ltd, London.

Barraclough, J. (1999) *A Practical Guide to Psycho-oncology*, 3rd edn. John Wiley & Sons Ltd, Chichester.

Berlins, M. (2007) They are either victims or foul-mouthed bullies. Why are we in such a panic about children? *The Guardian* (International Edition), 28 March, p. 12.

Birenbaum, K. (1995) State of the science: family research in pediatric oncology nursing. *Journal of Pediatric Oncology Nursing*, **12**, 25–28.

Blubond-Langner, M. (1980) *The Private Worlds of Dying Children*. Princeton University Press, Princeton, NJ.

Briggs, S. (2002) *Working with Adolescents*. Palgrave, Basingstoke.

Chesler, M., Weigers, M. & Lawther, T. (1992) How am I different? Perspectives for childhood cancer survivors on change and growth. In: *Late Effects of Treatment for Childhood Cancer* (eds D. M. Green & G. D'Angio), pp. 151–158, Wiley & Sons, New York, NY.

Cooper, L. B. (1998) Potentially fatal illness. In: *Comprehensive Adolescent Health Care*, 2nd edn (eds S. B. Friedman, M. M. Fisher, S. K. Schonberg, & E. M. Alderman), pp. 142–146. Mosby, St Louis, MO.

Department of Health (1991) *Welfare of Children and Young People in Hospital*. Department of Health, London.

Department of Health (1995) *The Report of the Expert Advisory Group on the Commissioning of Cancer Services*. Department of Health, London.

Department of Health (2006) *Transition: Getting it Right for Young People: Improving Transition of Young People with Long Term Conditions*. Department of Health, London.

Doyle, N. & Kelly, D. (2006) So what happens now? Issues in cancer survival and rehabilitation. *Journal of Clinical Effectiveness in Nursing*, **9**, 147–153.

Drew, S. (2003) Self-reconstruction and biographical revisioning: survival following cancer in childhood or adolescence. *Health*, **7**, 181–199.

Eccles, J., Midgley, C., Wigfied, A. *et al.* (1993) Development during adolescence: the impact of stage-environment fit on young adolescents' experiences in schools and in families. *American Psychologist*, **48**, 90–101.

Eiser, C. (1996) The impact of treatment: adolescents' views. In: *Cancer and the Adolescent* (eds P. Selby & C. Bailey), pp. 264–275. BMJ Publishing Group, London.

Gibson, F. (1997) Adolescents with cancer: is it the location or philosophy of care which matters? *Journal of Cancer Nursing*, **1**(4), 200–207.

Hamburg, B. A. (1998) Psychosocial development. In: *Comprehensive Adolescent Health Care*, 2nd edn (eds S. B. Friedman, M. M. Fisher, S. K. Schonberg, & E. M. Alderman), pp. 38–49. Mosby, St Louis, MO.

Hayout, I. & Krulik, T. (1999) A test of parenthood: dilemmas of parents of terminally ill adolescents. *Cancer Nursing*, **22**, 71–79.

Hedstrom, M., Skolin, I., & Von Essen, L (2003) Distressing and positive experiences and important aspects of care for adolescents treated for cancer. Adolescent and nurse perceptions. *European Journal of Oncology Nursing*, **8**, 6–17.

Heiney, S. P., Wells, L. M., Coleman, B., Swygert, E. & Ruffin, J. (1990) Lasting impressions: a psychosocial support program for adolescents with cancer and their parents. *Cancer Nursing*, **13**(1), 13–20.

Hinds, P. & Martin, J. (1988) Hopefulness and the self sustaining process in adolescents with cancer. *Nursing Research*, **37**(6), 336–339.

Hinds, P. S., Quargnenti, A., Bush, A. J. (2000) An evaluation of the impact of a self-care coping intervention on psychological and clinical outcomes in adolescents with newly diagnosed cancer. *European Journal of Oncology Nursing*, **4**(1), 6–17.

Hokkanen, H., Eriksson, E., Outi, A., & Sanna, S. (2004) Adolescents with cancer: experience of life and how it could be made easier. *Cancer Nursing*, **27**, 325–335.

Hollen, P. & Hobbie, W. L. (1993) Risk taking and decision making of adolescent long term survivors of cancer. *Oncology Nursing Forum*, **20**(5), 769–776.

Hooker, L. (1997) Information needs of teenagers with cancer: developing a tool to explore the perceptions of patients and professionals. *Journal of Cancer Nursing*, **1**(4), 160–168.

Jacobs, T. (1990) There is no age time: early adolescence and its consequences. In: *Child and Adolescent Analysis: Its Significance for Clinical Work* (ed. S. Dowling). International Universities Press, Madison, CT.

Kelly, D. & Edwards, J. (2005) Palliative care for adolescents and young adults. In: *Handbook of Palliative Care*, 2nd edn (eds C. Faull, Y. Carter, & L. Daniels), pp. 317–331. Blackwell, Oxford.

Kelly, D. & Hooker, L. (2007) Evidence based cancer policy: the needs of teenagers and young adults. Editorial. *European Journal of Oncology Nursing*, **11**, 4–5.

Kelly, D., Pearce, S., & Mulhall, A. (2002) Adolescent cancer – the need to evaluate current service provision in the UK. *European Journal of Oncology Nursing*, **7**, 53–58.

Kelly, D., Pearce, S. & Mulhall, A. (2004) 'Being in the same boat': ethnographic insights into an adolescent cancer unit. *International Journal of Nursing Studies*, **41**, 847–857.

Klopfenstein, K. J. (1999) Adolescents, cancer and hospice. *Adolescent Medicine*, **10**, 437–443.

Lawler, J. (1991) *Behind the Screens: Nursing, Somology and the Problem of the Body*. Churchill Livingstone, London.

Leonard, R., Coleman, R., & O'Regan, J. (1996) Social problems of adolescents with cancer. *Journal of Cancer Care*, **5**, 117–120.

Lewis, I. (1996) Cancer in the adolescent. *British Medical Bulletin*, **52**(4), 887–897.

Luna, B., Thulborn, K., Munoz, D. *et al.* (2001) Maturation of widely differentiated brain function subserves cognitive development. *NeuroImage*, **13**, 786–793.

Lupton, D. & Tulloch, J. (1998) The adolescent 'unfinished body', reflexivity and HIV/AIDS risk. *Body & Society*, **4**, 19–35.

Maguire, P. (1996) Psychological and psychiatric morbidity. In: *Cancer and the Adolescent* (eds P. Selby & C. Bailey), pp. 136–146. BMJ Publishing Group, London.

Mulhall, A., Kelly, D. & Pearce, S. (2001) Naturalistic approaches to health care evaluation: the case of a teenage cancer unit. *Journal of Clinical Excellence*, **3**, 167–174.

Mulhall, A., Kelly, D., & Pearce, S. (2004) A qualitative evaluation of a teenage cancer unit. *European Journal of Cancer Care*, **13**, 16–22.

National Association for the Welfare of Children in Hospital (1990) *Setting Standards for Adolescents in Hospital*. National Association for the Welfare of Children in Hospital, London.

Neville, K. (1996) Psychological distress in adolescents with cancer. *Journal of Pediatric Nursing*, **11**(4), 243–251.

Neville, K. (2000) The impact of cancer on adolescent development. *European Journal of Cancer Nursing*, **3**(4), 253.

Nichols, M. (1995) Social support and coping in young adolescents with cancer. *Pediatric Nursing*, **21**(3), 235–240.

Novakovic, B., Fears, T., Wexler, L. *et al.* (1996) Experiences of cancer in children and adolescents. *Cancer Nursing*, **19**, 54–59.

Pendley, J., Dahlquist, L., & Dreyer, Z. (1997) Body image and psychosocial adjustment in adolescent cancer survivors. *Journal of Pediatric Psychology*, **22**, 29–43.

Platt, H. (1959) *The Welfare of Children in Hospital*, HMSO, London.

Powell, K. (2006) Neurodevelopment: how does the teenage brain work? *Nature*, **442**, 865–867.

Ramfelt, E., Severinsson, E., & Lutzen, K. (2002) Attempting to find meaning in illness to achieve emotional coherence: the experiences of patients with colorectal cancer. *Cancer Nursing*, **25**(2), 141–149.

Rauste-Von Wright, M. (1989) Body image satisfaction in adolescent girls and boys: a longitudinal study. *Journal of Youth and Adolescence*, **18**, 71–83.

Ritchie, A. (1992) Psychosocial functioning of adolescents with cancer: a developmental perspective. *Oncology Nursing Forum*, **19**(10), 1497–1501.

Royal College of Nursing (1994) *Caring for Adolescents*, Royal College of Nursing, London.

Schilder, P. (1970) *The Image and Appearance of the Human Body: Studies in the Constructive Energies of the Psyche*. International Universities Press, New York, NY.

Schilling, C. (1993) *The Body and Social Theory*, Sage, London.

Schmied, V. & Lupton, D. (2001) The externality of the inside: body images of pregnancy. *Nursing Inquiry*, **8**, 32–40.

Sontag, S. (1991) *Illness as Metaphor*, Penguin Books, London.

Souhami, R., Whelan, J., McCarthy, J., & Kilby, A. (1996) Benefits and problems of an adolescent oncology unit. In: *Cancer and the Adolescent* (eds P. Selby & C. Bailey), pp. 276–283. BMJ Publishing Group, London.

Stuart-Clark, A. (1953) The nursing of adolescents in adult wards. *Lancet*, **1**(2), 1349.

Viner, R. & Keane, M. (1998) *Youth Matters: Evidence-based Best Practice for the Care of Young People in Hospital*. Caring for Children in the Health Services, London.

Weekes, D. and Kagan, S. (1994) Adolescents completing cancer therapy: meaning, perception, and coping. *Oncology Nursing Forum*, **21**(4), 663–670.

Whyte, F. & Smith, L. (1997a) A literature review of adolescence and cancer. *European Journal of Cancer Care*, **6**, 137–146.

Whyte. F. & Smith, L. (1997b) An exploratory study of the health care needs of the adolescent with cancer. *NT Research*, **2**(1), 59–69.

Young, B., Dixon-Woods, M., Windridge, C. & Heney, D. (2003) Managing communication with young people who have a potentially life threatening chronic illness: qualitative study of patients and parents. *BMJ*, **326**, 305–308.

Zebrack, B. (2006) Young adult cancer survivors. Shaken up, getting back, moving on. In: *Sexuality and Fertility Issues in Health & Disability* (eds R. Balen & M. Crawshaw), pp. 221–234. Jessica Kingsley Publishers, London.

Chapter 3
The Impact of Cancer on Parents and Families

Anne Grinyer

Introduction

This chapter examines the challenges faced by parents when their adolescent or young adult son or daughter is diagnosed and treated for cancer. The transitional life stage of the age group in question has a significant impact on the young adults' ability to manage the illness and, consequently, their families are also likely to be profoundly affected by the life stage issues of their sons and daughters.

When adolescents and young people are diagnosed with serious illness – or, indeed, any illness at all – parents are faced with many challenges, not least of which is that of renegotiating their relationship with their son or daughter, one that is already likely to be undergoing change at this life stage. Having been responsible for their health and welfare throughout their childhood, parents are – in this transitional stage of their son's or daughter's life – beginning to distance themselves and allow the young person to make their own health-related decisions and to manage their own lives. In other words parents are engaged in facilitating the independence that is so characteristic of this age group (Brannen *et al.*, 1994).

Apter (2001) called this generation of young people 'thresholders' and argued that there is, from the age of 18 years at least, an expectation that they will be in the process of becoming mature and self-sufficient. However, any newly acquired maturity and self-sufficiency may be fragile and only sustainable as long as it is not threatened by problems that the young person is not equipped to deal with. As Apter (2001) noted, while these thresholders may appear to be mature enough to have their problems under control, caught halfway between dependence and independence, they are rarely mature enough to solve them. Thus, the diagnosis of a life-threatening illness in this age group clearly presents a challenge for the young person, who may not be equipped with the life skills to deal with the diagnosis, treatment decisions, and illness management, and for their parents, who have been attempting to facilitate their sons' and daughters' independence from them.

Thus, even without the overriding concerns about survival, the disruption to family dynamics can present problems within the family structure and impact particularly upon the parents but also on other members of the family. This chapter considers some of those issues relating to the young people's life stage, and the particular difficulties that affect the family and the parents' ability to manage the renegotiation of relationships that are already undergoing change effectively.

Making this research possible

The issues raised here are based on narrative data collected from the parents of young adults with cancer, most of whom died from their illness. The parents of a young man called George, who died from osteosarcoma, instigated the research by setting up a charitable trust in his memory after his death. George had been diagnosed at the age of 19 years while a student living away from home at university. It was his parents' struggle with managing not only his illness but the additional disruption and difficulties caused, they believed, by George's age and life stage that led to the research being undertaken after his death. During his illness, George's parents found little in the way of either published research or professional expertise on the effect of transitional life stage on a cancer diagnosis, and the hope was that the outcome of research in this area would generate data from parents that could in turn help inform policy and practice and be used by other parents undergoing similar experiences.

The research approach

The call for contributions was made by Helen, George's mother, who put out an appeal for narratives from parents through the cancer network in publications and by word of mouth, though it was clear that any contributions would be sent not to Helen but to me as the named researcher at my university address. The decision to ask parents to respond via this 'narrative correspondence' approach (Thomas, 1998, 1999a,b) was taken on the basis that this would be asking them to engage with distressing recollections of their son's or daughter's illness in an ethical and sensitive manner. It would be less intrusive than other methods such as interviews or focus groups and would locate control of their participation with the parents. Thus, they could pick up and put down their account, writing only when they felt able in a style and at a length that suited them, without the pressure of a pre-arranged interview or visit from a researcher.

This method produced narrative accounts from the parents of 28 young adults, most of whom had died – only seven had survived the illness. The risk of using such a method was that a particular socio-economic group would be over represented: however, the details supplied by the participants suggested that this was not the case, and parents from a wide variety of backgrounds were represented.

The ages of the young people ranged from 15 to 25 years and the tumour types, treatment regimes, and illness durations varied. Some of the accounts had been written specifically for the research, but others had been written as journals, diaries, or letters during the illness. It was clear from some of the accompanying letters that the parents (predominantly mothers) who had written the narratives welcomed the opportunity to share their writing and experiences with others, and that contributing to the research reduced the sense of isolation frequently experienced during the illness. Those whose son or daughter had not survived said that participation in the research made them feel that something good might result from the tragedy of losing their son or daughter.

An ongoing relationship was established with the participants, and they were informed of all project-related activities and sent copies of any publications. However, despite this continuing informal contact, it was thought important to understand the longer-term effect of participation. Thus a follow-up study of the parents 4 years after the inception of the research and a year after the publication of a book based on the narrative data was undertaken. The results indicated that, while participation had been painful, it had primarily been experienced as thera-peutic. No one regretted their involvement and all welcomed the outcome and took pride in the contribution. Indeed many spoke of the research outcomes as being a tribute or lasting memorial to their sons and daughters (Grinyer, 2004b).

Fuller accounts of the methods and ethical issues involved in such sensitive research have been published elsewhere (Grinyer and Thomas, 2001, 2004; Grinyer, 2002a,b, 2004a,b).

Renegotiating relationships within the family

During adolescence and young adulthood, relationships with parents are, in any case, in a state of renegotiation (Brannen *et al.*, 1994; Lynam, 1995; Apter, 2001). When life-threatening illness is added to the equation the result may be confusion and even crisis for all concerned. As we have seen, this age group are neither children nor are they yet fully adult, they are neither independent nor do they want to acknowledge being dependent. They are in the midst of establishing themselves in relationships outside the home and family, in careers, and in achieving educational attainments. So what happens when they are suddenly faced with a cancer diagnosis?

Most young people, however independent they believe themselves to be, will not have the infrastructure in their lives to manage such a serious condition. Thus they are likely to be thrown back into dependence on their family of origin. If they are away at university they will probably have to suspend their studies and return to their parents' home, whereas if they are living in a shared flat or house and working they will usually have to take leave from their job and again return to their parents' home. Even if the change is not as far reaching for those still living at home, any degree of autonomy or independence attained will be compromised with the advent of the illness (Grinyer, 2002a).

The parents' accounts of their experiences in such circumstances contained many examples of how their sons and daughters had to relinquish their newly established and insecure independent status. This causes problems not only for the young people, who resent their life trajectories being disrupted in this way, but also for their parents, who have established different patterns and relationships based on their son or daughter leaving home – even if it was only during term time. However, a return home to be cared for cannot be equated with university vacations. The illness necessitates a dependence, emotional, physical, and financial, on the family that few parents are prepared for. The loss of their fragile and newly established independence also causes anger and resentment in the sons and daughters in addition to the fear for their lives. Thus family relationships are easily thrown into crisis.

Fluctuating dependence and independence

One of the issues articulated by the parents were the difficulties encountered, not only because of a return to a dependent state, but the nature of that dependence. In many cases the young adult needs the kind of physical care associated with infancy. Thus, during the acute stages of their illness and treatment, they may need assistance with washing, dressing, eating, and, in some instances, with going to the toilet. They may have soiled the bed during the night and need to be 'changed' like an infant. Such a return to infantile dependence is clearly profoundly disruptive of family dynamics and relationships, particularly during young adulthood.

Yet in contrast, during periods of remission or partial recovery, attempts to hang onto vestiges of independence can result in behaviours that challenge parents' notions of how a sick child 'should' behave. Young adults may take risks with their health in order to experience as many of the pursuits associated with their age group as they can manage. They go to rock festivals and camp out and they drink too much and stay out late at parties. In an extreme example of such behaviour that seeks both to regain independence and to experience life to the full, a mother recounted that her son travelled across the world and spent his final weeks many thousands of miles from his parents with friends from university who agreed to travel with him. Such bids for independence and 'normality' result in acute anxiety for parents, who may be forced to stand by helplessly while fearing that the activities entered into with such determination by their sons and daughters will jeopardise their chances of recovery or shorten their lives.

Taking control of their body

In addition to the sometimes extreme attempts to demonstrate that they could still undertake the 'normal' activities of adolescence and young adulthood, many of the young people in the study were distressed by the physical manifestations of the illness. For example, the loss of hair caused by chemotherapy, the weight gain resulting from medication, and the scars from operations were all experienced by the young people as symbolic of their separation from their peer group at a time when belonging is of fundamental importance. In some cases this results in young adults with cancer making attempts to regain control of their bodies in ways that challenge their parents. Thus parents may have to endure watching their son or daughter having a tattoo or piercing, which for the young person is symbolic of taking some control over a body over which they have lost control.

Thus it can be seen that, in a variety of ways, there is a loss of corporeal control to both the illness and to medical procedures at a stage when young adults have only recently begun to have autonomy over their bodies. This impacts not only on how they feel about their appearance, but also on the substances they ingest and the activities they undertake. It may be that their behaviours become more determined or extreme than had they not had the illness. At the very least, such activities now take place while under the renewed – and often resented – return to dependence on their parents. Thus, rather than such behaviour being out of sight, the parents are now confronted with it at close quarters while also attempting to provide the healthiest lifestyle in the hope that this will contribute to recovery.

Sharing intimate moments

Not only is the physical manifestation of the illness difficult for the young people to handle, so too is the effect of the illness on their ability to become parents themselves. Many young adults with cancer will be faced with the prospect that, if they survive the illness, their future fertility may be damaged. The legacy of some cancers may also affect sexual function, and future relationships may prove problematic as a result. The recognition of such a profoundly distressing prospect necessitates the need for parents to engage in discussion about issues that would under other circumstances remain unaddressed between parents and their young adult children. For example, parents may need to become involved in arrangements for the donation of sperm before chemotherapy or other treatments that may result in the sterility of young men. For some mothers, particularly when acting as a single parent, the discussion of such an intimate and private issue may be experienced as embarrassing. Again this demonstrates a challenge to family dynamics and relationships resulting directly from the illness or its treatment. While the prospect of sterility applies to both young men and young women, the parents in the study (most of whom had sons) tended to focus on the difficulties this presented to the young men. This may have been because there were more options at the time of diagnosis in terms of future procreation. There is, for example, the relatively uncomplicated option of sperm donation for young men, while egg harvesting for young women may not be a realistic prospect if urgent treatment is necessary. However, there may be an unfounded presumption that parents understand the processes involved in such procedures. In terms of sperm donation, it became clear during discussion with a health professional that some parents presumed the process was surgical but, in the case she was recalling, the son was too embarrassed to clarify the procedure to his mother.

However, the need to address issues of a sexual nature may extend beyond that of fertility to sexuality. In one instance a parent contributing to the research wrote of how she had attempted to arrange a visit from a prostitute to her son who (it transpired during the taking of his medical history) had never experienced sexual intercourse. Although her son was never well enough to engage in such activity, the fact that such matters needed to be discussed so overtly between mother and son may challenge many parents' notions of what is deemed appropriate between the generations. It is also unlikely that such details of her son's sexual experience – or lack of it – would ever have been confronted had it not been for the illness.

Even amongst parents whose son or daughter has been having an openly sexual relationship prior to the illness, the failure of such a relationship coupled with the intimate physical care frequently required to be given by the parents (usually the mother) may leave neither party in any doubt as to the long-term implications for future sexual encounters. This may prove distressing and disruptive of family dynamics.

It seems that many young adults' sexual relationships crumble under the strain of the illness, as partners are frequently not able to manage the degree of care required. Relationships at this life stage are often not sufficiently established and have neither the material nor emotional resources to be sustainable. The failure of such relationships coupled with the need to return to their family of origin adds to the distress felt by the young person and, consequently, to that of their parents, who are coping not only with the illness-related stress, but with the emotional impact of the break-up.

Financial dependence

Young adults may not only become physically and emotionally dependent on their parents, but in many cases they also become financially dependent. In addition to having relinquished any income of their own, their return home for care often results in a parent (usually the mother) giving up her own job to provide that care. Thus the family's income may be halved at a stroke at a time when expenses are rising, as caring for a sick person is expensive. For example, special food may need to be bought. While the young person may, when they feel well enough, be engaging in activity that can threaten their health, their parents will be trying to maximise the chances of recovery by purchasing organic produce or food that is both expensive and time-consuming to prepare. Such offerings may be rejected in favour of a more 'junk food'-based diet, which is so often eaten by students and young people who do not tend to spend much time in food preparation or be concerned with nutritional values or additives. Thus expensive provisions may be wasted, but this does not stop the urge to make them available and encourage their consumption. Again it is clear that such a scenario may cause friction and arguments between parents and children reminiscent of earlier childhood.

Many other 'hidden' expenses are also encountered. More fuel may be used both to keep the house warm and for extra laundry. Travelling to and from hospital appointments may be costly, as will accommodation for inpatient visits if the treatment centre does not make provision. Treats for young adults also tend to be more expensive than for younger children, thus money may need to be found for expensive holidays or outings. The parents in the study reflected that such expenditure, while draining of scarce and dwindling resources, would be worried about at a later date. Yet the parents' accounts suggested that the financial impact of the illness continued to be felt long after the illness was over or their son or daughter had died, but, at the time, it was of course very low on the list of anxieties and money was found to make life as pleasant as possible.

There were, however, examples from the parents in the study of situations in which they felt torn between the need to tolerate what they perceived as money wasting activities and the need to allow their son or daughter to do whatever made their life more tolerable and gave them hope for the future. The young adults – again attempting to regain control – may spend a great deal of (their parents') money on phone calls or Internet usage. One young man spent considerable sums on purchasing 'alternative' and unproven 'cures' from the Internet. While his parents both feared for the safe usage of such cures and also had concerns about the expense, their son was defensive about the medication and it appeared to give him hope.

Such activities also have an effect on siblings, who in some instances may resent the amount of attention and money being spent on their sick brother or sister and feel a mixture of neglect and anxiety. Parents too can feel torn between the amount of time and resources that they need to devote to their sick son or daughter that may take attention away from their other children, whose needs and concerns are also likely to be increased at a time when the whole family is under pressure and stress. Some parents expressed concern that they had to make a choice, either accompanying their son or daughter to hospital – sometimes a costly trip many miles from home – or being with their other children. Whatever decision was taken, feelings of guilt resulted and the parents said that, wherever they were, they felt as though they were 'in the wrong place', either having left their other children at home or leaving their sick son or daughter in hospital.

Relationships within the family

Thus it is clear that not only are relationships with the sick son or daughter thrown into crisis, so are relationships with other children in the family. The resentment, guilt, grief, and anxiety experienced by the siblings is again likely to extend beyond the duration of their brother's or sister's illness – whatever the outcome of the illness. Siblings are likely to fear for their own health as well as to carry continuing concerns about their surviving brother or sister. For those who have been bereaved at such a young age, the resulting loss and insecurity may follow them into adulthood. Again, such effects need to be managed by parents, already dealing with their own grief and loss, but needing to support their surviving children through the transitional life stage they too are likely to be at.

Parenting roles

That there should be an emotional impact on all members of the family appears self-evident. Nevertheless, evidence from the parents in the study suggested that the effect is far reaching and long lasting, extending to all relationships within the family unit and changing parental partnerships on an ongoing basis. In general it appears that there are clearly defined roles that mothers and fathers take in response to the illness. Typically, the mother will take the caring role – it will after all usually be the mother rather than the father who has given up work. It will be she who engages emotionally with the son or daughter, she who bears most of the burden of intimate physical care, and she who is more likely to want to talk about her feelings either during or after the event.

In contrast, fathers tend to adopt a much more pragmatic and practical role in relationship to the management of the illness. They tend to take responsibility for transport arrangements, the hire of equipment and its installation, they may do research on the illness and treatment options, and, when not engaged in such illness-related activity, they may retreat into their professional work role, thus appearing to distance themselves from emotional engagement.

That the majority of parents who responded to the appeal for narratives were mothers is not surprising, as it is they who are more inclined to reflect on the experience and want to make some sense out of it by talking the issues through. Indeed, there were some participants who only contributed their story on the basis that their husbands were not informed of their participation. It seemed that, in some cases, the fathers – just as grief stricken at the loss of their son or daughter – adopted the strategy of 'closing the door' on the chapter in an attempt to move on.

The difference in male and female responses to dealing with the illness and, in some cases, death was that husbands and wives – although sharing the same loss – were the least equipped to support each other. Some marriages may not survive such an event as each partner fails to understand the other's reactions and also has the least resources to draw on as the basis to offer support. However, even if the majority of marriages survive, resentments and recriminations after the illness is over may act as a barrier between partners, each failing to understand the response of the other and in turn feeling misunderstood and misjudged.

Place of death

Given the probable age of parents of young adults, there may be an expectation that if the son or daughter is unlikely to survive the illness, the death can and 'should' be managed at home. While the elderly spouses of older cancer patients may not have the physical or material resources necessary to care for a husband or wife dying from cancer at home until the end, parents may well feel that they are expected to manage such an event at home. There has been a growing awareness that home deaths are desired by the majority but achieved by the minority, and a consequent assumption that an increase in the provision available for home deaths would be desirable and beneficial. This may be the case for some families, but the expectation that parents should be able to cater for such an event may exert intolerable pressure on a family already struggling under the strain.

Some of the parents' accounts relating to deaths greatly valued the opportunity and the support that enabled the death to take place at home, while others indicated that facing the prospect of a home death was unacceptable to them. While there appears to be no 'right' or 'wrong' place for a young person to die, some parents found that, when their son or daughter had died at home, the place of death became a focus for grieving and remembering. However, other parents spoke of deaths being well managed in both hospital or hospice environments. Indeed, it may be preferable to turn a room in a hospice into an individual space with posters and personal items from home, rather than to turn the front room at home into a hospital ward with alien equipment and the paraphernalia of the medical environment. Such decisions will be intensely personal ones and will also relate to the son or daughter's preference and the manifestation of the illness. However, it seems that whatever the family's decision and/or ability to cope, they should be supported in their choice and not feel after the death that they could or should have acted differently.

Negotiating relationships outside the family

The changing nature of relationships discussed thus far has been situated within the family. However, the diagnosis of cancer in young adults has a wider impact and can in addition affect relationships outside the family. Once in the medical setting, many of the issues discussed thus far permeate and shape parents' encounters not only with their son or daughter, but also with the health professionals engaged in their care. During young adulthood, young people will usually have begun to take responsibility for their own health and, if living away from home, will have decided if and when to seek medical treatment. Even those living at home and taken to the general practitioner's surgery by their parents (usually mother) will tend to be unaccompanied by them during the consultation. However, when cancer has been diagnosed all such previously negotiated patterns are likely to be thrown into crisis. Parents will want to accompany their son or daughter, but their son or daughter may or may not wish to be accompanied. The question then arises as to who is given the medical information and how decisions about treatment regimes are negotiated. Young adults have the legal right to make their own treatment decisions and, if they wish, to exclude their parents from that process. This may be the first hurdle to negotiate after diagnosis. The participants' accounts showed that there are a variety of scenarios that may be encountered, and that confusion may occur on the part of both health professionals and parents on how to manage the situation.

Consultations with professionals

Health professionals admit that, in some circumstances, they do not know who they should be talking to – the patient or the parents. In the data submitted to the research it became clear that a wide range of practices were employed. In some instances the young person was clear that they wished to hear the information on their own and they would then choose what to divulge to their parents. It is clear that such exclusion was experienced as hurtful by parents – who, for example, were almost always responsible for transport to and from hospital appointments. Such assistance was both accepted by and taken for granted by their son or daughter, thus demonstrating significant dependence on the parents. However, on arrival for an appointment or treatment the quest for independence might result in the parents' exclusion from the consultation or the withholding of information from them.

However, even when parents are fully informed their son or daughter can still make decisions related to treatments that the parents find distressing. They may, for example, choose not to opt for radical surgery or aggressive chemotherapy, preferring instead to take a less interventionist approach. For a parent to stand by and watch what they may believe is their young adult child taking the 'wrong' decision presents a great challenge.

In contrast, some parents successfully conceal the seriousness of the diagnosis from their son or daughter in order that he or she will agree to aggressive and unpleasant treatment that might not prove life saving. When parents seek the collusion of medical staff to conceal information from their son or daughter, they are in a constant state of anxiety in case someone lets the information slip. When added to the distress already experienced as a result of the diagnosis, this lack of clarity serves to exacerbate the situation and on occasions causes tension and dissent within the family unit.

Family social networks

During such a stressful period parents may be reliant on a supportive social network to provide friendship and understanding and also, on occasion, practical assistance, perhaps with the care of younger siblings during hospital visits. However, it seems that life-threatening illness in the young can also be profoundly disruptive of such relationships outside the family. Parents who think they can rely on friends may discover that their friends back away, unable to cope with the distressing nature of the illness and the resulting change in the family's life. Friends may not know how to relate to the family's changed circumstances or may feel unsure of a welcome should they offer help, and thus the offer is unforthcoming. However, the parents, whose primary focus is the survival of their son or daughter and the management of the illness, are not likely to have the inclination or energy to start worrying about how friends are feeling. Thus long-standing friendships can fail at the very time they might be expected to provide much needed support.

Other friends who attempt to offer support appear to have a gift for saying the 'wrong thing' to parents, who have probably become very sensitive to the slightest nuance. Indeed, when saying or doing the wrong thing is so easy, it seems that this may be why some friends, insecure over what their contribution 'should' be, decide that withdrawal is the better option. That withdrawal may be gradual, and friends who start out offering support and help may find that it is hard to sustain over a lengthy period. Many of the illnesses experienced by the young adults are extended, with acute periods and remissions, again requiring friends to be sensitive and adaptive in their contribution, perhaps not knowing from one week to the next what may be required from them. Even after the illness is over – whatever its outcome – it seems that friendships damaged during the illness can never be resumed on the same basis.

The damage to the parents' social network may be coupled with the dwindling of their son's or daughter's circle of friends. In the same way that sexual relationships amongst this age group may not survive the illness, friends may not know how to relate to a seriously ill peer and, while many may offer support initially, the duration of the illness may make such a commitment unsustainable. This may occur not least because the lives of peers are moving on at this life stage. They will be going away to university, travelling, taking employment opportunities elsewhere, and setting up households of their own. Not only does this result in the friendship circle diminishing, it also impacts upon the young adults with cancer, who see the lives of their friends moving on while their own life trajectory has been disrupted. Thus parents have to fill the gap: their own friendship circles having been damaged, they also need to compensate for the loss of those of their sons or daughters.

The implications for policy

The particular challenges discussed above indicate the need for professionals engaged in the care of young adults with cancer to be sensitive to the transitional life stage issues of young adulthood. However, policy and resource implications need to underpin the implementation of any such provision. Thankfully cancer in young adults is relatively rare, but the result is that there are few specialist units that cater for the needs of the age group. Among the exceptions are the Teenage Cancer Trust wards, but these are few and far between and the majority of young adults with cancer do not have a chance to be treated in such an environment.

There is a growing realisation that this is an age group that needs special provision: this is evidenced in part by the fact that hospices for this age group – though still limited in number – are being established. In addition, the setting up of specialist treatment centres such as the Teenage Cancer Trust wards is indicative of the need for services that are age group appropriate. Both of these initiatives are largely funded by charitable donations.

However, the All-Party Parliamentary Group on Cancer does not have a specific subgroup on young adults. In addition the National Institute for Health and Clinical Excellence guidelines on cancer services combine 'child and adolescent' cancer though clearly the issues are very different. This lack of specialist focus indicates that policy making needs to catch up with charitable provision in this area and that there is scope for Government to take greater responsibility for such services. The resources required and the consequent funding implications are matters of national interest. While treatments may be improving, and survival becomes increasingly likely, this needs to be accompanied by a commitment to appropriate provision in the setting of care.

It has also been increasingly recognised that social care is an integral part of supporting those with cancer. However as Cardy (2005), a former chief executive of Macmillan Cancer Support, says, despite the fact that statistically more people are living longer with cancer, the gap between health and social care remains largely unaddressed. The focus on treatment and 'cure' means that even those patients who survive their cancer are never 'cured' of the social and emotional effects – Cardy (2005) included the financial impact of the illness in this definition. As the cancer patients in this discussion are teenagers and young adults, they tend to be financially dependent upon their parents (Grinyer, 2002a). Thus the financial strain can be acutely experienced by the family and needs to be recognised as an issue in any care package.

Without adequate recognition of the social needs of cancer patients and their families, and an integrated multidisciplinary approach to care, non-medical professionals working with the young adults and their families may find their role marginalised by medical professionals who see only the illness and the imperative of medical intervention. Indeed it seems that, in some cases, the medical staff do not understand why, for example, a social worker may be helpful, as this role can be associated with 'problem families'. The families in such circumstances may not be 'problem families' in the sense that is usually understood; however, they will become families with problems if they are not given the support needed to address the challenges to family life discussed in this chapter. Thus there is a need for support for families of young adults with cancer, who usually take on much of the care burden in their own homes.

Directly relevant to the families' needs is the health of the mothers: issues relating to this were embedded within the original narratives and were the focus for a follow-up study. It was clear from their responses that many had experienced health problems themselves, largely unspecific, chronic, and low grade. Their own health concerns were largely ignored, incorporated into their lives, and assumed a position low on the agenda. The mothers in many instances tried not to worry about their symptoms until their son's or daughter's illness had been resolved. However, as Hirst (2004) noted, care giving should be on the political agenda in order to reduce health inequalities, and should be regarded as a public health issue. There is no doubt that the health of carers may be compromised both physically and psychologically and that, as Hirst suggests, key Government departments need to assess the impact of their policies and programmes on carers and to consider measures intended to reduce care-related health inequalities.

Thus it appears that a multidisciplinary approach incorporating teamwork from disciplines both medical and non-medical needs to be adopted in order to provide a holistic approach that incorporates the medical, psychological, and social needs, not only of the patients, but also of those who act as their carers.

Final thoughts

We can see that the impact of life-threatening illness during young adulthood has profound consequences for parents in ways that extend beyond the anxiety that relates to the outcome of the illness. All relationships both within and outside the family are changed and all aspects of life that may, up until that time, have been taken for granted are thrown into crisis. The threat of being predeceased by one's children in modern industrialised society appears profoundly 'unnatural' and challenges deeply embedded cultural notions of the order in which such life events 'should' occur.

Not only are parents confronted with the unthinkable prospect of their son or daughter not surviving their illness, they are also faced with the daunting task of managing relationships within the family that, already in flux, are thrown into even greater turmoil. The normal anxieties and concerns over young adulthood and its attendant risks are exacerbated, and relationships within the family may suffer as a consequence: parents' understandable desire to protect their sons and daughters meeting the resistance of young adulthood. The usual flash points in parent/teenager relationships are writ large, with the resultant potential for conflict over many aspects of lifestyle and treatment choices. The parents' main aim is to protect their sons and daughters and to preserve or extend their lives, whereas the young people also need to reclaim lost independence and engage in activities associated with this age group that can run counter to parental agendas. It may even be that such behaviours are engaged in with more determination than had the illness not been an issue.

We have seen that, not only are the effects of the illness on the family far reaching, they are also long lasting and wide ranging. Yet because, thankfully, cancer amongst young adults is relatively uncommon, parents have felt isolated in their attempts to cope and blamed their family dynamic for the ensuing problems. For the same reason – although the average healthcare provider rarely sees it – there has been little experience of the illness in this age group on the part of many professionals. As a consequence they do not know what advice to give in relationship to the non-medical management of the illness. Nor do many professionals have the experience that would allow them to reassure parents that the immense difficulties encountered are 'normal' under such circumstances. The aim of this research and the purpose of the dissemination of its findings have been to contextualise the experience of caring for a young adult with cancer within a wider framework that recognises the very specific features and challenges presented. If awareness of the issues amongst both non-medical and health professionals and parents can be increased, the experience of the cancer journey may be improved for all parties. However, the message also needs to be heard by policy makers, so that provision for resources that go beyond the confines of medical care can be put in place to address the emotional and social needs of the young adults with cancer and their families.

Finally, the preceding discussion of the difficulties could be interpreted solely as profoundly bleak – indeed, it is a bleak prospect to accompany a son or

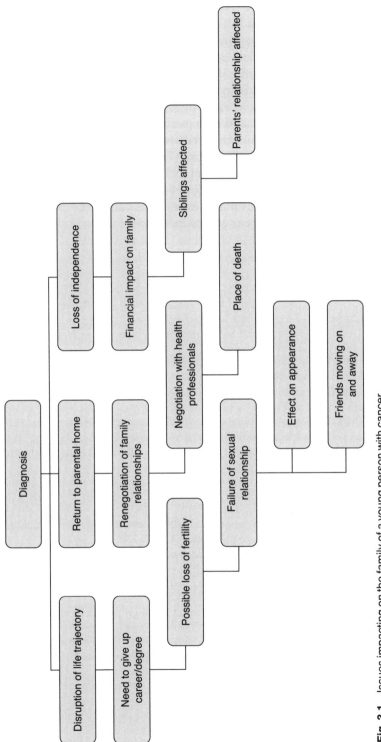

Fig. 3.1 Issues impacting on the family of a young person with cancer.

daughter on the cancer journey. Yet the 'flip side of the coin' is that the challenging behaviour of the young adults represents their indomitable spirit. This is matched by the corresponding tolerance of their parents, and these responses to the situation must not be overlooked as positive features. Thus, out of the experience, however traumatic, can be drawn many examples of love, compassion, courage, and strength that bring the best out of all those involved – and this can act as a foundation for the rebuilding of life after the illness. The family may not be the same, but with the support and understanding of those around them, and the knowledge that what they have endured would test the most robust of family structures, there can be hope for the future.

Figure 3.1 summarises these issues and the possible series of challenges and life events that may result from the diagnosis of cancer. However, the interconnectedness and synchronous nature of the experience cannot be truly represented through what is primarily a linear depiction.

References

Apter, T. (2001) *The Myth of Maturity: What Teenagers Need from Parents to Become Adults.* W.W. Norton and Co. Inc., New York.

Brannen, J., Dodd, K., Oakley, A., & Storey, P. (1994) *Young People, Health and Family Life.* Open University Press, Buckingham.

Cardy, P. (2005) Cancer crabbing. *Society Guardian*, 26 January (http://society.guardian.co.uk/cancer/comment/0,1398359,00.html).

Grinyer, A. (2002a) *Cancer in Young Adults: Through Parents' Eyes.* Open University, Buckingham.

Grinyer, A. (2002b) *The Anonymity of Research Participants: Assumptions, Ethics and Practicalities*, social research update. University of Surrey, Guildford.

Grinyer, A. (2004a) Young adults with cancer: parents' interaction with health care professionals. *European Journal of Cancer Care*, **13**, 88–95.

Grinyer, A. (2004b) The narrative correspondence method: what a follow up study can tell us about the longer-term effect on participants in emotionally demanding research. *Qualitative Health Research*, **14**(10), 1326–1341.

Grinyer, A. & Thomas, C. (2001) Young adults with cancer: the effect on parents and families. *International Journal of Palliative Nursing*, **7**(4), 162–170.

Grinyer, A. & Thomas, C. (2004) The significance of place of death in young adults with terminal cancer. *Mortality*, **9**(2), 114–131.

Hirst, M. (2004) *Hearts and Minds: the Health Effects of Caring.* Social Policy Research Unit, University of York, York.

Lynam, J. (1995) Supporting one another: the nature of family work when a young adult has cancer. *Journal of Advanced Nursing*, **22**, 116–125.

Thomas, C. (1998) Parents and family: disabled women's stories about their childhood experiences. In: *Growing Up with Disability* (eds C. Robertson & K. Stalker), pp. 85–96. Jessica Kingsley, London.

Thomas, C. (1999a) *Female Forms: Experiencing and Understanding Disability.* Open University Press, Buckingham.

Thomas, C. (1999b) Narrative identity and the disabled self. In: *Disability Discourse* (eds M. Corker & S. French), pp. 47–55. Open University Press, Buckingham.

Chapter 4

The Impact of Adolescent Cancer on Healthcare Professionals

Susie Pearce

Introduction

This chapter aims to bring together some new understandings of the impact of working with adolescents with cancer. There is currently a lack of research specifically examining the impact of working in adolescent cancer care. This is perhaps because the notion of the specific needs of adolescents and families with cancer is relatively new, together with the fact that the impact caring has on healthcare professionals has generally had a low profile in both policy and research circles.

My interest in this area stems from a career in cancer care and awareness, through clinical experience and through research, of the reciprocal nature of care. This places responsibility on healthcare organisations for supporting and nurturing professionals as they provide care for patients and families. Experience, together with the literature, strongly indicates that, although very often rewarding, caring for cancer patients is not without costs (Larson, 1992). When the setting of care involves adolescents or young adults with cancer, the nature of these age groups adds specific demands to the caring process.

An ethnographic study to explore the experience of adolescents, parents, and professionals within the adolescent cancer unit of an inner London hospital (Kelly *et al.*, 2004) portrayed some of the most relevant insights pertaining to this issue. The primary aim of the work was to describe how this care setting was perceived by those involved (Mulhall *et al.*, 2001). In-depth interviews with adolescents, parents, and professionals, including doctors, nurses, teachers, pharmacists, and an activities coordinator, together with non-participant observation, provided the original data for the study.

The interview data from the healthcare professionals interviewed in the study were reanalysed for this chapter. From this analysis the themes that emerged have provided a framework from which to explore and compare related theories that are introduced in this chapter. It is hoped that some of the uniqueness of working with adolescents with cancer will be highlighted and fresh insights may be provided for the reader so that they may compare them to their own work setting. To start this process, the impact of caring is examined against cultural meanings of cancer and adolescent cancer care.

Cultural meanings of care, cancer, and adolescent cancer care

If care is something that happens between people (Patterson and Zderad, 1976), regardless of the setting, it is not without its costs. Stress, burnout, or emotional labour are concepts that relate to the physiological, social, emotional, psychoanalytical, and ontological notions of what Weisman (1981) termed 'caregiver's plight'.

Since the experiences of both illness and care giving are always shaped by the culture of their occurrence (Kleinman, 1988), the individual and also healthcare professionals are not only just coping with the disease, but with the cultural interpretations and burdens attached to it (Delvaux *et al.*, 1988; Benner and Wrubel, 1989; Cohen and Sarter, 1992). In the case of cancer, the organisational, political, economic, and societal structure and values of care and caring are superimposed with the images and fantasies inspired by cancer. These tend to emphasise a disease that is poorly understood and is often perceived to be synonymous with death:

> Now it is cancer's turn to be the disease that doesn't knock before it enters, cancer fills the role of an illness as a ruthless, secret invasion . . . (Sontag, 1979, p. 5).

The distress and fear that the word 'cancer' seems to create (Weisman, 1981) is closely linked with existential threat. It is very difficult to perceive our own death, and so death remains a part of life that has evoked powerful protestations throughout the history of mankind (Pruyser, 1984). Despite advances in treatment and the ability to cure many cancers (and the corresponding discourse of cancer as a chronic illness), it remains a common perception that it is a fatal diagnosis (Wells, 2001). However, cancer in adolescence shows many of the characteristics of a chronic illness: long periods of treatment interspersed with remissions, cure, or eventual decline with the progression of the disease. Significant morbidity as well as long-term side effects can occur, particularly as a side effect of the treatment (Kelly *et al.*, 2004).

Societal perceptions of cancer were found to be reflected in nurses' attitudes towards cancer in a study of newly qualified non-specialist nurses (Corner, 1993). An overwhelming number associated cancer with death. Corner (1993) concluded that professional experiences of cancer, in terms of the often-negative outcome with the patient frequently dying, led to this pervasive feeling of the inevitability of death. Thus the experience fed pre-existing cultural beliefs. The effects of repeatedly caring for people who are dying is likened to the scarring effects of soldiers' experiences of war (Corner, 2002).

Although fundamental concerns around the notions of care and the impact of cancer are shared across specialities, certain patient groups will most likely evoke specific responses (Vachon, 1987). With children and young people there is a strong sense of unfairness and injustice at a life being ended prematurely. The supposition of caring for young people and their families through the transitional period of adolescence, compounded by the impact of cancer and its treatment, will have vast implications for care relationships and care settings. As one mother said about her first entry onto the adolescent cancer unit, 'It's not something anyone wants . . . having to go there with your child' (Kelly *et al.*, 2004, p. 851).

Other research and recent guidelines from the National Institute for Health and Clinical Excellence (2005) have highlighted the specialist nature of adolescent cancer care and the importance of specialist services and appropriately trained and experienced multi professional teams. It is not surprising that, since the cultural and structural notions of caring within society shape professional care giving, much of the theoretical and empirical literature pertains to nursing. Although this literature will underpin the messages within this chapter, the involvement of different disciplines is fundamental to the effective care of adolescents with cancer and their families. It goes without question, therefore, that the impact on all disciplines needs to be considered. It has already been mentioned that interview data from professionals who participated in the ethnographic study of an adolescent cancer unit will be used in this chapter to illustrate specific aspects of working in this field (Kelly *et al.*, 2004). The experience of care is grounded within the theories and conceptualisations of stress, burnout, and coping, and it is these terms that are most frequently cited in relation to the personal impact of caring (Gray-Toft and Anderson, 1981).

Theories of stress, burnout, and coping

There has been considerable research conducted into occupational stress over the years. Although the literature lacks consensus as to what stress exactly encompasses, it has recently become, without doubt, a 'social fact' (Pollock, 1988). Occupational stress traditionally has its roots in the industrial workplace rather than the public sector. As a parallel, burnout was developed to describe the vulnerability of the individual caregiver in stressful situations (Freudenberger, 1974). Stress and burnout do overlap and, whereas stress can be perceived either positively or negatively, burnout is exclusively negative and is a direct consequence of negative stress. Stress, support, and coping are interlinked and, in many ways, should be seen as integral components of one unified human experience (Bailey and Clarke, 1989; Benner and Wrubel, 1989). Stress, like caring, is the inevitable result of living in a world where people (and some things) matter (Benner and Wrubel, 1989). If stress is defined as the 'disruption of meanings, understanding and smooth functioning so that harm, loss or challenge is experienced and sorrow, interpretation or a new skill is required' (Benner and Wrubel, 1989, p. 59), then coping is what one does in order to manage such disruption. The extracts below describe the sensation of stress by a group of cancer nurses (Pearce, 1997):

> It's basically frustration, you get the odd physical symptoms, but basically it's frustration . . .

> A feeling of being out of control, a fuzziness – you can't think properly, you've probably got palpitations and a feeling of panic.

It feels like you are swimming against the tide all the time.

Like a treadmill, running round in a hamster wheel, just round and round.

In here (pointing to the chest) and it's very bad for you to keep all this repressed anger inside – its carcinogenic.

Just escalates throughout the shift and you pass on that vibe. One sentence is enough . . . Stress escalates and is passed on very quickly.

Seyle (1957), an endocrinologist, was particularly influential in stimulating research into the physiological process and physical impact of stress. He formulated the 'general adaptation syndrome' characterised by a non-specific but stereotypical response of the body. This comprises three stages: 'the alarm reaction', where an individual becomes aware of the stressful stimulus, 'the stage of resistance or adaptation', where homeostasis is gradually recovered, and 'exhaustion', where the recovery processes, under continuing stress, are unable to restore equilibrium. At this stage the stress response can cause long-term physical changes associated with the stress response. This is illustrated in Table 4.1.

From a cognitive behavioural perspective and the transactional approach of theorists such as Lazarus (1966), stress occurs when there are demands placed on

Table 4.1 Effects of stress on the individual

Stress reaction response areas	Short term	Medium and long term
Physiological/Somatic	Increased heart rate Increased blood pressure Increased adrenaline level Increased cholesterol level Electrodermal activity Headaches and palpitations	Psychosomatic complaints Somatic disease
Psychological	Fatigue Exhaustion Tension Insomnia Frustration Anger Irritability	Depression Anxiety Job dissatisfaction Burnout
Behavioural	Fluctuation of achievement Reduced concentration Increased errors	Increased consumption of cigarettes, drugs, and alcohol Absenteeism Relationship problems

Adapted from Zapf (1996, p. 70).

the individual that he or she cannot adjust to. Stress arises when the individual appraises and evaluates the situation as threatening. Such evaluation is based on an assessment of the situational demands and the individual's 'coping mechanisms' for dealing with such demands. Influences from the environment, such as available support resources, the individual's cultural background, and past experiences all play a part in how a stressor will be appraised and/or perceived (Benner and Wrubel, 1989; McNamara *et al.*, 1995).

Since there are strong links between individual experience and the social context, it is important to include the importance of context when trying to understand why one individual or group may find a particular situation stressful while others do not (Helman, 1994). Indeed, some research into stress has been criticised for decontextualising the causes of the stress (Young, 1980). For example, historically determined features of a culture or group, or structural arrangements within which individuals are embedded (such as being excluded from full participation in a social system) (Pearlin, 1989; Aneshensel, 1992), can contribute to resentment and stress. Some cultures will also protect against work-related stress by shaping what is constituted as 'success' as opposed to 'failure' in the workplace. High-achieving cultures, for example, will invoke more pressure on individuals to succeed and so lead to more stress (Helman, 1994).

Feeling valued (Pearce, 1998), cared for (Smith, 1992), and having the necessary resources (Savage, 1995) have all been linked by nurses to the experience of lowered levels of stress. In an ethnographic study on nursing intimacy, a lack of resources and its consequence for nurses in not being able to provide appropriate standards of care was found to create the most stress. This was caused by nurses struggling to sustain some form of equilibrium between their institutional role and personal aspirations and commitment to patients (Savage, 1995).

Caregivers to the critically ill, the mentally ill, the dying, and patients with life-threatening illnesses (such as cancer) have received the most attention in the reviews and research studies on stress and burnout in the last 20 years (Newlin and Wellisch, 1978). Particular interest has lain in the measurement and management of stress in cancer care professionals, originating from the early work of Vachon *et al.* (1978).

Tables 4.2 and 4.3 provide a selection of relevant studies in cancer care. Most of these have used quasi-experimental, cross-sectional, and retrospective designs to ascertain specific variables contributing to stress or to compare groups. Levels of support, education, feelings of helplessness, levels of job satisfaction, amount of job experience, inter-professional communication, available resources, individual characteristics, and the settings of practice are all attributed to the impact of working in cancer care. In turn these can have negative effects on interpersonal relationships and physical and psychological health. Most of the studies are limited by exploring stress from an individual rather than an organisational or context-specific perspective. Neither does the available research provide conclusive findings about the experience of stress. However, both the rewarding and demanding nature of cancer care work was reinforced in out study (Kelly *et al.*, 2004).

Table 4.2 Stress in cancer healthcare professionals (selected studies)

Study	Setting	Sample	Method	Findings
Ullrich and Fitzgerald (1990)	Thirteen cancer units	$n = 91$ nurses $n = 57$ physicians	Structured interviews with questionnaire developed from this comprising four areas: conflict situations, background, institutional variables, and health	Strong associations between situational stressors and psychosomatic complaints Nurses: interpersonal difficulties = physical distress Doctors: job dissatisfaction = malaise
Whippen and Canellos (1991)		$n = 1000$ oncologists randomly sampled	Questionnaire 60% response	Experience of burnout in 56% Significance between type of practice and burnout
Cull (1991)	Academic oncology unit	$n = 11$ nurses $n = 6$ doctors $n = 4$ paramedics	Delphi technique Poor response in third questionnaire = 6	Need to discuss issues raised Open problem solving group set up to maintain mutual support and communication
Kent et al. (1994)	Oncology centre	$n = 125$ medical, university, nursing, and support staff randomly selected	Critical incident sheets Maslach Burnout Inventory Hospital Anxiety and Depression Scale Intention to leave post Response $n = 48$ (38%)	Perception of inability to help patients scored higher on the Maslach Burnout Inventory Risk of clinical anxiety in 22% Recently considered leaving their job in 33%
Miller and Gillies (1996)	Seven HIV/AIDS and two oncology centres	$n = 203$ staff (all staff employed in units for more than 6 months)	Structured interview Maslach Burnout Iventory General Health Questionnaire	Low response rate for oncology Few overall differences between HIV/AIDS and oncology Sample partners reported over commitment to work in 39% Relationships suffered as a result of work reported in 25%
Isikhan et al. (2004)	Five oncology hospitals in Turkey	$n = 57$ nurses $n = 52$ doctors	Self-report Questionnaire Job Stress Inventory Ways of Coping Inventory	Signs of physical and psychological stress Levels considered serious Number of related variables Use similar strategies: most common was a self-confident approach

Adapted from Pearce (1997).

Table 4.3 Stress in cancer nurses (selected studies)

Study	Sample	Method	Findings
Yasko (1983)	n = 185 oncology nursing specialists	Jones Staff Burnout Scale for Health Professionals Self-report Questionnaire	Burnout score lower than other nurse sample Burnout related to inadequate support, high levels of stress, feelings of apathy and withdrawal, and dissatisfaction with role
Stewart *et al.* (1982)	n = 5 outpatient oncology nurses, n = 40 cancer, intensive care, cardiac, and theatres	In-depth interviews Questionnaire	Oncology nurses experienced more enduring stress
Ogle (1983)	n = 22 oncology nurses	Maslach Burnout Inventory	Moderate intensity of burnout: able to determine stage of burnout experienced
Jenkins and Ostchega (1986)	n = 152 oncology nursing society. Random sample	Staff Burnout Scale for Health Professionals Yasko Survey Tool	Oncology nurses not a greater risk of burnout Variables correlating with higher score: organisational problems, job stress, availability of support, and level of job satisfaction
Bram and Katz (1989)	n = 29 hospice nurses n = 28 hospital nurses	Staff Burnout Scale for Health Professionals Corwin's Nursing Role Conception Scale Work-related questionnaire	Oncology nurses significantly more stressed Different work-related variables correlated with burnout for each group with the exception of support
Razavi *et al.* (1993)	n = 72 nurses	Randomly assigned to a 24-hour psychological training programme / control group Assessed 1 week before and 1 week and 2 months after Semi-structured interview Semantic Differential Questionnaire Nursing Stress Scale Role play	Significant change to self-concept and occupational stress related to inadequate preparation after PTP, Psychological Training Programme

Table 4.3 (*Cont'd*)

Study	Sample	Method	Findings
Hinds *et al.* (1994)	*n* = 25 paediatric oncology, *n* = 9 new, *n* = 14 experienced	New nurses interviewed at 3, 6, and 12 months and experienced nurses interviewed once Guided interviews	Difference in stress between the two groups, with new nurses having fewer coping reactions: most common reaction was resignation
Papadatou *et al.* (1994)	*n* = 217 oncology nurses *n* = 266 general nurses	Maslach Burnout Inventory Hardiness Scale Ways of Coping Scale Life Style Scale Type A Behaviour Scale Job Stress Questionnaire General Information Questionnaire	No statistical difference in degree of burnout between groups, personality greatest prediction of burnout, and sense of control in personal life and in the work context found to protect against burnout
Wilkinson (1994)	*n* = 65 cancer nurses from six wards in two hospitals	Self-administered questionnaire, Spielberger State Trait Anxiety Inventory completed six times in 8 months	General anxiety no different from working females, newly qualified nurses more anxious, and most nurses satisfied: statistical difference in nurses' anxiety between wards
Pearce (1998)	*n* = 10 cancer nurses from three wards	In-depth interview of experience of stress in cancer nursing	Nature of stress, boundaries, 'difficult' relationships, not good enough, lack of time, valued, and gaining mastery
Mohan *et al.* (2005)	*n* = 25 nurses in non-specialist wards	Twenty-five surveyed Five in-depth interviews	Themes: emotional nature of care, lack of time, lack of knowledge, family, poor environment, and non-acceptance

Adapted from Pearce (1997).

Emotions and care work

Although caring is universal and can be thought of as one of the most basic elements of being human (Roach, 1984), it has, however, traditionally been seen as 'women's work'. Part of women's caring role in society is that they are deemed to be 'naturally good' at dealing with other people's emotions, an invisible and unacknowledged form of labour that is particularly evident (and therefore often invisible and unvalued) within the domestic domain (James, 1989). Unsurprisingly, the impact of professional care giving has also been examined within the framework of emotional labour (Smith, 1992; Kelly *et al.*, 2000).

Hoschild (1983b) first described this concept in *The Managed Heart: Commercialization of Human Feeling*, where she linked care feelings and emotions with the everyday work of flight attendants. Flight attendants' smiling, courteous, and caring demeanour has a monetary value – both for themselves and for the airlines. Thus, emotional labour does have value, as does physical labour, within the world of mass production. Similarly to Goffman's (1969) ideas of presenting a 'face' and maintaining congenial appearances in particular settings, whether we feel that way or not, Hochschild (1983a) suggested that such work requires people to learn to change feelings from the inside using a variety of methods so that the 'preferred' feeling shows on their face. These responses are socially constructed and termed 'feeling rules'.

Several authors have emphasised the emotional nature of the work involved in caring for the dying or those who are seriously ill. This is because of the strong emotions and feelings it creates. In her study of the emotional labour of student nurses, Smith (1992) found they would sometimes concentrate on the physical aspects of work to avoid coming into contact with the difficult, often painful work of engaging emotionally with those who were dying. Something of the 'love'/'care'/'use of self' was lost in this process, with boundaries and distancing being used as a way of coping. The feeling rules of a ward were shaped by the nursing hierarchy, with ritualistic ways of working, such as separating technical from emotional nursing work and delegating death work to the most junior staff, being common.

Field (1984) also highlighted leadership style as central to the ethos of patient care enacted on the ward. In his study of nursing on a general medical ward, strong and supportive leadership resulted in a different set of feeling rules to that of Smith (1992). Nearly all the nurses spoke of being emotionally involved with their patients – often to the extent of grieving after their deaths. Such involvement was felt to be unavoidable and inevitable. Nursing the dying was said by the nurses to be satisfying because it allowed them to implement their ideal standard of nursing care.

Each of these studies suggests that there are specific factors that will influence the extent and nature of emotional engagement in health settings. These include the emotional culture or 'feeling rules' of a ward or unit, which will be explored later in this chapter. The extracts below illustrate some of the emotions discussed by some of the healthcare professionals interviewed about their work on an adolescent cancer unit (Kelly *et al.*, 2004):

> Sometimes I don't like saying what I do because there's the stigma about cancer . . . and they think, Oh isn't that terribly depressing? Well, yeah, it's really sad and it's really stressful but it's also really positive. It is a really positive job.

> I think you know if we sat there and really thought about our patients and their real situation we would be paralysed, we just wouldn't be able to go out there and face them.

> I've never gone home and not felt very privileged.

The 'emotional self'

Interestingly, there may be different perceptions about the appropriateness of using the 'emotional self' in different health settings and for different professional groups, with or without what may be considered the medical/technical protection of objectivity. For the medical profession this has been described as the 'medical gaze' (Foucault, 1973), the observing/rational perspective on illness that reinforces the social power of medical knowledge. In an analysis of nursing work, the ritual and routine of nursing practice also created a sense of distance between the nurse and the patient (Menzies, 1988). In our research we found that some groups, such as non-medical professionals, felt more exposed emotionally:

> Draining, draining is a word that I would definitely use to describe this job . . . it's just the whole environment, the whole emotion is kind of transferred to you.

> You still get shocked, I will still get surprised and think, gosh I didn't think that would upset me. But then on the other hand if you cease to be upset in oncology then. . . .

> I think that if staff feel they can sit and cry or sit and say they find it really hard . . . we had a clinical discussion group . . . and it was just complete psychobabble going around the room, and I thought isn't this desperately sad but it's fine because they need to express that, I think that's what's really essential.

> Whereas the nurses they have a medical thing. They can go into someone and say can I do your whatever . . . and they have a reason for going into the room, but I don't and I go in and it's just me, just me and my personality.

Adolescence, the growing from childhood to adulthood, juxtaposed with cancer, constitutes a deep engagement with loss in a context of uncertainty, ambiguity, and anxiety. This can have a huge impact on adults in close quarters with teenagers, whether as parents or for those who work with them professionally (Briggs, 2002). Working with both the impact of cancer on teenagers and their families, whilst also managing the normal behaviour of teenagers, brings another level of complexity to the emotional work of adolescent cancer care. An

Table 4.4 Defences and reactions against anxiety encountered in everyday clinical work

Defence/Reaction	Definition
Defences	
Denial	An unconscious defence mechanism by which an aspect of the self or a painful experience is denied
Suppression	A conscious attempt to forget, deny, or avoid thinking about something unpleasant
Repression	An idea may unconsciously be repressed owing to its unpleasant nature: it may be an idea or feeling that conflicts with our view of ourselves and what is acceptable
Splitting	Involves separation of good and bad aspects of the self and others or between good and bad feelings
Projection	Externalising unacceptable emotions and then attributing them to others or to an object
Projective identification	Projecting feelings and important aspects of one's self onto others so that person owns and feels qualities and impulses that are not their own
Reactive formation	Going to an opposite extreme to obscure unacceptable feelings, e.g. acting happy to hide unhappiness
Rationalisation:	Justifying an unconscious impulse or giving a good reason for something but it is not applicable to the situation
Conversion and psychosomatic	Unacceptable feelings may be converted into physical symptoms
Reactions	
Phobic avoidance	Avoiding situations that arouse unpleasant or unbearable feelings
Displacement	Being afraid to express feelings to a person who provoked them and deflecting them elsewhere
Regression	Regression to a more childlike and dependent way of behaving in order to cope with unpleasant emotions
Sublimation	Unconscious drives are allowed partial expression in modified, socially acceptable, even desirable ways
Depersonalisation	The state where an individual feels him-/herself to be unreal: as if separated from feelings or other people by a glass screen
Confusion	Disorientation in time and place

Adapted from Brown and Pedder (1991).

adolescent cancer nurse gave an example of this work (Kelly *et al.*, 2004), with perhaps a suggestion of the possible contradictions it may raise:

> Losing their hair, Hickman lines, weight loss, not using make-up, not feeling pretty, feeling tired all the time with the chemotherapy . . . are they going to be able to achieve what they should have done, are they going to be impeded in life because of the treatment we have given them? We still have the responsibility to allow them to realise that they can't lie on the bed in their clothes talking to somebody outside the ward and bitch about another patient and their mum, that is not acceptable behaviour and has to be policed somehow . . . do you see what I mean?

Unconscious feelings in adolescent cancer work

Not surprisingly unconscious processes in individuals and organisations can contribute to the emotional work and the impact of caring. By its very nature, working with adolescents, combined with the suffering of cancer, is likely to be an extremely powerful experience for professionals. Work that has its roots in the Tavistock Clinic suggests that organisations specialising in human services may develop specific institutional defences against the intensity of the impact of care, whether it is adolescent care (Briggs, 2002) or any other form of care for that matter (Obholzer and Zagier Roberts, 1994). This is an issue that may have relevance for cancer care more generally. Table 4.4 illustrates some of the psychodynamic defences that may be witnessed in clinical practice (Brown and Pedder, 1991). These are listed for readers to consider in relation to how they might react to the suffering of adolescents and young adults.

When anxieties are too deep and dangerous to allow confrontation, psychic defences are used by the individual and over time are built into socially structured defence systems. The psychic defence process goes back to infancy and the psychic phantasies of the 'paranoid–schizoid position' (Klein, 1959) when the mother contains the early intolerable emotions of the infant. This process is similar for teenagers when intense emotions need to be contained by adults, whether they are biological parents or parental figures such as professionals (Briggs, 2002).

The seminal work of Menzies (1988), in her study of nursing systems of work in a London hospital, demonstrated that the same may happen when dealing with the anxieties raised by working closely with suffering and illness in professional caring relationships. This issue was explored in Menzies' (1988) study, which was commissioned by senior nursing staff concerned at the numbers of nurses leaving the profession and the impact this was having on the quality of patient care. What Menzies (1988) found in the late 1950s is still widely perceived to be relevant to the systems of nursing and health care today (e.g. Bailey, 2001; Corner, 2002; Rafferty and Traynor, 2002).

In a similar fashion to a mother figure, a nurse or healthcare professional may be unable to bring together the opposing feelings of pity, compassion, and love with the feeling of revulsions and distaste of working with the 'profane', that is with illness and death. Winnicott (1947), in the concept of the 'good enough mother', drew attention to the mass of complex feelings a mother and also a professional may have in relation to their child or patient. Menzies (1988) also found that the splitting of 'good' and 'bad' feelings by the nurse towards the patient was projected outside into some of the rituals of the ward routine that helped to separate the physical and emotional care. This removed both the close relationship with suffering and the anxieties that closeness and intimacy can create. The rituals and routines that developed included the frequent moving of nurses from ward to ward and the reduction of accountability by checks and counterchecks and delegation to superiors (Menzies, 1988).

However, these systems for defending anxiety contributed to a secondary type of anxiety. They deprived healthcare professionals of the necessary assurances and satisfactions that derive from providing good care, working effectively in teams, and the capacity to master anxiety and change. Thus,

> Anxiety tends to remain permanently at a level determined more by the phantasies than the reality . . . (Menzies, 1988, p. 75).

Working in adolescent cancer care means working with serious illness and death and has the potential to trigger intense emotions. In terms of institutional adolescent care settings, Briggs (2002) highlighted how difficult and often forgotten feelings from the professionals' own adolescence may be projected back onto the adolescent patient as part of the adults' own defence. In this way the power of adolescent emotionality may affect professionals who work with them, and has the potential to evoke defence systems such as impulsiveness, individualisation of methods of work, reliance on charismatic leaders, huge overestimation of the work, or, alternatively, defences against the power of adolescent emotionality through controlling the environment, strong boundary formation, and complete separation from the notion of adolescent pain (Briggs, 2002).

Healthcare settings can be seen to act as mirrors of the emotional tone that defines them – an 'anxious' or stressed team or unit will probably inject this anxiety into everyone involved. As the nurse said earlier, stress is contagious. Organisations need to be aware of their role as 'containers' for anxiety in a similar way that some professionals may be for the adolescent and family with cancer (Briggs, 2002). This emphasises the importance of developing and maintaining supportive yet 'emotionally aware' environments of care (Walker, 1994).

Mastering intense feelings

Whilst needing to contend with the intense emotions of both cancer and adolescence, with the right supportive environment the professional and the team can use their feelings to work with understanding and to practise therapeutically. It is crucial that, in painful and stressful work, staff have the opportunity to think about their anxieties and the negative and positive effects of these emotions

(Mawson, 1994). A clinical discussion group is an example of how to achieve open discussion. The role of multidisciplinary team meetings and other vehicles for reflective practice (Schon, 1983) and clinical supervision should also be considered. Through this individuals and teams may be better able to understand reactions, such as 'projection' or 'splitting', and to discuss ways of containing the anxieties of teenagers and their families, both from an individual and from a team perspective.

Maintaining boundaries

The importance of maintaining flexibility within a rigorous framework of working with boundaries is important in all aspects of care, but perhaps more so within adolescent care where there is the potential for workers to be swept along with the intense emotionality of the work (Briggs, 2002).

Another reason for the importance of a sound internal support structure in adolescent cancer care, particularly in specialist units, relates to the informality of the physical environment, which may not provide the external structures or boundaries of a more conventional health setting. The examples below from our study illustrate the importance placed on boundaries in adolescent cancer care:

> To an outsider I think we come over as being very informal and very relaxed but on the inside there is very much a structure and a kind of, there are certain expectations with the work.

> You know they don't want to particularly be here, they are here because they have got cancer. Their friends and important people are out there, they are not here. . . . We're not a youth club . . . that doesn't mean we can't strike a balance and meet their needs as adolescents, and I think that is the difference.

The boundaries within a team and unit structure and the boundaries of interpersonal working are interlinked as the former can help to create the framework for the latter. The development of boundaries is imperative to be able to care professionally. For some, detachment may equal survival, particularly in environments where people die. However, some degree of involvement will be necessary in order to be caring (May, 1993). In addition, while involvement is therapeutic and beneficial, over-involvement has been revealed as inherently dysfunctional (Turner, 1999).

The disruption of boundaries may be experienced as stressful when a professional identifies with one particular patient. Some examples from our work may be helpful here:

> When people try and make a patient their patient, when they become unprofessional, cross professional boundaries, then the ward's informality can become a problem.

> You just can't develop close bonds with patients because you just wouldn't survive, you'd eventually burn out, you would eventually lose the capacity to

care for them. There is another element as well, you can't burden someone who is already coping with something they never thought they would have to deal with in their life. It may be a diversion, but we can't have cancer patients worrying about members of staff.

Bowlby's (1979) 'attachment theory' is one way of conceptualising the propensity of human beings to make strong affectional bonds with others. Although developed in infancy, attachment behaviour continues throughout life. Similarly to all relationships, strong emotions of anxiety, despair, anger, and guilt will arise when a close nurse–patient relationship is threatened by separation or death. Since the motivation and reasons for the work we choose is largely unconscious, it is important to be aware of and to reflect on this choice occasionally in our practice (Vachon *et al.*, 1978; Zagier Roberts, 1994). However, once again this emphasises the importance of creating a safe place for people to work, where they are able to discuss and work through their feelings – including strong feelings that may not initially be consciously recognisable. Some insight may already be present, as participants in our study showed:

> I come and do my job. You do have coping mechanisms and there has been a shift away from me and the patients to enable me to carry on. I can't get involved with them myself . . .

> Boundaries make the ward a safer place. I think if patients get mixed messages it can be very confusing for them and very difficult. I think you have to be very clear about what we can offer. It doesn't mean we don't cry, it doesn't mean we don't get distressed . . .

The multidisciplinary team, particularly the leaders, need to be aware of clear guidelines for boundary formation: such as dealing with issues on the unit and identification of risk factors for boundary-related issues. Related to boundaries is the facilitation of defined tasks and roles of individuals within a team. This is particularly important when roles may overlap in diverse teams, such as in the care of adolescents with cancer. However, all this should be considered alongside Briggs' (2002) warning about boundaries acting as barriers to emotionality in themselves.

Multidisciplinary team working

A multidisciplinary team is 'a group who share a common health goal and common objectives, determined by the community's needs' (World Health Organization, 1984). Multi-professional team working is now a key feature of cancer services, in part to ensure there is appropriate care throughout the patient journey. A complex arrangement of services may be required for children and young people with cancer as will many disciplines and professional groups, as well as the crossing of organisational and institutional boundaries (National Institute for Health and Clinical Excellence, 2005). For adolescents this may include specialist treatment centres, district general hospitals, the community, and voluntary organisations, and it will involve different medical specialists, nurses, community nurses, general practitioners, specialist nurses, liaison nurses, teachers, pharmacists, psychotherapists, counsellors, play and activities coordinators, complementary therapists, physiotherapists, occupational therapists, social workers, voluntary workers, and so on. This is a long list of people who must communicate effectively in order to achieve a sense of teamwork and open debate.

Effective team working is central not just to the patients' and families' experience of cancer care, but also to the effect of cancer care on the professionals – both as individuals and as a group. Since hospitals are staffed by diverse occupational groups, each with their own cultures, career structures, internal divisions, and hierarchies (Allen, 1997), there is ongoing debate about professional roles and boundaries, perhaps most notably between doctors and nurses. In her investigation of the social processes of gender and other power relations, primarily through the standpoint of nurses, Wicks (1998) found a 'clash' in some situations where nurses were torn between 'obedience' to doctors and their view of what is necessary to ensure the comfort of their patients. This was a finding supported by other studies (e.g. May, 1993; Field, 1984; Savage, 1995), and may impact on areas where conflict arises from the desire to achieve cure and the desire to care and palliate, particularly towards the end of life. Stress can arise for all concerned where clashes exist between individual values and expectations and the reality of what is possible (Ramirez *et al.*, 1995).

Despite the potential for conflict, nurses and doctors and other members of the multi-professional team can find common ground and work together as a team with genuine pleasure (Wicks, 1998). As the literature pertaining to the anxieties triggered when working with adolescents with cancer suggests, effective team working is imperative for the functioning of a therapeutic environment (Gunderson, 1983) and the development of effective and high-quality patient care. As one professional on the adolescent cancer unit stated, 'If the team isn't healthy or working well the ward doesn't work well . . .'

Table 4.5 highlights some of the key elements for good team working (Firth-Cozens, 1998). Essential components include reflection, adaptation, and full participation, where everyone is a member of the team and all the skills of a team are recognised and valued. Communication, support, and information, against a background of truthfulness, through the multidisciplinary team meeting, creates the framework for this. As one of the senior medical staff also stated in our research:

> The weekly meeting is key to showing the involvement of everybody and I would hope that their views are listened to . . . the ward works well in terms of allowing people to feel that they have a voice, and I don't always know which grade nurses are, but they all seem to ask things . . . My job is made easier by a well polished team . . . I would regard myself as no more than a component in the process.

Effective leadership is essential in helping the healthcare team recognise its primary goal, maintain its values and philosophy, and help build a coherent sense of purpose. Ensuring that the environment is supportive and enabling whilst

Table 4.5 Strategies to encourage good team working

Clear team goals and objectives
Clear accountability and authority
Diversity of skills and personalities
Clear individual roles for members
Shared tasks
Regular internal formal and informal communication
Full participation by members
Reflexivity
Diversity
The confronting of conflict
Monitoring of team objectives
Feedback to individuals
Feedback on team performance
Outside recognition of a team
Two-way external communication
Team rewards

working 'diplomatically' with the wider organisation and external bodies (Engel, 1994), often in the context of competing needs and changing circumstances, is also vital. This in turn can shape the wider culture of care. Participation in wider organisational processes and in meetings for the raising of issues and problems that a team or unit may be facing is also crucial for the development of effective and empowered individuals and teams (Jones, 2003). All of this helps to promote support and coping.

Care and support

Whilst the caring professions are not always good at caring for themselves or for each other, the lack of support for all staff and the under-provision of care for a profession with a mandate to care seems staggering (Rafferty and Traynor, 2002). The quotes below illustrate the importance of supporting and caring for each other in adolescent cancer care (Kelly *et al.*, 2004):

> It always concerns me how you support staff through this and how you actually make sure that they remain invigorated and don't feel damaged by the whole process . . . particularly for junior medical staff, who are a species resistant to any concept of support.

> We all give a lot but I think it is important that people feel that their giving is being appreciated. And I think that if appreciated by their colleagues they don't demand it as much from their patients.

Empathy is essential when individuals and the group confront the ambiguity, uncertainty, and anxieties stirred by their work involving cancer. Understanding oneself, others, and the dynamics of the group are central to effective participation in a team, the management of the self and of others, and, indeed, the provision of good quality care to the patients and families (Pearce *et al.*, 2001). More empirical evidence is needed, but there can be no doubt that caring for staff is directly related to the quality of patient care provided (Miller, 2000).

There is a lack of studies and, indeed, policy and organizational initiatives that explore and attempt to address the complexities of caring in healthcare organisations. As Miller (2000) suggested in his book exploring stress and burnout in human immunodeficiency virus/acquired immune deficiency syndrome (HIV/AIDS), there needs to be a differentiation between both chronic and acute stress, the former needing to be addressed by long-term and often multifaceted interventions and individual, interpersonal, and organizational causal factors and strategies. Table 4.6 gives examples of some of the strategies that are important to think

Table 4.6   Care and support strategies for individuals and teams

Care	Support
Professional supervision	Clinical supervision Performance review Mentorship
Emotional support	Therapeutic counselling One-to-one and group debriefing Normalisation of the expression of stress and acknowledgement of the impact of loss
Team working	Regular multidisciplinary team meetings Team building time Education and workshops on inter-professional working Clinical discussion groups

Self-care and nurturing	Family and friends support
	Exercise, relaxation, and meditation
	Holistic therapies, e.g. massage and yoga: these techniques
	    can be individually accessed or access offered via the
	    organisation
	Outings and fun time (outside of work and with work
	    colleagues)

Environmental	Pleasant environment, e.g. clean, light, and bright Quiet staff areas Adequate facilities, e.g. changing room, kitchen, and canteen

Management	Training, education, and skill development opportunities
	    including stress management
	Appropriate resources in terms of staff numbers and
	    equipment
	Pre-employment orientation
	Limitation of work hours/Scheduling of work breaks and
	    holidays

about as individuals and as teams working in adolescent cancer care. As the National Association for Staff Support (1992) highlighted, staffs' individual rights need to be valued and respected: recognition of the nature of stress and the need for emotional support is at all times important.

Concluding thoughts

In the published study by Kelly *et al.* (2004) one of the most significant conclusions was the importance of effective care being provided within a supportive environment which acknowledges the wider social and cultural needs of both the adolescents and their families – and also the staff who are caring for them. The sense of mutual support, or what we termed the 'therapeutic milieu', was a central finding and suggests further attention is required both in the adolescent cancer field, but also in cancer care and, perhaps, the professional caring world more generally. This is true of research, policy development, and in the development of effective models of multi-professional care.

The chapter has gone full circle, starting with the cultural meanings of care and finishing with practical strategies for self-care and the care of the team and unit. As Benner and Wrubel (1989) suggested, caring itself is not the cause of stress. Rather it is the loss of caring that causes sickness or burnout. We recover when we return to care and to our relationships to ourselves and with others. Reflection on practice, boundaries, and emotions, support groups and supervision, complementary therapies, counselling, and relaxation strategies, and effective management, environments, resources, and leadership are some of the ways that individuals, teams, and organisations can not only make caring for adolescents with cancer easier (Mackereth *et al.*, 2005) but can also ensure the development of sustainable care.

References

Allen, D. (1997) The nursing–medical boundary: a negotiated order? *Sociology of Health and Illness*, **19**(4) 498–520.

Aneshensel, C. S. (1992) Social stress: theory and research. *Annual Review of Sociology*, **18**, 15–38.

Bailey, C. (2001) Cancer, care and society. In: *Cancer Nursing: Care in Context* (eds J. Corner & C. Bailey), pp. 26–46. Blackwell Science Limited, London.

Bailey, R. & Clarke, M. (1989) *Stress and Coping in Nursing*, Chapman & Hall, London.

Benner, P. & Wrubel, J. (1989) *The Primacy of Caring: Stress and Coping in Health and Illness*. Addison-Wesley, Menlo/Park, CA.

Bowlby, J. (1979) *The Making and Breaking of Affectional Bonds*. Routledge, London.

Bram, P. & Katz, L. (1989) The study of burnout in nurses working in hospice and hospital oncology settings. *Oncology Nursing Forum*, **16**(4) 555–560.

Briggs, S. (2002) *Working with Adolescents: a Contemporary Psychodynamic Approach*. Palgrave Macmillan, Basingstoke.

Brown, D. & Pedder, J. (1991) *Introduction to Psychotherapy*, 2nd edn. Routledge, London.

Cohen, M. Z. & Sarter, B. (1992) Love and work: oncology nurses' view of the meaning of their work. *Oncology Nursing Forum*, **19**, 1481–1486.

Corner, J. (1993) The impact of nurses' encounters with cancer on their attitudes towards the disease. *Journal of Clinical Nursing*, **2**, 363–372.

Corner, J. (2002) Nurses' experiences of cancer. *European Journal of Cancer Care*, **11**, 193–199.

Cull, A. (1991) Staff support in medical oncology: a problem solving approach. *Psychology and Health*, **5**, 129–136.

Delvaux, N., Razavi, D., & Farvacques, C. (1988) Cancer care: a stress for health professionals. *Social Science and Medicine*, **27**(2) 159–166.

Engel, C. (1994) A functional anatomy of teamwork. In: *Going Interprofessional: Working Together for Health and Welfare* (ed. A. Leathard), pp. 64–67. Routledge, London.

Field, D. (1984) 'We didn't want him to die on his own' – nurses' accounts of nursing dying patients. *Journal of Advanced Nursing*, **9**, 59–70.

Firth-Cozens, J. (1998) Celebrating teamwork. *Quality in Healthcare*, **7**(Suppl.), S3–S7.

Foucault, M. (1973) *The Birth of the Clinic: Archaeology of Medical Perception*. Vintage, London.

Freudenberger, H. (1974) Staff burn-out. *Journal of Sociological Issues*, **30**, 159–165.

Goffman, E. (1969) *The Presentation of Self in Everyday Life*. Penguin Books, London.

Gray-Toft, P. & Anderson, J. (1981) Stress among hospital nursing staff: its causes and effects. *Social Science and Medicine*, **15**a, 639–647.

Gunderson, J. (1983) *Principles and Practices of Milieu Therapy*. Jason Aronson Inc., Hillsborough, NJ.

Helman, C. G. (1994) *Culture, Health and Illness*, 3rd edn. Butterworth Heinemann, Oxford.

Hinds, P., Quargnenti, A., & Hickey, S. (1994) A comparison of the stress response sequence in new and experienced paediatric oncology nurses. *Cancer Nursing*, **17**(1), 61–71.

Hochschild, A. R. (1983a) Emotion work, feeling rules and social structure. *American Journal of Sociology*, **85**(3), 551–575.

Hochschild, A. R. (1983b) *The Managed Heart. Commercialization of Human Feeling*. University of California Press, Berkeley, CA.

Isikhan, V., Comez, T., & Danis, M. Z. (2004) Job stress and coping strategies in health care professionals working with cancer patients. *European Journal of Oncology Nursing*, **8**, 234–244.

James, N. (1989) Emotional labour: skill and work in the social regulation of feelings. *Sociological Review*, **37**, 15–42.

Jenkins, J. F. & Ostchega, Y. (1986) Evaluation of burnout in oncology nurses. *Cancer Nursing*, **9**(3), 108–116.

Jones, A. (2003) Some benefits experienced by hospice nurses from group clinical supervision. *European Journal of Cancer Care*, **12**(3), 224–232.

Kelly, D., Ross, S., Gray, B., & Smith, P. (2000) Death, dying and emotional labour: problematic dimensions of the bone marrow transplant nursing role? *Journal of Advanced Nursing*, **32**, 952–961.

Kelly, D., Mulhall, A., & Pearce, S. (2004) 'Being in the same boat': ethnographic insights into an adolescent cancer unit. *International Journal of Nursing Studies*, **41**, 847–857.

Kent, F. G., Wills, G., Faulkner, A., Parry, M., Whipp, R., & Coleman, R. (1994) The professional and personal needs of oncology staff: the effects of perceived success and failure in helping patients on levels of personal stress and distress. *Journal of Cancer Care*, **3**, 153–158.

Klein, M. (1959) Our adult world and its roots in infancy. In: *Group Relations Reader* (eds A. Colomon & M. A. K. Geller), pp. 247–263. Rice Institute Series, Washington, DC.

Kleinman, A. (1988) *The Illness Narratives: Suffering, Healing and the Human Condition*. Basic Books, London.

Larson, D. (1992) The challenge of caring in oncology nursing. *Oncology Nursing Forum,* **19**(6), 857–961.

Lazarus, R. (1966) *Psychological Stress and the Coping Process.* McGraw-Hill, New York.

Mackereth, P. A., White, K., Cawthorn, A., & Lynch, B. (2005) Improving stressful working lives: complementary therapies, counselling and clinical supervision for staff. *European Journal of Oncology Nursing,* **9**, 147–154.

McNamara, B., Waddell, C., & Colvin, M. (1995) Threats to a good death: the cultural context of stress and coping among hospice nurses. *Sociology of Health and Illness,* **17**(2), 222–244.

Mawson, C. (1994) Containing anxiety in work with damaged children. In: *The Unconscious at Work: Individual and Organizational Stress in the Human Services* (eds A. Obholzer & V. Zagier Roberts), pp. 67–75. Routledge, London.

May, C. (1993) Subjectivity and culpability in the constitution of nurse–patient relationships. *International Journal of Nursing Studies,* **30**(2), 181–192.

Menzies, L. I. (1988) *Containing Anxiety in Institutions – Selected Essays,* Vol. 1. Free Association Books, London.

Miller, D. (2000) *Dying to Care? Work Stress and Burnout in HIV/AIDS.* Routledge, London.

Miller, D. & Gillies, P. (1996) Is there life after work? Experiences of HIV and oncology health staff. *Aids Care,* **8**(2), 167–183.

Mohan, S., Wilkes, L., Ogunsiji, O., & Walker, A. (2005) Caring for patients with cancer in non-specialist wards: the nurse experience. *European Journal of Cancer Care,* **14**(3), 256–263.

Mulhall, A., Kelly, D., & Pearce, S. (2001) Naturalistic approaches to health care evaluation: the case of a teenage cancer unit. *Journal of Clinical Excellence,* **3**, 167–174.

National Association for Staff Support (1992) *A Charter for Staff Support for Staff in the Health Care Services.* National Association for Staff Support, Woking.

National Institute for Health and Clinical Excellence (2005) *Improving Outcomes in Children and Young People with Cancer.* National Institute for Health and Clinical Excellence, London.

Newlin, N. & Wellisch, D. (1978) The oncology nurse – life on an emotional roller coaster. *Cancer Nursing,* **1**, 447–449.

Obholzer, A. & Zagier Roberts, V. (1994) *The Unconscious at Work: Individual and Organizational Stress in the Human Services,* Routledge, London.

Ogle, M. (1983) Stages of burnout among oncology nurses in the hospital setting. *Oncology Nursing Forum,* **10**(1), 31–34.

Papadatou, D., Anagnostopouros, F., & Mouros, D. (1994) Factors contributing to the development of burnout in oncology nursing. *British Journal of Medical Psychology,* **67**, 187–199.

Patterson, J. & Zderad, L. (1976) *Humanistic Nursing.* John Wiley, New York, NY.

Pearce, S. (1997) The experience of stress for cancer nurses: a Heideggerian phenomenological approach. Unpublished MSc dissertation, Institute of Cancer Research, University of London.

Pearce, S. (1998) The experience of stress for cancer nurses: a Heideggerian phenomenological approach. *European Journal of Oncology Nursing,* **2**(4), 235–237.

Pearce, S., Kelly, D., & Stevens, W. (2001) 'More than just money' – widening the understanding of the costs involved in cancer care. *Journal of Advanced Nursing,* **33**(3), 371–379.

Pearlin, L. (1989) The sociological study of stress. *Journal of Health and Social Behavior,* **30**, 241–256.

Pollock, K. (1988) On the nature of social stress: production of a modern mythology. *Social Science and Medicine,* **26**, 381–392.

Pruyser, P. W. (1984) Existential impact of professional exposure to life threatening illness. *Bulletin of the Menninger Clinic,* **48**(4), 357–367.

Rafferty, A. M. & Traynor, M. (2002) A case study of the functioning of social systems as a defence against anxiety. In: *Exemplary Research for Nursing and Midwifery* (eds A. M. Rafferty & M. Traynor), pp. 111–141. Routledge, London.

Ramirez, A., Graham, J., & Richards, M. (1995) Burnout and psychiatric disorders among cancer clinicians. *British Journal of Cancer*, **71**(6), 1132–1133.

Roach, M. S. (1984) *Caring: the Human Mode of Being. Implications for Nursing*. Faculty of Nursing, University of Toronto.

Savage, J. (1995) *Nursing Intimacy: an Ethnographic Approach to Nurse Patient Interaction*. Scutari Press, London.

Schon, D. A. (1983) *The Reflective Practitioner*. Jossey-Bass, London.

Seyle, H. (1957) *The Stress of Life*. McGraw Hill, New York.

Smith, P. (1992) *The Emotional Labour of Nursing*. Macmillan Press Ltd, London.

Sontag, S. (1979) *Illness as Metaphor*. Penguin Books, London.

Stewart, B., Meyerowitz, B., Jackson, L., Yarkin, K., & Harvey, J. (1982) Psychological stress associated with outpatient oncology nursing. *Cancer Nursing*, **5**, 383–387.

Turner, M. (1999) Involvement or over involvement? Using grounded theory to explore the complexities of nurse–patient relationships. *European Journal of Cancer Care*, **3**(3), 153–160.

Ullrich, A. & Fitzgerald, P. (1990) Stress experienced by physicians on the cancer ward. *Social Science and Medicine*, **13**(9), 213–218.

Vachon, M. (1987) *Occupational Stress in the Care of the Critically Ill, the Dying and the Bereaved*. Hemisphere Publishing, Washington, DC.

Vachon, M., Lyall, W., & Freeman, S. (1978) Measurement and management of stress in health professionals working with advanced cancer patients. *Death Education*, **1**, 365–375.

Walker, M. (1994) Principles of a therapeutic milieu: an overview. *Perspectives in Psychiatric Care*, **30**(3), 5–8.

Weisman, A. D. (1981) Understanding the cancer patient: the syndrome of caregiver's plight. *Psychiatry*, **44**, 161–168.

Wells, M. (2001) The impact of cancer. In: *Cancer Nursing: Care in Context* (eds J. Corner & C. Bailey), pp. 63–86. Blackwell Science Limited, London.

Whippen, D. A. & Cannellos, G. P. (1991) Burnout syndrome in the practice of oncology: results of a random survey of 1000 oncologists. *Journal of Clinical Oncology*, **9**(10), 1916–1920.

Wicks, D. (1998) *Doctors and Nurses at Work, Rethinking Professional Boundaries*. Open University Press, Buckingham.

Wilkinson, S. M. (1994) Stress in cancer nursing: does it really exist? *Journal of Advanced Nursing*, **20**, 1079–1084.

Winnicott, D. W. (1947) Hate in the counter-transference. In: *Collected Papers: Through Paediatrics to Psychoanalysis*, pp. 194–204. Hogarth Press, London.

World Health Organization (1984) *Glossary of Terms Used in the 'Health for All' Series*, Nos 1–8. World Health Organization, Geneva.

Yasko, M. (1983) Variables which predict burnout experienced by oncology nurses. *Oncology Nursing Forum*, **6**, 109–116.

Young, A. (1980) The discourse on stress and the reproduction of conventional knowledge. *Social Science and Medicine*, **14B**, 133–146.

Zagier Roberts, V. (1994) The self assigned impossible task. In: *The Unconscious at Work: Individual and Organizational Stress in the Human Services* (eds A. Obholzer & V. Zagier Roberts). pp. 110–121, Routledge, London.

Zapf, D. (1996) Stress factors at work and mental health. In: *Current Topics in Occupational Health: Knowledge and Research Needs*, pp. 68–78. The European Commission, Luxembourg.

A Young Person's Experience 2
Life During Treatment

Kelly Denver

Cancer. The very word immediately conjures up images of death and sadness. The result of this was that, following my diagnosis in February 2001, I had little idea of what treatment would bring. Images of ailing parents or tiny, helpless children in hospital beds, bald and sick, filled my mind, but something inside me refused to visualise myself in their place. As a result, upon entering Weston Park Hospital, Sheffield, for my first treatment, I was still completely unaware (or in denial) of what was about to happen.

My diagnosis of non-Hodgkin's lymphoma meant I needed an 18-week programme of chemotherapy that was designed to destroy my immune system and with it the cancer. Embarrassingly, at the initial diagnosis I was not told that lymphoma was a type of cancer and thus spent several days at school feeling relieved that it was less serious than I had imagined.

My consultant had warned me that I would be likely to lose my hair and so, most unwillingly, I had my shoulder length brown hair cut into a 'bob'. I hated it. Hated it with a passion. In hindsight, this was entirely unrelated to my new appearance, but to the fact that it had been forced upon me. I felt as though I was walking around with a sign attached to my forehead that read 'I've got cancer'. That was not an exclamation that I was happy to make.

Although I would only have 1 day of treatment every 3 weeks the impact upon my body would be severe: my A levels were suspended and schooling effectively stopped. It was a weird feeling, knowing that I would never go back and to realise the agonies of the teenage mind are tiny, compared with what lay ahead.

Sitting in the outpatient's reception area with my mother, my 18-year-old self felt decidedly out of place amongst the predominance of elderly people, and I stared at the same page of my book for 20 minutes to avoid meeting their gaze. I did not want to see their curious looks, wondering whether the patient was my mother or I, and to look at them was a reminder of what I would become – pale, sunken, and bald.

My name was called for a blood test and then an hour's wait ensued whilst the results were tested in the laboratory and I was deemed fit for treatment. The outpatients' treatment area was a bright room, in which plastic-covered armchairs lined three walls and the fourth acted as a dispensing counter. I was expecting to be given four drugs, but little could have prepared me for what followed. First, I was given and was highly thankful for an injection of an anti-sickness drug through an intravenous cannula. 'Great,' I thought, then the itching hit me, about half a minute before the nurse said 'Some patients do experience a tingling sensation, don't worry.' It only lasted about 5 minutes and was gone as quickly as it had come, but I had the ominous feeling that this was only the beginning.

Second, I was presented with a small saucer containing what looked like 16 tiny red sweets – if only – they were steroids and I was asked to swallow them as quickly as I could so that I could move on to drug number 2. I looked from my mother to the nurse and then down at the not-so-innocent tablets. 'She has got to be kidding,' I thought, 'I can't even take a paracetemol.' Apparently, however, if your mother distracts you sufficiently anything is possible. Luckily, the other three drugs were via the intravenous cannula and directly injected so no more tablets were involved, much to my relief.

I'm not sure why, but I expected to feel sick immediately following the treatment, but, except from feeling a little shaken by the whole experience, I left with anti-sickness tablets and a blood test appointment for 2 weeks in the future. However, 3 hours later I began a night during which I learned what it was like to feel really dreadful! I slept on a mattress next to the toilet that night wondering if it was possible to be sick *all night* or whether I would eventually go to sleep. Although I began to feel better soon after, the next week was spent confined to bed, taking anti-sickness tablets and the daily steroids and treating a walk downstairs as heavy exercise, so shocked was my body by the onslaught of the chemicals.

After my first treatment I was transferred onto an 18-month treatment scheme, of which the first 3 months would be spent in hospital. This was because a second biopsy had shown the tumour to be more resistant and high grade than originally suspected, and normal life simply went out of the window. I was given the choice to remain on the previous regime, but to me the answer was obvious: if the longer treatment meant life, I would grab hold of it with both hands.

Thus far I have given a distinct impression of negativity about my treatment, which actually does me a disservice. It was a time when my ability to stay upbeat and positive about my situation was challenged repeatedly. However, following the shock of the initial stages of treatment and the acceptance of the changes that would occur in my life, I stepped decidedly onto the path of recovery and ignored all thought of an alternative ending.

The first 3 months consisted of treatment almost every day, but often I was allowed to go home if my blood counts were high enough. My mother had stopped working to keep me company and I remain eternally grateful to her. Looking back, I can remember only odd snippets from this time, as my body was struggling against the evils of both chemotherapy and the cancer. Certain drugs had 'weird and wonderful' side effects and, even though my regime was very rare, my lymphoma nurse kept me informed of what I should expect: on the other hand, other drugs left their names firmly imprinted upon my memory. L-asparaginase or, as my mum referred to it, 'asparagus', seemed like a harmless injection and yet every morning, for the 7 days I had it, I suffered car sickness and was in the hospital toilet for an hour before I could emerge for the injection. Harmless? I think not!

Another little fiend was cytosine arabinoside. To take this drug I was connected, via my Hickman line, to a drip stand for 7 days and 7 nights. Aside from the fact that changing my tops became something of a circus act, this drug was so successful in killing cells that, 24 hours after finishing it, I was readmitted to hospital with a non-existent blood count and a temperature of 40°. Over the next 2 weeks, I fought the neutropaenic septicaemia that had invaded me with antibiotics, paracetemol, many blood and platelet transfusions, and a flannel on my head. This was the only time during my treatment when I acknowledged the chance that I might die – and the possibility that it would be something other than cancer truly humbled me.

The hardest aspects of these 3 months were the boredom and isolation induced by the hospital situation. Being treated, aged 18 years, in an adult cancer hospital, I was in a minority and met very few people of my own age. Usually treated in a bay of six, there was one television between us all and I rarely had it – although my mum did bring me one in from home when I was in for long spells. But there was very little else in the way of distraction: white walls, drab curtains, and a few flowers. Had it not been for the constant support of my mum I think I would have lost all sense of personality and become a representative of my symptoms, but I read, listened to music, and attempted art – all in the name of sanity.

Friends visited, but the ward atmosphere was not conducive to friendly chats and my bald, skinny appearance was not aided by the homogeneity of appearance that surrounded me. 'Friends': an interesting subject in the context of chemotherapy. I have to admit to only telling the bare minimum when I was first diagnosed, as I didn't know how to cope with the new situation, let alone how to protect others when I told them. A few people did visit: some took me out for a drive, others came to watch a film with me, and some just rang often to see how I was. Strangely, they were not necessarily the friends that I had thought would be there to support me. Many of them found the thought and the sight of a cancer patient too much and we drifted apart. However, the boys seemed to rise to the challenge by visiting with pictures from school parties and the gossip I yearned for to distract my mind from the mundane. It did upset me to lose touch with some people, but others were brought into my life, who have proved to be great friends.

Following these 3 months I took my A levels at home – amazingly getting three grade As, which made the future seem hopeful rather than stunted by my illness. Not, however, until I had started on the 15-month maintenance regime that required 1 week of treatment every 3 weeks. Some of the drugs were beginning to make me feel less sick, but the thought of others such as thioguanine (12 tablets per day for a week) was enough to make me nauseous. The only way I could take them was with strong blackcurrant juice, although this flavour now induces nausea by association. My least favourite treatment, however, was the lumbar puncture that came round every 13 weeks. This was a painful procedure and I felt very vulnerable lying on my side with the consultant injecting methotrexate into my spinal column, even though my mum tried to distract me with crosswords!

This period spent at home was the best test of perseverance. The time away from hospital reminded me just how much I didn't want to go back, and I found myself crying more and more as each round of treatment neared. In addition, because I was having less chemotherapy I was less dozy and more aware that I was slow. I had also been whispering for so long from tiredness that I could no longer shout, and I found these things hard to accept. At about the halfway mark I became very low, as I could not remember the person I had once been, but I couldn't yet picture a future. A short and unwilling spell on Prozac gave me the boost I needed, however and I started going to the gym when I felt well enough, just to get out of the house. I think at this point I became aware of what I was missing. All my friends were at university and, although I didn't feel jealousy, I did feel left behind and that made me feel lonely. I didn't want to be a burden to them when they came home.

Throughout the 18 months of treatment I felt most worried about the effect that my illness was having upon other people. I have always felt that being the patient is easier than watching, as there is less of a feeling of futility. Having initially stopped working, my mum had returned part time and had to leave me for several days a week, which I know worried her. She was my emotional support, with the patience of an angel. Dad found his role in the injections and flushing of my Hickman line, but for my younger sister I think I was just a 'pain'. She was doing her A levels and wanted to have friends over, yet my lowered immunity often prevented this. If she got a cold, she was relegated to the other side of the house and, if I needed attention, I had to have it. With hindsight, I can see that it must have been quite stressful having to be the healthy child. It has taken time to rebuild our relationship and she can now understand that I needed a lot of emotional support during that time, but that at no time did I mean to take time or attention away from her.

Finishing my treatment was a bittersweet moment. I was glad to be finished, but terrified to leave the folds of the hospital, only to return for check-ups at ever-increasing intervals. I also found reintegration very hard. I had lost so much confidence throughout my treatment through not being able to discuss my feelings with other young people with the same experiences that I no longer really knew how to interact with my own age group. I took a gap year, working in schools to build up my confidence and now, 4 years later, I am finishing my geography degree and hoping to become a teacher, but I still fear those check-ups: in fact it gets worse every time I visit as I settle into life beyond cancer and I think it always will.

Chapter 5
Supportive Care for Adolescents and Young Adults During Cancer Treatment

Neale Harvey and Alison Finch

Introduction

When we were asked to write this chapter the first question that occurred to us was, what do we mean by supportive care for the teenager or young adult with cancer? What does the term encompass? What are its dimensions, both in terms of the concept of supportive care, but also in relation to the dimensions of the concept of adolescence or young adulthood? This musing led us to ask the question is supportive care different for these populations and, if so, what is different, why is it different, and how is it different? This provided us with some structure, at least to the questions posed. To begin this exploration we would like to return to our opening question. What do we mean by supportive care for the young person with cancer? To address this question adequately we feel it necessary to subject it to some further analysis:

1. What does the term supportive care mean?
2. What issues impact most profoundly when considering the supportive care needs of young people with cancer?

Supportive care: how is it defined?

Discussions around the supportive care needs of children with cancer can be found in the literature dating back to the 1960s and possibly earlier (Siegelman, 1964; Djerassi, 1967). This element of cancer care was then and largely still is generally associated with the amelioration of the side effects and symptoms associated with cancer and its treatment, for example pain, nausea and vomiting, oral care, cancer-related fatigue, and so on. However, contemporary usage of the term supportive care can be demonstrated to be inconsistent both in its definition and application: this is compounded by the continued interchangeable use of supportive care, palliative care, and symptom control, as selected definitions

---

Box 5.1   Selected definitions of supportive care

1. Supportive care is designed to help patients and their families cope with non-curable disease and its treatment. This care includes diagnosis and treatment, which results in improvements, continuing illness, or death. It also covers bereavement. It helps patients to maximise the benefits of treatment and to live as well as possible with the effects of the disease (National Council of Hospices and Specialist Palliative Care Services, 2002; cited by Morgan, 2003).

2. Supportive care is the term for interventions used for supporting the patient through the anticancer treatment period. Outcomes in cancer are dependent not only on the safe and effective delivery of treatment, but also on the timely and effective management of the acute and longer term side effects. Improvements in supportive care have played a key role in increased survival (National Institute for Health and Clinical Excellence, 2005).

3. Definitions of supportive care on the World Wide Web:

    *   Care given to improve the quality of life of patients who have a serious or life-threatening disease. The goal of supportive care is to prevent or treat as early as possible the symptoms of the disease, side effects caused by treatment of the disease, and psychological, social, and spiritual problems related to the disease or its treatment. Also called palliative care, comfort care, and symptom management (www.stjude.org/glossary).
    *   Treatment given to prevent, control, or relieve complications and side effects and to improve the comfort and quality of life of people who have cancer (www.seniormag.com/conditions/cancer/cancerglossary/glossary.htm).
    *   Treatment aimed at reducing the clinical signs of disease, e.g. providing fluids to correct dehydration (members.lycos.co.uk/furbabies/glossary5.html).
    *   http://www.google.co.uk/search?hl=en&lr=&oi=defmore&q=define:supportive+care.

---

illustrate (Bisset *et al.*, 2001; Regnard and Kindlen, 2002; www.google.co.uk, search: 'define: supportive care') (see Box 5.1).

The National Council of Hospices and Specialist Palliative Care Services (2002) definition has been variously cited (Morgan, 2003; National Institute for Health and Clinical Excellence, 2004). Indeed, the Morgan (2003) citation explicitly limits the realm of supportive care to those with a 'non-curable disease' (Box 5.1). As the 5-year disease-free survival for teenage cancer patients can range from 40% to 90%, dependent on diagnosis (Cancer Research UK, 2004), it could be argued that this would imply that those 'cured' are not 'eligible' for supportive care? However, it should also be noted that the National Council of Hospices and Specialist Palliative Care Services (2002) scope extends beyond the boundaries of the patient and includes support of the family through treatment, death, and bereavement. This contrasts sharply with the National Institute for Health and Clinical Excellence (2005a) publication *Guidance on Cancer Services: Improving Outcomes in Children and Young People with Cancer – The Manual*, which limits supportive care to interventions for side effects during the treatment period,

---

Box 5.2   Improving outcomes guidance in children and young people with cancer

Domains of supportive care
   Febrile neutropenia
   Central venous access
   Blood product support
   Pain management
   Management of nausea and vomiting
   Nutrition
   Oral and dental care

NICE (2005a).

---

choosing to place broader dimensions of care under the heading of a care pathway (Box 5.2). Entering the term 'supportive care' into a popular search engine on the World Wide Web affirms this dimensional dichotomy of philosophy or intervention (www.google.co.uk, search: 'define: supportive care') and, in the nursing discourse, this was exemplified by Redmond's (1996) review of symptom management and Richardson's (2004) holistic discussion, both of which were framed as supportive care. Such muddied waters suggest that it is necessary to interrogate and deconstruct the term, asking what each word, supportive and care, means. Hanvey (2006) considered this:

> *The New Oxford Dictionary of English* defines support as; 'bear all or part of the weight of: hold up', supportive as; 'providing encouragement or emotional help' and care as; 'the provision of what is necessary for the health, welfare, maintenance and protection of someone or something' (Pearsal and Hanks 1998, p. 1865 & 275). This suggests investment of considerable agency to bear all or part of the weight in the provision of what is necessary for the health, welfare, maintenance and protection of the teenager with cancer whilst providing encouragement or emotional help. However this raises further questions. What does this agency consist of and what are supportive behaviours or actions? But, most importantly, what are the needs they aim to meet? (pp. 7–8).

Defining supportive care

We want to make it clear from the outset that it is not our intention in this chapter to discuss evidence-based supportive interventions for symptom control. Rather we would direct interested readers to the National Institute for Health and Clinical Excellence (2005b) publication *Guidance on Cancer Services: Improving Outcomes in Children and Young People with Cancer – The Evidence Review*, which provides a comprehensive evaluation and grading of the extant literature. The above discussion suggests that the effective delivery of supportive care for young people with cancer has the potential to be vast in its dimensions and complex in its scope. Therefore, to elucidate what such interventions may look like it is important to first establish our philosophical or epistemic position.

Clinicians in various disciplines continue to view the randomised controlled trial (RCT) as the gold standard for research and, therefore, the generation of new knowledge (Rolfe, 2000). However, we believe that, in order to comprehend the dynamic dimensions of supportive care needs in adolescent cancer successfully, such a reductionist approach would be of limited value. The evidence that we have chosen to present should be viewed from a post-modern perspective of 'little narratives'. These are not narratives in the sense of a narrative discourse: rather, in this context, the term narrative is used to describe each way of knowing amongst the competing discourses. This epistemic position challenges the dominance of the RCT as *the way* of knowing and promotes a plurality of discourses that do not compete but complement, thereby enabling a richer understanding of phenomena (Rolfe, 2000).

As vehicles for discussion we will present vignettes from our own practice. The chosen vignettes exemplify particular challenges or issues that teenagers, their friends and family, and ourselves as healthcare professionals have faced as we negotiate the path of each cancer journey. The supportive approaches employed are intended to promote mental health, a sense of normality, functional coping, choice and control, decision making in response to disease, treatment modalities, and hospitalisation. A philosophy of care that was developed by staff caring for adolescents at University College Hospitals London underpins this approach (Box 5.3).

In order to provide a logical structure and comprehensive framing to this chapter, attention will be given to each of the developmental tasks outlined in Box 5.4. At this point we again reinforce that we do not claim to provide absolutes: rather, each vignette should be viewed as a reflection of the reader's

---

Box 5.3   Teenager Cancer Trust unit: philosophy of care

You deserve the right to be recognised as individuals with unique and changing needs.
We recognise that your cancer diagnosis affects not only you but also your family and friends.
Our policy is one of honesty, openness, and informed consent. You can expect to be cared for with respect and dignity.
The care planned by your team will aim to meet your needs and also foster personal control, understanding, and growth of independence.
We will strive to allow equal access to services provided: therefore, you should not feel disadvantaged due to differences of race, colour, ethnicity, gender, language, sexual orientation, religious belief, physical ability, age, or football team!
All care provided should be clinically effective based on research wherever possible and provided by competent and professional practitioners.
We will always endeavour to do our best for you.

This revision circa June 1998.

Box 5.4 The developmental tasks of adolescence

- Forming a clear identity
- Accepting a new body image
- Gaining freedom from parents
- Developing a personal value system
- Achieving financial and social independence
- Developing relationships with members of both sexes
- Developing cognitive skills and the ability to think abstractly
- Developing the ability to control one's behaviour according to socially acceptable norms
- Taking responsibility for one's own behaviour

Based on Havighurst (1952) from Russell-Johnson (2000).

---

own experience. Some points may resonate more than others and the generalisability of each vignette will be unique to each reader (Popay *et al.*, 1998). Where possible we will draw on appropriate theory to analyse data and attempt to draw out emerging meanings, patterns, and themes.

The young person and cancer

To identify and respond effectively to the needs of young people with cancer it is important to consider the often complex issues facing any young person. For it is within this context that the event of cancer occurs. Definitions of adolescence are many and varied, each attempting to capture and convey the essence of the concept succinctly. From selected historical definitions it is possible to identify key words, such as 'change' (Lore, 1973), 'transition' (US Department of Health Education and Welfare, 1979, cited by Taylor and Müller, 1995, p. 3), and 'develops' (Pearsal and Hanks, 1998, p. 23). This suggests a temporal movement from one state to another. Indeed, theorists have attempted to make sense of this journey from childhood to adulthood that we have come to accept in Western society as adolescence (Hall, 1904, cited by Gross, 2001; Erikson, 1968; Coleman, 1993). Chronological definitions have also been widely used although there is also much variance and little corroboration in these (Leonard *et al.*, 1996; Souhami *et al.*, 1996; Viner and Keane, 1998; Gross, 2001). In health care this has resulted in claims that go as far as to state that it is 'clearly impossible' (Leonard *et al.*, 1996, p. 117) to set age boundaries: rather, they are set for the 'practical purpose' (Souhami *et al.*, 1996) of service planning (Viner and Keane, 1998). This confusion and difficulty of definition supports the view that, as a concept, adolescence is unstable (Coleman, 1993; Barnes, 1995): an ill-defined[able] (*sic*) social construct, more *grey* than *black and white*. It is therefore essential to explore the qualities and context of this period of transition.

Adolescence and transitions

Hall's (1904, cited by Gross, 2001) seminal treatise of adolescence is regarded as the starting point for the use of the term transition in describing the adolescent experience (Conger and Galambos, 1997; Coleman and Hendry, 2000). Whilst this term is applicable at a rather high level of abstraction, concerns remain that attempts to clarify specific transitions or stages have yet to achieve wide agreement (Coleman and Hendry, 2000). It could be argued that this continued debate could actually be a reflection of the intrinsic idiosyncratic nature of adolescence in Western society as discussed above: it is not a static concept. This continual drift was exemplified by the work of Chisholm and Hurrelmann (1995) as they plotted the timing of key milestones of transition to adulthood in a historical context (Fig. 5.1). However, in the absence of agreed transitions or stages it is important nonetheless to explore the 'work' that is occurring for the adolescent during this time.

Havighurst (1952, cited by Russell-Johnson, 2000) identified the key tasks of adolescence (Box 5.4). The apparently small number of these tasks belies their complexity, not just as individual tasks, but their interrelatedness and co-dependency, which we hope to illustrate in this chapter. But how indeed are these tasks accomplished?

As mentioned previously, several theoretical models have been suggested to explain the process of development through adolescence: how and when such tasks are accomplished. Graber and Brooks–Gunn (1996) supported the view that adolescence is indeed a period of transition, but argued that to consider it as one long transition would be 'broad and sweeping' (p. 768). Rather, they

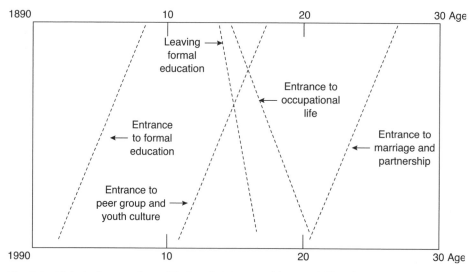

Fig. 5.1 Historical comparison of timing of status transition to adulthood.

suggested that key life events should be considered as separate transitional periods that are characterised by universal developmental challenges. These challenges demand a modification of the approach to and development of skills to cope with biological, psychological, or social change. Whilst Graber and Brooks-Gunn (1996) discussed the impact of negative life events on the progression through transitions, such as drug taking and smoking, they did not consider the impact of chronic illness or indeed a life-threatening diagnosis. It is also important to consider that a cancer diagnosis is not an isolated event: rather, the diagnosis marks the start of a process often referred to as *the cancer journey*. This journey *must* run alongside the process of transitions of adolescence, as neither journey can be put 'on hold'. Therefore, it is important to consider the impact a cancer diagnosis has on the adolescent's ability to modify their approach to and development of skills to cope with the biological, psychological, or social change brought on by that diagnosis. But what of the young adult with cancer? What help might they need to achieve developmental and personal goals?

Beyond adolescence

It is also important to explore what we mean when using the term *young adult*. Whilst the Viner and Keane (1998) definition of adolescence accommodated a flexible upper age range into the early twenties, recent discussion has proposed a chronology of 16–26 years (Barton, 2006). The difficulty defining this group and the resulting dichotomy has implications in the following ways:

1. If the professions engaged in the care of these patients do not communicate using language that is technically consistent, then it becomes difficult to move discussion and strategy forward.
2. Whilst the strategic development, design, and delivery of care should be informed by such discourse, it must also recognise legal boundaries, e.g. the age of majority.

It is not our intention, however, to devalue or denigrate such work. Rather, this discussion seeks to advance discourse by raising such questions. These issues are fundamental and foundational to young and emerging sub-specialities; exploration is needed to help organisations develop cogent arguments on how best to meet young persons' needs. For the purpose of our continued discussion we will use the term young person to encompass both adolescents and young adults.

The zeitgeist of youth is in motion as it responds to socio-cultural influences. This can place ongoing developmental tasks and the social context at odds. The prolonged dependence on the parental role, due to increasing numbers in higher education, student debt, and high house prices, must ultimately have implications for the timing of key tasks, such as achieving social and economic independence, gaining freedom from parents, and, ultimately, establishing an adult identity. The relationship between the young person and their environment or context in which the development is occurring is central to the growing theoretical perspective of developmental contextualism (Coleman and Hendry, 2000).

This school of thought subscribes to the notion of 'goodness of fit', which states that the individual and the context are inseparable. 'Goodness of fit' enables a consideration of the degree of congruence between the needs and aspirations of the individual and the nature of the social or physical world: the developmental outcome is therefore dependent on how well these two systems match. It is quite possible that the young person may have continuing developmental challenges that are context related. Application of this notion in the cancer context emphasises the potential dissonance that can be created, not only to the aspirations of the individual, but also to their social and physical world. Therefore it is vital that we, as healthcare professionals, develop an active awareness of patients' aspirations and context, to help support the interruption created by a cancer diagnosis.

Supporting the tasks of adolescence: forming a clear identity

Being diagnosed with cancer at a time when a young person is taking steps to establish their own identity outside of the family and lay down aspirations for their future life threatens their journey towards an emergent independent self. How individuals endeavour to deal with their experiences beyond our encounter at their bedside is intrinsic to developing an understanding of the patient experience (Richardson, 2004). Yet our involvement with young people and families outside hospital may be limited, in some sense shielding us from the emotional toll that extends beyond the clinical context of their situation.

Cancer shapes and redefines life's meaning, becoming a permanent and significant marker in the young person's personal biography of life. Life thereafter is seen to take on a new identity both for the individual and their family (Lewis, 2006), the uncertainty of the disease compounding existential fears for what is at risk and what may be lost or not realised. What we will later describe as one of 'the most challenging ironies of cancer, in adolescence is the development of abstract cognitive thought. Having an awareness of 'being' and recognition for one's future potential drives the excitement of youth: this is reinforced by familial and societal expectation. Cancer, however, dares to challenge immortality, significantly threatening future aspirations. Adolescents describe the feeling of life being 'put on hold', the fulcrum of a certain future shifting into unpredictability and the unknown:

> The last 2 years at school have all been about the future, working hard, achieving good grades, then university and a career. I want to get on with my future, but my life plan has now been snatched away from me. I now have 'no plan' except to get better . . . but even that's out of my control (Ross, aged 18 years, following a diagnosis with acute myeloid leukaemia, personal communication).

Life thereafter often becomes a metaphorical 'battle' against the odds, with the young person thrust back into the heart of family life. *Their* cancer subsequently becomes the family's concern. Patenaude (2000) suggested that teenagers and young adults may worry about how to exert and develop their independence at a time when family cohesion is mandated by the physical and psychological demands of their illness. Whilst grounded in a family systems context, this chapter addresses such issues from the young person's perspective, with the intent of fostering *their* personal growth and a sense of control. In this sense our work complements Chapter 3 by Anne Grinyer, which explores the impact of cancer on parents.

The perception of cancer has shifted since the work of Sontag (1979) from one of covert shame to 'an evil enemy to be battled with ferocity and pride' (Mason, 2006, p. 11): societal expectation denotes that pain and suffering is met with defiance and that strength of character emerges through adversity. Surviving cancer therefore becomes a lifelong battle that is 'just as bad as the stigmatising paradigm it has replaced' (Mason, 2006, p. 11). Even at a 5-year disease-free marker 'the battle' is not 'won'. Living beyond the sword of Damocles (Koocher and O'Malley, 1981), a metaphorical sword suspended by a single hair that hangs over the head of cancer survivors, is suggestive of a life always tinged by the uncertainty and fear of a cancer's return.

The ever-present threat of an unknown future is most usually problematised with a negative connotation in extant literature (Parry, 2003). Yet from our practice we bear witness to immense strength of spirit, resilience, and maturity amongst young people living with a cancer diagnosis. Greater awareness of life's purpose and an existential sense of 'being' in the world are seen to develop alongside emotional maturity far exceeding a young person's chronological years. A sense of unity is often fostered that transgresses age:

> I remember the first time I spoke with someone older . . . there I was just out of school alongside a father of 45. Yet I saw in him what I could see in me (Ross, aged 18 years).

As a consequence of this heightened awareness of being, our patients may feel that they are on a different emotional level from their friends. Prolonged periods of hospitalisation may also impact on social contact with peers, a situation that is often intensified with an increased physical and psychological dependence on parents and the immediate family. Returning to the dependence of childhood, the antithesis of independence and maturity, may also be observed in our practice. This observation reinforces how the nature and treatment of cancer impinges uniquely on each young person's ability to express their sense of self.

Accommodating a changing or new body image

The physiological changes of puberty in many ways mark the beginning of adolescence, resulting in greater interest and anxiety about one's physical self-concept (Gross, 2001). The demands that physiological and hormonal changes impose on the young person require intense negotiation and psychological adjustment, but it is the very nature of adolescent development that makes this a difficult and often unsettling task. The sense of 'flux', the fluidity of perception and emotion experienced during this period, challenges the teenager's evolving sense of identity and self-concept. These changes or fluctuations in self-image can confuse or impair self-perception, impacting on self-esteem (Richie, 2001).

The term 'body image' is often used interchangeably with terminology such as self-esteem and self-concept. Though a highly subjective and multi-faceted construct (Rosen *et al.*, 1991), its use invariably assumes commonality of definition and meaning. References are often made to 'negative' or 'positive' body images (Burt, 1995), yet application of this terminology fails to 'distinguish the multiple dimensions that comprise subjective aspects of body appearances' (White, 2000, p. 184). These dimensions, comprising perceptions, thoughts, and feelings about such elements as body size, competence, and function, are in many ways inseparable from feelings about the self he or she asserts (White, 2000).

Body image is, therefore, different from but a significant dimension of self-concept. Gross (2001) discussed two differing body images in adolescence, the way the young person thinks they look and the ideal of the way they would like to look. This conflict, coupled with a constantly changing self-concept, poses a considerable challenge to the healthy adolescent. For the young person diagnosed with cancer, concerns about physical appearance, heightened body awareness, and body ideal may be further intensified as illustrated in the vignette (Box 5.5) below.

Body image is embedded in the total experience of cancer (Gibson *et al.*, 2005). It is also a fundamental feature of puberty and adolescence, imprinting on the young person's identity and future sense of self. Yet in this context how often do we overhear casual attempts at reassurance that focus on the temporality of a patient's treatment-related losses?

Box 5.5   I'll be the brunt of friends' jokes

Kerry, aged 15 years, was recently diagnosed with acute myeloid leukaemia. She admitted that, when she started treatment, her biggest fear was alopecia. Kerry had always worn her long blonde hair loose around her shoulders, which she felt 'defined me . . . who I am', but had her head shaved after getting fed up of finding loose hairs on her pillow. 'Not having hair doesn't really bother me much anymore,' she assured her parents and staff. Kerry used to be worried that people might laugh or that she'd be the brunt of jokes, but has surprised herself with her ability to adapt. 'I used to wear a hat, but now I just don't worry,' she now confidently remarks.

Kerry then concedes that, since her diagnosis, she has not been out beyond the hospital reception and worries about going out socially when she is well enough to go home. She feels safe on the ward and within the confines of the hospital, explaining that most people she has seen around 'don't look normal', which she finds comforting. 'It's having to see my friends again that I worry about most. Mum says not to worry too much, it'll grow back soon enough . . . I suppose it will. The one thing that I wasn't prepared for though was that I'd lose all my body hair . . . now that really bothers me.'

In the vignette (Box 5.5) Kerry asserts that she has got used to losing her hair and does not feel the need to conceal her baldness under a hat. Indeed, Kerry gives the impression that she feels relatively at ease with this aspect of her physical appearance. As we read further, however, it is apparent that this sense of confidence is self-limited to the boundary of the hospital's physical environment. Amongst her peers baldness now potentially isolates her, singling her out as different from her friends, at a time when acceptance and conformity is generally regarded crucial to the maintenance of self-esteem. Within the security of the ward, however, Kerry's physical appearance can and does fulfil a need to feel accepted, corroborating with research undertaken on an adolescent unit identifying how 'Baldness seemed to represent a mark of belonging' (Kelly *et al.*, 2004, p. 852).

To an onlooker Kerry's hair loss signifies her status as 'a cancer patient', robbing her, like other individuals, of any privacy they may wish to keep about their illness (Freedman, 1994; Evans, 1997). Beyond the immediate ward environment her physical appearance may attract questioning stares from the curious or sympathetic looks from others. Faced with a very physical assault on her developing self-image, Kerry is faced with having to negotiate her new 'cancer'-focused identity and interaction in the social world (Woodgate, 2005).

Alopecia, a very visible sign of cancer, acts as a constant reminder of the disease for the person and those close to them (Wells, 2001; Richer and Ezer, 2002; Kuzbit 2004). An altered body image, however, transcends the 'visible' to recognise the impact of internal bodily change on self-perception and psychosocial wellbeing. For girls who have developed a woman's body, specifically by growing breasts, body hair, and commencing menstruation, cancer and its treatment-related symptoms may exacerbate an already profoundly disorientating experience (Lanyado, 1999). Personal symbols of adult femininity and sexuality may be compromised, as eyebrows, eyelashes, and pubic hair may be lost (Evans, 1997). Loss of body hair and muscle bulk, and the worry of infertility, may similarly threaten the masculine 'body ideal' and sense of self.

This conflict between the 'ideal self' and the 'real self' can impact negatively on psychological wellbeing and self-esteem (Woodgate, 2005), which in turn may have a negative effect on coping, although evidence to support this supposition is lacking. Research into body image remains to date focused on a general weight-related appearance, with few attempts to understand cancer-associated appearance changes (White, 2000). We must therefore draw on our own clinical experience to help shape and enhance understanding and practice. It is important, however, that we do recognise such gaps in the evidence base relating to the 'everyday issues' facing young people with cancer and challenge ourselves to translate this experience into research enquiry.

Cancer treatment is by its very nature intensive and protracted (Leonard *et al.*, 1996), with chemotherapy, radiotherapy, and many invasive and possibly mutilating procedures having to be tolerated (Evans, 1996). In addition to the aforementioned hair loss, there is a whole directory of additional physical side effects that can challenge the adolescent's sense of self. A puffy face, weight gain, and feelings of persistent bloating and restlessness associated with steroid treatment may exacerbate the sense of 'living in a stranger's body' often cited by young people. Other physical side effects, such as skin pigmentation changes, scarring, tremors, immobility, and weight loss, may contribute to feelings of self-consciousness and isolation from peers (Allen, 1997; Whiteson, 2003). Tunnelled central venous access lines, implanted ports, and nasogastric tubes may be further endorsed with significant meaning (Daniels, 1996), not only through their physical effect on appearance and restrictions on lifestyle, but as a psychological reminder of the new cancer self. Young people can struggle to respond to this, cancer's depersonalising upheaval.

Internally mediated changes may be equally as upsetting and disorientating as those that are outward and physically apparent (Evans, 1997). Tiredness, muscle weakness, and lack of concentration can restrict the activity that a young person confidently engages in and may be perceived as additional confirmation of being different from others, particularly peers. Vinca alkaloid-induced peripheral neuropathy, myocardial damage and weakness associated with anthracycline use, emotional fragility exacerbated by high-dose steroids, and use of norethisterone medication to suppress menstruation are just a few examples of other internal changes that threaten self-image and self-esteem (Zeltzer, 1993; Enskär *et al.*, 1997; Hockenberry-Eaton *et al.*, 1999; Gibson *et al.*, 2005).

The significance of symptom management on body image and self-concept

The impact of a cancer diagnosis is often amplified once treatment has begun and the young person starts to experience symptoms (Woodgate, 2005). Nausea, vomiting, diarrhoea, constipation, uncontrolled pain, and mucositis often present huge discomfort and embarrassment for a young person, making it hard to retain their dignity and a sense of control (Evans, 1997). Treatment-related fatigue may also burden young people, 'making everyday life a struggle' (Gibson *et al.*, 2005, p. 656) and compounding feelings of failure and dissatisfaction with oneself. Good symptom management, however, may restore some semblance of control for the individual, advancing their perception from 'being a passenger in your own body' (Matt, aged 17 years) to feeling secure and connected again.

Woodgate (2005) undertook a qualitative study with 15 adolescents aged between 12 and 18 years in an attempt to understand adolescents' perceptions of how cancer affected their sense of self. Most significant to these young people was the distress and suffering experienced from clinical symptoms and their experience of physical and mental bodily change (Woodgate, 2005). Such a finding has a clear message for clinical practice: some disease- and treatment-associated symptoms and side effects may be clearly unavoidable (for example, hair loss or weight gain), but others (such as nausea or stomatitis) can often be well managed and should be addressed within the context of supportive care at its most elementary stage. Good pre-emptive symptom management has a critical role in helping to develop a positive sense of self.

The interrelatedness of the physical symptoms, emotional impact of the illness, and adolescents' evolving self-concept invariably means that to separate the illness from the individual's identity would be fallacious. Instead the illness becomes embedded in the personal identity and sense of self. Yet this does not necessarily signify acceptance or successful accommodation by the young person, who may struggle to reconcile these demands with their 'pre-cancer' self.

In our experience young people fear losing themselves irrevocably amidst a tangled web of disease, symptoms, and bodily change. They feel under pressure to act with maturity and stoicism whilst simultaneously craving the nurturing support and encouragement of friends, family, and professional staff. Young people in this position often struggle to reassure others that they are in essence still fundamentally the 'same old person' within. Woodgate (2005) concurred with this: her study indicated that it was important for those involved in adolescents' lives to respond to them like they were the same person, whilst taking subtle account of their difference from others. As healthcare staff we have an important role in both meeting this challenge and questioning to what extent our practice accommodates this. An exploration of the actions that may be undertaken in order to support young people's accommodation of changes to self-concept is presented in Table 5.1. Detailed are some of the possible effects of a cancer diagnosis on a young person's emergent identity and sense of self, as well as offering suggestions for professional engagement that may be perceived as supportive.

Physical appearance, sexual attraction, and social acceptance are of special importance during adolescence and young adulthood. Disease- or treatment-related changes in appearance vary in their prominence, permanence, controllability, and extensiveness (White, 2000). Grouping these changes or symptoms together under the heading 'altered body image' may therefore risk derogating the complexity of each individual's unique experience. For example, the temporality of treatment-related changes may provide hope for many young cancer patients of a future closer to their body ideal. For the adolescent facing salvage or loss of a limb or anatomical structure, however, an unavoidable permanence to their situation is presented. Such individuals risk losing their sense of the (pre-cancer) self in a more profound way (Shell and Miller, 1999):

> Whenever I look in the mirror I know I'll never see John without cancer again (John, aged 20 years, post-limb salvage surgery).

In this context the skilled support of a cohesive multidisciplinary team becomes even more crucial to the individual's task of preparing for, adapting to, and re-negotiating their new identity in the world. In particular, sustaining feelings of hopefulness and restoring body image may be extremely difficult when future life plans are shattered by disability (Hinds and Gattuso, 1991; Hinds *et al.*, 1999). A young person with an amputation, for example, is faced not only with the loss of anatomical function, but their lifestyle and future career may also be under threat. For a young person with testicular cancer the affected anatomical structure is

Table 5.1 Possible impacts of cancer on self-concept: supporting young people through altered physical appearance and emotional and internally mediated changes

Impact	Support
Feelings of vulnerability and perceived difference, which can be debilitating	Facilitate a trusting environment in which it is safe to share experiences and ask questions
Feeling misunderstood	Be willing to listen to young people's accounts of their symptoms, as they are the experts in explaining how they feel: symptoms that can be controlled should be managed, advancing self-perception from being 'a passenger' to being 'in control'
Not being consulted about decisions relating to a person's self	Respect the individual and their decision-making capacity: facilitate informed decisions and choices wherever possible to foster a sense of control
Fear or embarrassment may deter young people from asking questions	Prepare young people honestly for their experiences, anticipating, where appropriate, their need to ask questions that may feel difficult or awkward
Feeling 'at odds' with change	Promote the normalcy of routine, the constancy of which may be helpful at a time of physical and emotional change: be prepared to challenge routines in equal measure
Being different	Adolescence and young adulthood is a time when the security gained from conforming to a trend or particular genre is self-assuring and comforting for the young person: try to reassure that this need not change
Feeling isolated from peers	Where appropriate encourage relationships with other patients of a similar age: having someone to relate to and identify with may counterbalance feelings of isolation
Infringement of physical and emotional space	Respect the young person's need for privacy: allowing time alone to reflect on feelings and self-concept can be perceived as painful, but may also be therapeutic
Being witness to others' symptoms and suffering	The ward environment provides an open, visual display of the cancer experience: help support young people through this rather than hiding such realities

symbolic of masculinity and sexual performance (Gurevich *et al.*, 2004), whilst potentially impacting on fertility and hopes of future parenthood.

Cancer diagnosis and treatment requires renegotiation with different aspects of the self. At the same time, individuals will be required to renegotiate external relationships as they traverse the path of their cancer journey. The following section explores this process in more detail.

Negotiating a new relationship with parents

Living with a cancer diagnosis is a family concern (Coscarelli, 2000). It imposes change not just on the individual, but the whole family, etching an imprint on both individual and family identity and ways of life. The entire family unit is seen to experience life with the illness (Shaw and Halliday, 1992; Newby, 1996; Robinson and Janes, 2001). This often requires individual members having to redefine relationships and make adjustments to their familial and societal roles. It is the interactive and reciprocal nature of the individual and family experience that suggests viewing cancer within a family systems model or perspective is both meaningful and cogent. At the foundation of this theoretical perspective is a belief that an individual cannot be considered in isolation from their wider social world.

Healthcare professionals may often consider their primary commitment or focus to be their patient, but the needs of other family members should not be overlooked, just as the interdependent relationship between the parents and their son or daughter should not be disregarded. Whilst it is right to concentrate on meeting the psychological and developmental needs of the young person, a more comprehensive approach to care would traverse relationships between them and their surrounding familial and social system. Moving towards this 'family-centred' nursing care often poses a significant challenge to the inexperienced professional. Yet embracing this concept remains important into early adulthood, and our supportive role to both the young person and their family is central to effective therapeutic care. With this in mind the following section explores three vignettes that focus on a young person's relationship with their parents at a time when they were undergoing treatment for cancer.

The development of a life-threatening illness has been identified as a parent's worst fear (Thompson, 1990). Cancer is an inherently emotive word that is often associated with fears of death, re-occurrence, uncertainty for the future, disruption in lifestyle, short-term losses, forced adjustments to family life, and personal anxiety or distress (Northouse, 1992; Lewis, 1996; Lewis *et al.*, 1996). It is not unusual for parents to attempt to shield their child from the impact of the diagnosis and treatment, irrespective of their son or daughter's age. In comparison with younger children, however, adolescents may experience 'a fuller and more adult sense of the potential loss and its meaning' (Adams-Greenly *et al.*, 1986, p. 134).

For a young person, being diagnosed with cancer during their adolescent years can place an immediate halt to their journey towards an independent adult life.

One newly diagnosed 17 year old described himself being 'in time neutral', the uncertainty of his situation making him unable to look to the future, his feelings compounded by a sense of powerlessness and of being suspended in time, orbited by his parents and health professionals. Yet he took comfort from feeling that there was a sense of temporality to his situation. Other young people, however, have articulated that, from the point of diagnosis, their relationships with family and friends changed irrevocably. For more detailed discussion of the impact of adolescent cancer on parents see Chapter 3.

The emerging independent self

All young people, irrespective of illness or disability, must negotiate the path to an emergent, independent self. As we have described, adolescence is a time when the development of identity and individualisation is of particular relevance, played out through renegotiating one's role in the family and in developing relationships outside of the home environment. The physical impact of a cancer diagnosis and its subsequent treatment poses a stress that stifles an emerging independent life, particularly as increased dependency on others often becomes necessary when one is feeling ill. Low self-esteem and depression associated with the cancer is not uncommon and may compound the sense of dependency on others. Treatment and symptoms that impact on central nervous system function affecting cognition and cognitive development will pose an additional threat to present and future independent life.

Hospitalisation impacts significantly on parent–adolescent relationships. Living each day with a parent in confined physical and emotional space will be unfamiliar for any young person, but with increasing age and maturity a mother or father's continued presence during a hospital admission may further threaten a young person's independence and the fragile sense of self. Physical ill health and disability inevitably involves others in order to meet the basic activities of living, and it is often the parent rather than the nurse who responds to the need for help with washing, dressing, and toileting. This 'infantile dependency on parents' (Grinyer and Thomas, 2001, p. 166) may not only evoke feelings of frustration and lack of control, but the physical intimacy that such care demands may raise its own difficulties. A young person's initial embarrassment experiencing a symptom such as diarrhoea with a parent present, for example, may be superseded by resigned acceptance of the need for their help.

Jack (Box 5.6) had been admitted to an adult ward. Standing nearly 183 cm tall and with the physical characteristics of a grown, and man some of the staff caring for him could not quite make sense of this situation. Jack was physically mature and was, they felt, to all intents and purposes, 'adult-like'. It was hard for them to understand why he wanted his mother with him, especially as he was clearly angry with her. The incongruity between the manner in which Jack appeared physically and the way he felt had perhaps not been appreciated (Neven, 1997).

Jack felt scared, vulnerable, and physically unwell. He therefore quickly accepted his mother's wish to remain with him and found himself taking a more

---

Box 5.6 Sharing my 'bedroom' with Mum

Jack was 16 years old when he was admitted to hospital with relapsed acute lympho-blastic leukaemia. A keen footballer, Jack had recently started to spend weekends away playing with his team. Jack hadn't coped at all well with the shock of relapse and sudden hospitalisation. In response to this his mother decided take leave from work in order to remain at hospital with her son during the day. Jack's mother then spent each night on a mattress at the bedside. After a month in hospital the strain of this arrangement had become evident.

Jack had been taking daily steroids as part of his treatment programme. His perpetual hunger, continual snacking, and subsequent rapid increasing size became difficult for him to cope with. Jack had always been physically strong, but now he felt cumbersome. He felt like a stranger in his own body and was frustrated by his clumsiness and 'sloth-like' self. Jack had become increasingly aggressive towards his mother: it was not unusual to hear him shouting at her and he had on one occasion hit out at her whilst in a rage.

---

passive role in the relationship, not having the mental strength or drive to assert autonomy or participate in decisions about his care himself. Development of autonomy is a critically important task in adolescence (Conger and Galambos, 1997), yet the dichotomous relationship between emergent autonomy and the desire to remain in the safety and comfort of childhood can be difficult for all young people to negotiate. As seen here, the desire to assert oneself juxtaposed against the need to feel protected is often intensified when faced with a life-threatening illness.

All behaviour carries meaning. Jack's frustration and anger towards his mother was self-evident. Whilst there could be clinical explanations for this (e.g. the side effects of steroids), one must also consider the possibility that it emanated from a very real fear that he was losing his identity and former sense of self, compounded by the experience of their living together in a single hospital room for many weeks. By shouting at his mother, Jack may have been attempting to assert himself and re-establish a degree of control. Neven (1997) corroborates this: in her observation of mother–son relationships she described how a young male may feel that he has no option but to be cruel to his mother, because it represents the only way to create separation. Months later Jack spoke to us about this time, explaining that he felt totally consumed by his mother's presence:

> Mum was crowding out my space . . . it was too much. I know she was trying to take care of me but . . . I mean it's not normal at my age to have your Mum hang out in your room with you . . . and there she was with me 24/7 (Jack, aged 16 years).

Often a mother's intuitive feeling is to remain with her child in hospital, irrespective of the son's or daughter's age or gender. As healthcare staff we may find that we have more conscious, preconceived ideas about who should stay and for how long, according to the patient's age and stage of physical or emotional development. Relationships between young people and their parents, of the same or opposite genders, evolve and readjust continuously throughout the adolescent transition into adulthood and there is, therefore, no absolute guidance that can be offered. Enabling periods of physical and emotional space in the relationship, however, is suggested to help maintain and foster each individual's identity, independence, and autonomy.

We recall one parent who left her 14-year-old son alone on his very first night in hospital. She explained that this was a deliberate decision in order for her son to build rapport and gain the trust of staff independent from herself. She also expressed belief in the importance of him having his own 'thinking time'. This struck staff as a very brave and selfless act, as she was clearly distressed at leaving her son facing a new diagnosis of cancer alone on the ward. Others worried that he would feel isolated and upset. Yet, as a result of periods alone to reflect on his situation, this young person felt he had become more self-sufficient, and staff noted that he had greater control over his situation in comparison with some peers on the unit.

From early adolescence, young people do have the capacity to be alone, but parents often worry that, if they are left with their own thoughts, their children will dwell on their situation. Having time to 'just be', however, represents what Neven (1997) described as 'vital to being able to negotiate sad, unhappy and difficult experiences' (p. 159).

Although emotionally demanding, this may help the young person identify and articulate how they inherently feel, in contrast to the suppression of feelings, which is a risk in situations where a parent is continually present. At its most pragmatic level, having time apart from a parent whilst in hospital also provides opportunities to meet other young people and develop relationships with staff.

Trying to reconcile the situation

Life, of course, must continue beyond hospital, and the interface between the cancer world and normal life is often brought into sharper focus when hospital visits are balanced with the family's daily life. One of our older patients, Mark, aged 18 years, recently commented that 'it's hard for my parents, but I'm living this night and day, through times when they are not here with me in hospital.' He sensed that his parents felt guilty for the situation he had to endure. Each time his parents and grandmother visited they showered him with gifts. Yet he found that he no longer attached importance to materialistic gain, respecting and placing greater value on 'a decent shower and a night's sleep in my own bed'.

The following vignette (Box 5.7) illustrates the extent of the potential disruption of a cancer diagnosis on the family system. Sarah's family's values upheld the need to help out around the home in order to earn pocket money. With the exception of Christmas and birthdays, Sarah had to save independently for non-essential treats herself. Since being diagnosed with cancer, however, her parents had showered her with an abundance of gifts – an example of how illness challenges established patterns of behaviour within the family.

Box 5.7   Nothing's too expensive . . . if it will help make you better

Sarah was 15 years old and hospitalised with a new diagnosis of sarcoma. Her parents took turns to stay with her and meticulously attended to every detail in her care: clean towels, fresh pyjamas, a timetable for oral medications . . . They were noticeably keen to maintain some kind of control in what was an uncertain and unfamiliar situation. Staff noticed that Sarah's dad regularly returned to the hospital with gifts: a portable DVD player, a new mobile phone, and a bracelet she had admired whilst shopping with her mum. Her dad also offered to buy Sarah a special pair of gold earrings that she had been saving up for. Sarah's response to this offer was that they 'were too expensive', to which her Dad's response was 'nothing's too expensive if it will help make you better.'

'A pair of earrings isn't really going to make me better now is it,' Sarah retorted.

Parents' feelings of helplessness and inadequacy engendered by situations such as Sarah's can evoke a true sense of feeling 'out of control'. Treats are attempts, not only to provide distraction from the boredom of hospital life, but may also be an attempt to remedy the sense of impotence experienced. Parents very naturally wish to remove or redirect their son's or daughter's pain and suffering and gift giving may be an attempt to achieve this (Grinyer and Thomas, 2001). However, in Sarah's experience such behaviour appeared contradictory to established family values and beliefs.

Gift giving and/or the fulfilling of wishes are perhaps less emotionally draining ways of demonstrating affection. For the parent of the young person with cancer it is an obvious means of 'making things better', at least for that moment in time. Faced with an uncertain future, it is easy to see how spending can easily be justified, with the financial burden of this being considered immaterial.

Many young people with cancer have said that they do like to feel special at times (Woodgate, 2005), but that, fundamentally, they also want to feel that they are the same person. The experience of living with cancer sometimes makes this balance difficult to achieve. Readers may note rapid maturation amongst young cancer sufferers (Steefel, 2000) and a heightened sense of 'being in the world' is often also described in association with chronic illness experiences. Young people in this situation may place greater value on peer relationships and gifts of time and sentiment, rather than those of materialistic value. As a result, the status and acclaim previously associated with the latest fashion, information technology, or other 'must have' possessions may no longer be considered with the same respected standing.

The ethics of supportive care

Truth and disclosure in the context of cancer is a complex issue (Wilkinson, 2002). As professionals we each have our own perspective on the best way to manage a

---

Box 5.8   To tell the truth?

Ayesha, aged 14 years, remained in hospital 3 months after an allogeneic bone marrow transplant. Her recovery had been complicated by bacterial, fungal, and viral infection and by graft versus host disease of the liver. Ayesha was acutely unwell, septic, and in advancing organ failure. Whilst her team hoped she would survive, a shift in emphasis from active intensive treatment to palliation had become clinically indicated.

Ayesha's mother had raised her alone. She had remained with Ayesha throughout the transplant and indicated to staff that she recognised the significance of her daughter's steady deterioration. When the medical team spoke with Ayesha's mother, accompanied by her nurse, they gently explained the potential futility of continuing intensive treatment. Her mother agreed and a difficult discussion exploring treatment boundaries and palliation ensued.

At the close of this conversation Ayesha's mother requested that the medical and nursing staff did not tell her daughter that she was expected to die, stating that she believed this would be too emotionally painful for Ayesha to cope with. The healthcare team were faced with a difficult dilemma: did they collude with her mother and withhold this information from their patient or did they uphold the ethical principle of veracity (truth telling) and share with Ayesha knowledge of her likely imminent death?

---

situation: this is in part influenced by our own belief structure and personal and professional experience. We may inherently feel that the truth should always be told, yet each situation has its own unique circumstances and characteristics.

In this situation (Box 5.8), to advocate that Ayesha was told of her imminent death would not have been in accordance with her mother's expressed cultural beliefs or personal wishes. Her mother essentially believed that Ayesha would not be able to cope with the news and that she should therefore not be burdened with the knowledge that she was dying. In the vignette we see 'mum' trying to influence the team to collude with her and share custodianship of the truth. She appealed to the staff's professional judgement, presenting the argument that it would not be in her daughter's best interests to know of her clinical status, believing it would engender more harm than good. Ayesha's mother's emotional connection with her daughter's situation, however, posed a challenge to reasoned thought and decision making.

Balancing subjective motives with more objective reasoning can be attempted, yet the ethical principles of non-malfeasance (to do no harm) and beneficence (to invoke good) are inextricably difficult to delineate from each other in this situation (George, 2006). It is similarly difficult to ascertain the extent to which withholding information can be considered a beneficent act. This young person's situation was particularly challenging for the healthcare team to negotiate, as Ayesha's mother's wishes were in conflict with what many staff felt was both 'proper' and ethically 'the right thing to do'.

Ayesha, being aged 14 years, was legally a minor. Her mother had made key decisions about her treatment pathway up until then, but generally involved her daughter, as she felt this helped engender greater control and self-sufficiency. Death, however, challenged the collaborative relationship that mother and daughter had fostered. Like many young people living with cancer, Ayesha's life experience belied her age: she possessed maturity and emotional depth of character rarely seen in someone of 14 years of age. Arguably, she demonstrated the intellectual and emotional capacity to understand her situation. Nonetheless, how important was it that Ayesha knew she was going to die?

Staff felt particularly aggrieved that, by colluding with her mother, Ayesha would be denied the opportunity to talk with family, friends, and staff in the knowledge that she was dying. Key members of the nursing team firmly believed she should have had a choice and control in her own terminal care, but this was going to be problematic as the treatment's shift in emphasis from curative to palliative had not yet been explicitly communicated in her presence. Ayesha, meanwhile, began to ask questions about her wellbeing, and was increasingly frightened as the symptoms changed or progressed. Ayesha's mother responded to her daughter's articulated fear with reassurance that all would be well. She considered it imperative to maintain this reassuring guise believing that Ayesha would then enter the terminal phase of her condition without being scared of death. Yet Ayesha started to witness a steady stream of tearful visitors and whispered conversations, acts that perhaps indirectly served to reinforce the clarity of the truth that had not been openly discussed.

Ayesha died more suddenly than anticipated, 3 days after the initial discussion detailed in the vignette (Box 5.8). Her mother took comfort in the belief that her daughter died peacefully, unaware of her imminent passing. An interprofessional meeting to explore this ethical dilemma had been planned, and it still went ahead, although, rather than focusing on whether Ayesha should have been directly informed of her situation, it offered structured reflection on the team's involvement and decision making. Pivotal to the discussion was consideration of the relative importance of a cohesive approach to care and the extent to which this had been fostered.

Certain members of the healthcare team had always maintained that continued disclosure was indeed in the patient's best interests. One professional had organised some time alone with Ayesha to assist in the team's decision making. During their meeting, as Ayesha did not ask any questions, it was surmised that she had in effect chosen not to hear the truth. There could be a number of interpretations of this encounter.

One account could be that Ayesha instinctively knew she was going to die, yet chose not to raise this with her mother or staff in an attempt to protect both herself and others from further pain and distress. Co-dependent relationships of this nature have been substantiated in other research (Hilton and Gustavson, 2002; Finch, 2003). In both studies adolescents were seen to be conscious of modifying their behaviour with the intent of protecting both the self and others in light of the seriousness of their families' illness.

The ethical principle of veracity is complex by its very nature. In situations such as that of Ayesha, there is no right or wrong path to follow, as the subjectivity of the patient, their family, and our professional team influences the decision-making process. As professionals, we cannot also presume to always understand what is in the patient's best interests. It may be important to enable the family, as a partner in care, to therefore help lead and shape the decision-making process. Having the confidence in parents and family to know how their son or daughter would feel may assist the healthcare team in acting in their *proper* interests.

This situation illustrates the complexity inherent in each individual case and emphasises the need for multidisciplinary team discussion and cohesive team working in order to help resolve or, at best, contain such issues towards the best or, rather, the proper interests of all concerned. When one judges another culture through the lens of one's own, it is difficult, if not impossible, not to superimpose our 'alien' values on to that other culture. This is a complex issue that is not possible to explore in detail here. In the next section we will examine another ethical dilemma: issues of competent decision making.

Developing a personal value system

The development of cognitive skills and social awareness are necessary for developing moral thinking. Indeed, it has been argued that much of moral theory stems from the work of Piaget (1932; Coleman and Hendry, 2000). A significant focus of the work examining moral development has been conducted using hypothetical dilemmas that aim to measure the moral sophistication of the individual. Piaget (1932) identified two principal stages of moral development: an early stage of objective judgement, which was focused on consequence, and a later stage, where a subjective judgement was made based on intention. Kohlberg (1981) elaborated on this work and identified six stages against which moral thinking could be measured. However, Gilligan (1982) made a significant criticism of Kohlberg's (1981) work. Gilligan (1982) argued that the theoretical dilemmas used bore little resemblance to the real life dilemmas adolescents face and, furthermore, that they did not take account of other contextual factors such as gender. Therefore, when an adolescent finds themselves cast as the protagonist in a real and complex dilemma, what challenges does it raise for them and the team and what form of support is required? The following section examines the challenge of developing a supportive care strategy in response to a real ethical dilemma using ethical theory.

Consent

Consent is an accepted and fundamental part of professional practice. The concept of informed consent to treatment has received significant attention in the UK (Department of Health, 2001a–c). A formal record of consent is usually only obtained for major procedures or treatments, as consent for care usually happens informally and is implicit rather than explicit. This consent occurs through negotiation and is dependent on the practitioners's interpersonal relationships with their

---

Box 5.9   A refusal of care

As a 16-year-old young man, John was diagnosed with an osteosarcoma of his sacrum that extended into the nerve plexi. He also had multiple bilateral pulmonary meta-stases. Due to his extensive disease and several failed attempts to control his disease with chemotherapy, the team aimed to palliate his symptoms and, hopefully, allow him to die in a dignified manner, free from pain and distress.

John's social history was difficult and complex. He had been adopted at 3 weeks old and lived at home with his adoptive parents and one brother. Recent life had been difficult due to persistent bullying at school and, because of this, he had not attended school for several years and spent much of his time alone at home. Whilst on the unit a psychiatric assessment concluded that he was an intelligent boy who found the engagement forced by his situation difficult. He was not felt to be suffering from any psychiatric illness and was deemed competent. Continued contact with the psychi-atrist was recommended to support both John and the staff through this 'difficult time'. Both the palliative care and acute pain teams were involved in his management from admission. Despite continued attempts to control his pain it increased as his disease progressed. The pain affected his ability to mobilise and he found the experience of his pain and resulting physical restriction very difficult to cope with, often becoming fear-ful and distressed. This manifested in loud screaming and shouting when any attempt was made to negotiate his care. These distressed cries often filled the ward, which was upsetting for other patients and parents. John began to refuse all care offered, fearing exacerbation of his pain on movement. The nursing staff became very concerned that they were now unable to negotiate or maintain basic care, as he was refusing to leave his bed or allow his soiled sheets to be changed. His room was malodorous, which again was very distressing and offensive to the other patients on the ward.

This presented the team with the following dilemma. If they provided John with care in the absence of consent they risked accusations of the 'tort of battery' regardless of good intent (Kennedy and Grubb, 1994, p. 87). Alternatively, by respecting his refusal, they would be failing to prevent the foreseeable risk of his developing pressure sores, infection, and possible sepsis. The nursing staff, as the direct care providers, had identified that both the actions were imperatives of the UK Nursing and Midwifery Council (2002) *Code of Professional Conduct*. They believed that they had an obligation to perform both of these actions (duties), but they could not do both in this circumstance: a clash of duties existed (Beauchamp and Childress, 2001).

---

patients, responding to their individual needs by involving them in the decision-making process (Department of Health, 2001a–c; Sainio and Lauri, 2003). Sainio and Lauri (2003) reported that there has been little exploration in the literature of cancer patients' participation in nursing care decisions. This view is clearly valid, as much text and journal information deals with patients' consent or refusal for surgical or invasive treatments or procedures (Kennedy and Grubb, 1994; Pape, 1997; Jones, 2000; Edozien, 2001). Therefore, when one is faced with what appears to be *competent* refusal of basic care, there is little evidence to draw upon to inform the situation. How, then, does one establish a morally congruent path that upholds professional conduct, but also acknowledges and accommodates a young person's developing personal value system within a supportive care context? Here we examine the dilemma through the application of key ethical theories that illustrate the complexities involved in such circumstances.

Ethical theories

Applying duty-based ethics (deontology) in this situation demands that the guiding principle is that the intervention is judged to be right or wrong irrespective of the outcome achieved. In this case, both conflicting tenets of the nurse's code of conduct are duties of equal measure and, according to this school of thought, both should be upheld. Therefore, it first appears that duty-based ethics have little to offer in resolving this conflict. However, stepping outside the professional conflict and applying the rule of law, it was possible to achieve some resolution. Although John was legally able to consent to treatment at 16 years of age (in the UK), as he was under 18 years of age, a refusal of treatment could legally be overridden by his parents (Department of Health, 2001b,c). This decision provided the team with one duty, guided by law, allowing them to minimise foreseeable risk to John. However, this raised further concerns about John's autonomy (Box 5.9). Cancer patients often face issues that restrict their autonomy (Gadow, 1989): one should consider how overriding autonomy could be considered as a supportive care strategy in this context.

The presence of the emotion of fear can be viewed as a coercive and manipulating factor in John's decision-making process, and it raises questions about the validity of John's refusal. In order to consent and, therefore, to refuse, three criteria must be satisfied: (1) capacity, that is the ability to intellectually process information and make a decision, (2) information, that is having the necessary information to comprehend the arguments at hand, and (3) voluntariness, that is that the decision is made freely without pressure or coercion (Beauchamp and Childress, 2001; Kennedy and Grubb, 1994; Kamm, 1996; Jones, 2000; Edozien, 2001). In John's case he had been assessed as having the capacity to make such decisions. The team had informed John of the risks related to his refusal, therefore providing information. However, due to the coercive influence of his pain and resultant fear it is possible to question the condition of voluntariness. If the ability to act without controlling influences was not met, it could be argued that his refusal was non-competent.

Viewing this dilemma through the lens of utilitarian ethical theory, our concern shifts to that of the outcome achieved rather than the means of getting there. In this context one could argue that maximising the good for the many could involve overriding John's refusal. This would maintain his dignity (good), allow the nurses to perform one of their obligations (minimising risk), his parent's wishes for him to be cleaned would be met (good), and the malodour from the room would be significantly reduced, thereby improving the environment for the other patients (good). However, by ignoring the rules and concentrating on the outcome there is a potential that this perception of what constitutes *the many* may be misguided. The team not only have a responsibility to John and the patients directly under their care, but also to their professional bodies and to society in general. By failing to acknowledge and accommodate their professional rules and the law, they could potentially break their fiduciary responsibility to society and leave themselves open, not only to professional discipline, but also to criminal prosecution (Kennedy and Grubb, 1994; International Council of Nurses, 2000; Thompson *et al.*, 2000; Nursing and Midwifery Council, 2002; Tschudin, 2003). Therefore, focusing solely on outcomes fails to address the issue, as overriding a patient's wishes in this sort of situation would have the potential to undermine the public view of the profession. So how does one balance such ethical challenges whilst keeping the supportive needs of the patient central?

The four-principle approach put forward by Beauchamp and Childress (2001) does not claim to be an ethical theory in the traditional sense. It is based on 'considered judgements in the common morality and medical tradition' (Beauchamp and Childress, 2001, p. 37). They described the use of these principles as a method of specifying, deliberating, and balancing dilemmas when direct application of ethical theory has the potential for furthering the conflict or is unable to provide a clear resolution. This approach differs from duty-based ethics and utilitarianism, as there is no single absolute principle to judge or justify the moral worth of actions. Rather, the four prima-facie principles must be weighed in the balance through the application of experience and judgement. Developing a working knowledge of how to apply the principles of respect for autonomy, beneficence, non-malfeasance, and justice in practice is essential in the provision of supportive care that accommodates the developing personal value system of the young person. It requires that healthcare professionals maintain sensitivity with such complex issues if they are to support an individual's moral development successfully as they negotiate consent, choice, capacity, etc. The objective should not be to judge what is in the young person's best interests, but rather to try to meet their proper interests (George, 2006). This requires one to reflect on one's own ethical context in the situation and one's values, personal beliefs, biases, duties, responsibilities, and, indeed, liabilities. It is also important to note that making decisions for those considered non-competent cannot guarantee the 'right' outcome, as such decisions provide imperfect procedural justice (Beauchamp and Childress, 2001). Therefore, the involvement of families, guardians, courts, and health professionals must be considered to ensure a fair, reliable, but always imperfect outcome (Beauchamp and Childress, 2001). Once the decision to provide care was made, John was informed. He accepted that the care was necessary and was able to negotiate all of his care successfully under sedation until his death 6 weeks later.

Achieving financial and social independence

As we alluded to in our introduction, the concept of adolescence can be considered unstable as it responds to social and cultural changes (Chisholm and Hurrelmann, 1995). We also discussed the notion of goodness of fit between the young person's needs and aspirations and their context. As we have said

---

Box 5.10   I want my life back

Pat was 18 years old when she was diagnosed with a large retroperitoneal sarcoma. Shortly before her diagnosis she had left the family home, moving into a small flat. She had a job, her own money, and her own space. However, as her treatment progressed she had become very dependent on her parents to take her into hospital and care for her whilst she was at home. This had meant that she rarely stayed at her flat and spent most of her time out of hospital back at the family home. Throughout her treatment her mum and dad had been very supportive. However, Pat often perceived this as them fussing around her and interfering in her life. After a prolonged period of treatment with chemotherapy and surgery she was about to complete her final course of chemotherapy. In preparation for her discharge we were reflecting on her situation and her hopes and fears for the future. Although we discussed many issues she was clear: 'All I want is to get all of this over so that I can get my life back.'

---

previously, this raises concerns about the potential dissonance that a cancer diagnosis can exert on both the needs and aspirations of the young person, but also on their own sense of context. This can be particularly pronounced when they have begun to establish their financial and social independence. Such independence can range from holding down a part-time job to earn extra pocket money to having left the family home and asserting full financial and social independence. Cancer has implications for both circumstances, as the young person may need to give up their part-time job or the financial, social, and interim care needs may make it difficult for them to continue to live independently. Here (Box 5.10) we recall one young person who felt cancer had invited her parents back into her newly independent life.

It would appear that, for Pat, her independence was intrinsic to her life and, thus, her identity – as if getting away from her parents' control was as important as beating cancer. In one study that explored the transition of leaving home, it was argued that leaving is related to events that can track far back into the young person's and parents' history (Stattin and Magnusson, 1996). It is therefore very difficult, if not impossible, for those of us who meet the young person and their parents at such a time in life to grasp the complexity of their context in its broadest sense. However, we should be aware that feelings such as those expressed by Pat may have a validity that we cannot personally perceive. This is essential if we are to accept and value them as true to their experience. Conversely, we could possibly view Pat as being ungrateful for the support her parents had bestowed on her. However, this view could be considered as narrow, subjective, and unhelpful. This emphasises not only the importance of family relationships on how the young person seeks to assert their independence, but also suggests that other important relationships may have some role to play in how they move towards financial and social independence. Therefore, supportive care strategies should be cognisant not only of the time of life at which cancer occurs, but should be informed by what has gone before and make provisions for the young person's vision of their future. In the next section we consider the impact of cancer on developing relationships.

Developing relationships

Relationships with peers of both sexes play an important role in the development of adult identity. These relationships enable the young person to explore their thoughts and feelings in relation to a broad range of issues, such as social awareness, roles and behaviour, romance intimacy, and sexual identity. These can be seen to act as prototypes for future adult relationships (Conger and Galambos, 1997). As the young person moves from the dependent yearnings of childhood and strives for independence there is a need to achieve some separation from their parents. This is required not only to assert independence, but also to begin to negotiate an adult relationship with their parents: peer relationships can provide the space for exploring and affirming this. Furthermore, peer relationships have an equal orientation to the young person, whereas parents' orientation usually places the young person in a subordinate role, and subsequently peers can provide 'support, companionship and [serve to] reaffirm self-identity' (Coleman and Hendry, 2000, p. 140).

A cancer diagnosis can precipitate a dislocation from a teenager's social world. By this we mean that, although the relationship may still exist, the quality and function of it is affected by the diagnosis. This can manifest in a variety of ways, some of which will now be explored.

Peer relationships

Prolonged spells in hospital put the adolescent out of touch with the day-to-day happenings in their social world. Having access to peers over the Internet is helpful, but the young person may be restricted in doing so. For example, fatigue brought on by cancer and its treatment can last up to 4 weeks after each course of treatment (Gibson *et al.*, 2005). As many chemotherapy regimens are on cycles of 2–4 weeks this illustrates how pernicious and debilitating cancer-related fatigue can become. However, cancer-related fatigue is not restricted to physical fatigue, and mental and emotional fatigue brought on by worries can be just as debilitating. Whilst management of the symptoms of physical fatigue has only begun to be explored (Gibson *et al.*, 2005) the implications for emotional and social wellbeing also require consideration. Furthermore, adolescent patients have reported that their diagnosis has a stigmatising and isolating effect (Kelly *et al.*, 2003): therefore, one must always consider how their peers may respond when they do re-establish contact.

As we will discuss in Kim's story later (Box 5.12), being popular and attractive did not prevent her friends from 'abandoning' her soon after diagnosis. Whether this was to do with their fear of cancer, her reduced contact and availability, or her change in physical appearance is unknown. However, it is possible that a combination of such influences acted as a catalyst. In the case of Kerry (Box 5.5) her baldness defined her as different from her peers, but it was also the mark of belonging on the unit. This illustrates one of the very challenging aspects of peer relationships for these patients. Whilst a sense of shared understandings or 'being in the same boat' is an expected need of the adolescent (Conger and Galambos, 1997), this requires an understanding of what it is like to be in 'the boat', and this in itself may be an over-demanding expectation for peers 'back home'. However, peer relationships also form on wards and units between patients who *do* have a shared understanding of their circumstance. These relationships are at one and the same time vital and perilous. Vital as we have said for the shared understanding and all that brings, but perilous as each has an uncertain future and the impact of relapse, disease progression, and death cannot be over-emphasised. Indeed, the gestalt of this shared experience can persist into survivorship. We recall one patient talking several years after his successful, albeit harrowing, matched unrelated donor transplant about the impact his cancer experience had on him. He told us that he felt a sense of arrogance towards people who had no idea of what he and his friends (other cancer patients) had been through, and that probably the worst thing they had experienced was a messy break-up with a girlfriend. At the time it seemed that he really gained a mature perspective on what was important in life, something that set him apart. That was until his relationship broke down and we realised that he was not immune from the devastating effects that such a circumstance brings. Regardless of what he had been through before, he could still be hurt. Therefore, it is also important to consider what romantic or intimate relationships are occurring during this time.

Romantic relationships

The onset of puberty places the development of secondary sexual characteristics central to the development of the adult sexuality or sexual identity. However, the physical changes of puberty do not themselves deliver the sexual identity: social and emotional development are also intrinsic (Coleman and Hendry, 2000). Furthermore, it has been suggested that the pursuit of romance and intimacy or falling in love is part of the quest for identity (Zani, 1993; Moore and Rosenthal, 1998), supporting the colloquial notion of the 'other half'. That is, one's other half is as much about one's sense of self-definition as it is about one's partner, and vice versa. Romantic relationships can act as a mirror to the emerging adult, thereby allowing a reciprocal and intimate exploration of the self (Coleman and Hendry, 2000). However, this can present a challenge for the young person with cancer, as their partner may feel ill-equipped to explore not only what the diagnosis means to the patient, but also what it means to them. Furthermore, there are data to support an inverse relationship between intensity and longevity between opposite sex (romantic) and same sex (platonic) relationships (Feiring, 1996). Therefore, if the effects of a cancer diagnosis can threaten platonic peer relationships, 'prototype' romantic relationships would appear to be particularly fragile. It is also important to consider that, although they may be prototype relationships

---

Box 5.11   It's not supposed to be like this!

James was 16 years old when he was diagnosed with non-Hodgkin's lymphoma. He was admitted for work-up to treatment, part of which required him to store sperm prior to starting the proposed chemotherapy regimen. The team had just briefed James and his parents about the content of his 'work-up' when his father approached me asking to speak privately. He told me that he was very nervous about talking to James about storing sperm: although they were close, they did not have such intimate conversations. He was reassured that it would be usual for a member of the team to provide some written information, which would be supported by an explanation of the whole process. James would also have an opportunity to visit the laboratory and meet the staff before storing sperm. However, James's father was still distressed and we took some time out to explore this. The issue had really brought home to him the significance of the situation and what was at risk. He found the thought of supporting his son making such a profound decision about an unknowable future very upsetting. To him everything had become abnormal: this is not how it was supposed to be. James's father was able to be present during our discussion and, following a visit to the laboratories to meet the staff, James returned the following day and successfully stored his sperm. In our continued conversations James's father told me that, because James had successfully stored his sperm, he felt that James had secured his future: he just had to get through the treatment now.

---

for those without cancer, for the young person with cancer their importance may be significantly magnified. This reinforces the need to be aware of the challenges facing young people with same-sex sexual preferences, who may find disclosure and, therefore, the seeking and accessing of support difficult.

Sexuality is of course not only a social and personal challenge for the young person with cancer. Often before treatment begins it is necessary to broach the subject of fertility. Such conversations often force the considerations of parenthood onto an incongruous time of life. The young person may not be in or may never have had a romantic relationship. Supporting the young person through such issues is not without significant challenge. Whilst healthcare professionals have an important role to play in such discussions (Koeppel, 1995), the provision of such support is not always consistent or well defined (Quinn and Kelly, 2000). Providing this support may require that we address issues such as masturbation, whilst maintaining sensitivity to the individual's age, culture, and religious context (Quinn and Kelly, 2000). However, such issues also challenge the parents and their own hopes and fears for the future, which are highlighted in the vignette (Box 5.11).

Fertility

It is estimated that around 60% of childhood cancer patients can now achieve cure, which translates into 1:1000 survivors of childhood cancer in the general population (Hawkins and Stevens, 1996). This has emphasised the need to consider the preservation of fertility before commencing gonadotoxic treatment

(Wallace and Thomson, 2003; Edge *et al.*, 2006). However, patients are often faced with this issue soon after diagnosis, when anxiety is high, and this can affect their ability to think about fertility (Edge *et al.*, 2006). Furthermore, there is concern that there is an absence of information about how adolescents with cancer are treated or prepared prior to attempting sperm cryopreservation (Bahadur *et al.*, 2001), and a wide variation in practices in UK paediatric oncology centres has also been demonstrated (Glaser *et al.*, 2004). Indeed, it has also been shown that there are significant variations in clinicians' practices and patients' experiences. In one study only 51% of male cancer survivors aged 14–40 years reported that they had been offered sperm banking and just 60% were made aware of the possible effects treatment could have on their fertility before starting treatment (Schover *et al.*, 2002a). In a further study of physician attitudes it was reported that, although 91% of physicians felt that sperm storage should be offered to postpubertal males who were to receive gonadotoxic treatment, 48% of them failed to raise the issue (Schover *et al.*, 2002b). In the UK such facilities are known to be available in 20 out of the 21 paediatric oncology centres, with 85% of the study population actually being offered sperm storage (Glaser *et al.*, 2004). However, a recent study looking specifically at sperm banking in the adolescent and young adult population identified that, out of 171 patients who had received potentially gonadotoxic therapy, only 55 (32%) had a discussion of a semen cryopreservation documented in their medical records (Edge *et al.*, 2006). Only 55 (67%) were able to bank sperm successfully. Furthermore, these results supported an earlier study by Bahadur *et al.* (2002) that demonstrated a relationship between a failure to bank sperm and a younger age of around 15.5 years, and greater success from 16.7 years onwards. The use of patient information leaflets explaining the process of sperm banking to adolescents has been discussed (Quinn and Kelly, 2000): however, this has not been evaluated for effectiveness. In conclusion, Edge *et al.* (2006) poignantly cited Lance Armstrong:

> Conceiving a child was supposed to be wreathed in hope, not this sad, solitary procedure. I had no choice; I closed my eyes and did what I had to do (Armstrong and Jenkins, 2000, p. 38).

Fertility is not solely an issue for male patients, however. Whilst the indications and feasibility of ovarian tissue cryopreservation have been discussed (Fabbri *et al.*, 1999; Poirot *et al.*, 2003; Schenker and Fatum, 2004) and may preserve ovarian function in the future, currently the procedure remains experimental and clear guidance is not yet available (National Institute for Health and Clinical Excellence, 2005b).

Developing cognitive skills and the ability to think abstractly

The development of cognitive skills, and particularly the ability to think in the abstract, can be one of the most challenging ironies of cancer for the young person.

Box 5.12 'Popstars' and big sister

At the time of our discussion Kim was 15 years old. She had been through over a year of intensive chemotherapy, surgery, and radiotherapy for a Ewing's sarcoma of her left pelvis. Despite exhausting all treatment options, she had failed to achieve remission and she was working through the implications of this.

Her relationship with her mum, her mother's partner, and her younger brother had become especially close as her cancer journey progressed. Conversely, as a popular girl in a popular group at school she had initially struggled as those friendships fell by the wayside soon after diagnosis.

It was a warm late summer early evening and I had popped in to her room to see how things were: her face said it all. Her perilous situation had hit home, she knew she was dying, and she needed to talk. When the tears flowed they were angry, frustrated tears. Two things were upsetting her the most. One was the popular 'Popstars' television programme and the other was that her little brother was going to lose his big sister.

Kim told me that she found it too painful to watch or pay attention to the television show. But it seemed to her that it was everywhere she looked and everyone was talking about it. However, what upset her most was that she could see herself in the contestants: rather she saw what might have been, what could have been. In short she knew her potential and that hurt.

After some time she turned the conversation to her younger brother. Before her diagnosis he had been the archetypal 'little brat' in her eyes, but as the family regrouped in response to her diagnosis their bond strengthened and she began to value her role as his big sister. This had allowed her to develop a strong sense of her ongoing responsibilities and her grief was focused on not being able to fulfil the role as she saw it.

Whilst the ability to construct other than fact possibilities provides the individual with the capacity to map out and plan possible futures, for the young person with cancer this also delivers an insight into what is at risk, what is lost, or what may never be. The development of this skill therefore enables young people to confront and to measure the impact of their mortality. In their study Enskär *et al.* (1997) noted that adolescents contemplated death and dying from their disease from an early stage, rehearsing related activities such as writing a will. As none of the participants were dying they used the proposition of dying to help them articulate their hopes and promote positive thinking. This included constructing rewards or goals in their future. However, worries about the future and possible relapse have also been shown to persist into follow-up (Novakovic *et al.*, 1996), thus suggesting a continued awareness of mortality. What then for those, like Kim (Box 5.12), who are dying?

The above vignette illustrates how Kim's lost aspirations and goals provided a vehicle to articulate and explore her anger and frustration at the loss of her future. At the time it was not possible or, indeed, appropriate to ponder or explore the target of that anger. Nonetheless, it is now possible to consider that this anger was about her loss in its totality. Indeed, such loss can precipitate grief reactions such as feelings of helplessness and loss of control, yet in the teenager or young adult this is juxtaposed with a need and desire to foster autonomy, control, and independence. This loss of control can also be compounded by other impacts of a cancer diagnosis, such as increased attention from and reliance on the parental role (Gibson, 1997; Hokkanen *et al.*, 2004). It has been suggested that allowing the teenager to express their emotions and fears can foster some sense of control (Papadatou, 1989): however, providing such support must be handled very carefully and at the teenager's pace. Kim invited support through the disclosure of deeply personal and difficult issues. Indeed, having given this much reflection, we are sure that she was not seeking practical advice, but rather she chose someone she felt able to have present while she explored her thoughts aloud, someone to share her burden and hear her pain. Such a therapeutic presence, i.e. being aware of where a patient 'is at' and knowing when not to fill pauses with questions, has been reported by adolescent patients as a valued measure of expertise (Kelly *et al.*, 2003). However, it is clear that there were other issues that related to control in Kim's situation. Consequently, there is value in considering the situation further within the context of control.

Controlling their future

Throughout her treatment Kim had projected a strong sense of control, giving the impression of maintaining a predominantly internal locus of control: by this we mean control over future events continued to reside with her. However, repeated failures to achieve remission had moved the locus towards an external orientation (Rotter, 1966), where the control lay with others or, indeed, to chance or luck. Subsequently, over time, her sense of control had receded, as had her goal orientation. Correspondingly, this increased external locus of control may also have emphasised a need for or reliance on hope: an expectation of greater than zero of achieving a goal (Stotland, 1969). On the other hand, the content of her disclosure and who she chose to make it to were variables that she alone could control. Although this may seem obvious it is important, not least because this was a very significant conversation, but also it may have been a symbol of her unwillingness to give up, to remain goal orientated, and to have something to hope for: to be told it could come true.

Mention of hope exists in historical, mythological, and theological discourse and there is speculation that it is central to human existence (Cutcliffe and McKenna, 2005). Indeed, Cutcliffe and McKenna (2005) further argued that the therapeutic value of hope should translate into a duty for nurses to inspire hope in their patients. However, this raises a fundamental question. What if hope is unrealistic or there *is* a zero chance of achieving the goal? Is this false hope, non-therapeutic hope, or is the situation actually 'hopeless'? Perhaps, through our conversation, she was able to cast those once aspirations, then hopes, aside when it was apparent they would never come to pass. In Kim's case she sought new hopes that were realistic: she hoped to understand, to make peace, and to find some solace – and it was these that became her new goals.

It was clear that, for Kim, there was always something to strive towards, something to achieve. Indeed, this is a consistent theme when working with teenagers. There appears to be a need to maintain forward momentum in their life whilst they negotiate their cancer journey. Perhaps this in itself is a reflection of hope. This is especially true in terms of schooling and examinations. However, for the teenager with cancer, being able to stick to rigid school hours is particularly challenging. Interrupted sleep due to the side effects of treatment or cancer-related fatigue can impact significantly on their general quality of life. Indeed, although many healthcare professionals recognise the signs and impact of cancer-related fatigue this rarely translates into their treatment plans (Gibson *et al.*, 2005). It is essential that any such plan includes communication with and the support of the student's school, college, or university. Furthermore, such cancer-related effects are compounded by the physiological challenges of adolescence. In a large study across seven Minneapolis high schools, delaying the school start time by 90 minutes demonstrated significant benefits such as improved attendance, reduced sleepiness in class, and less student-reported depression (Wahlstrom, 2002). This suggests that supportive care needs not only to accommodate the impact of the disease and its treatment, but also a greater understanding of the already present physiological challenges facing all young people.

As mentioned above, the development of cognitive skills is an irony associated with cancer in this age group and one that must be handled carefully. But how might one do this? Facing one's mortality *must be* a profound experience (we use 'must be' as we can only imagine). It is an emotional, visceral experience as well as one of intellectual reasoning, bringing with it a maturity that should not be underestimated. We suggest that respecting this maturity must be central to supporting the teenager or young adult explore, plan, and hope for their possible futures. Flexibility is vital and routines should, as far as possible, respond to their needs. However, healthcare professionals must also be prepared to accept the responsibility to help the young person begin to explore such issues, as parents and friends are usually only accessed after treatment has been completed (Hokkanen *et al.*, 2004). On a personal level the most moving and challenging experiences of one's career can still arouse an emotional response several years on. As a confident and skilled practitioner this highlights an important need for the provision of support to staff who may be exposed to such challenging conversations. See Chapter 4 for further discussion on this point.

Developing the ability to control behaviour according to social norms and taking responsibility

The ability to control behaviour according to social norms and rules begins in childhood (Conger and Galambos, 1997). However, during adolescence this is explored and refined further, with more sophisticated social skills being learned through peer relationships with both sexes and developing new adult relationships with parents. However, the individual and their social context can only

---

Box 5.13   Bully for you!

Jenny and Helen were diagnosed at around the same time and hit it off straight away. As their chemotherapy cycles usually coincided they were able to support each other through the trials and tribulations of treatment. Their mothers always accompanied both of them and they too had developed an important supportive relationship. In between treatments both families kept in contact by telephone and became close. Shortly after they had been admitted Christine came to the unit for treatment. Again, her mum always accompanied her. Christine and her mum were quiet and reserved and, as her course of treatment was not in synchronisation with Jenny and Helen, they rarely spent much time with either of them. However, further into treatment synchronisation was lost and Jenny found herself in hospital without Helen's company. The team were quite sensitive to this and enabled regular contact with the ward telephone. However, during one such conversation one of the nurses heard Jenny making critical and offensive remarks about Christine and her mother's appearance and social background. What was very troubling was that Jenny was doing so openly, in earshot of other patients on the ward, and with her mother sitting listening to her conversation.

---

really define the perennial question of what is the 'norm' or, indeed, what is normal. This includes their family, culture, ethnicity, peer relationships, gender, religion, and social background. In a multicultural environment this requires a dynamic response to sometimes challenging dilemmas, as discussed earlier in Ayesha's case. Furthermore, peer relationships may allow the young person to explore and set new boundaries of behaviour in their social context. However, individuals such as John, who had been bullied and was isolated from such social experimentation, can lack the skills required for social interaction, thereby compounding their isolation and sense of being 'different' (Coleman and Hendry, 2000). As we have mentioned before, patients being treated for cancer can already feel set apart from their peers because of their appearance, but it can act also as a mark of belonging on a cancer unit. However, it is still important to consider exclusion, isolation, and bullying beyond such obvious circumstances. The above vignette (Box 5.13) considers the social context of a teenage cancer unit.

We as healthcare professionals have a role in monitoring and managing situations that involve bullying and harassment. Whilst attending hospital can be a challenging and frightening experience for young people we must ensure that it is at least safe from such behaviour. In the circumstances given above the nurse who heard the conversation sensitively but firmly challenged the behaviour and, fortunately, we did not see a repeat. However, it was a particularly challenging issue for the nurse concerned. Nonetheless, if units are to put forward philosophies of care that emphasise respect they must not be vacuous. Rather, they should come from shared values and beliefs that all the team have signed up to.

Reflecting on the above vignette the nurse concerned made an important observation about Jenny's response. She had understood and accepted the hurt that she could cause and was very sorry. However, her mother was visibly angry and, although she did not challenge the advice, she was obviously not pleased. This may have been because she felt exposed to criticism and censure because she had colluded with the bullying behaviour. However, Jenny took responsibility for her behaviour and made an honest effort to engage with Christine when it was appropriate.

The independence that young people strive for during this time as they seek to establish their identity requires that they also take responsibility. However, young people affected by cancer still must contend with all of the challenges that any other teenager has to face, including drugs, alcohol, sex, and the challenges of stereotypes. Young people with cancer can and do come from all walks of life with a myriad of issues at different stages of their personal development.

Meeting the challenges of supportive care in reality

The publications of the National Institute for Health and Clinical Excellence (2005a,b) regarding improving outcomes for children and young people are firmly set within the context of a multidisciplinary approach to care. However, the evidence review for the guidance identified only one 'good quality' RCT that demonstrated the benefit of such an approach (National Institute for Health and Clinical Excellence, 2005b). Furthermore, this benefit was an improved patient attitude towards the healthcare team, rather than any demonstrable improvement in their quality of life. The remaining seven pieces of evidence reviewed were classed as 'fair' to 'poor' quality. Nevertheless, as a practitioner it seems implausible to consider an approach to care of the teenager or young adult outside of such a paradigm. This brings us back to an important point that was raised at the beginning of this chapter, that of philosophical orientation, and forces us to raise the following question: is an RCT really the best or only way to obtain robust evidence to support such working?

Throughout this chapter we have presented a number of vignettes that illustrate the complex and engaging nature of what really is 'supportive care'. Whilst not explored in great detail here, discussion of each young person's personal and family circumstances was central to their care and also to the mutual support of each member of the team. Individual patients living with varying diagnoses will have a unique perception of the cancer's impact on their being in the world. In order to provide supportive care in its most holistic sense this demands a dynamic yet grounded patient-centred approach to care. Establishing this philosophical position, whether in a dedicated young people's or an adult or paediatric facility, can often pose a genuine challenge to the healthcare team. Our closing paragraphs explore this challenge in greater detail.

We have maintained throughout this chapter that the skilled involvement of the multidisciplinary team is central to the delivery of supportive care. Engaging in multidisciplinary team activity at its most fundamental level ensures that each patient is considered from a range of viewpoints and expertise (National Institute for Health and Clinical Excellence, 2005a), thereby encouraging shared learning and continuity of involvement. Team working in this way values and embraces the contribution of each individual staff member and enables a thorough exploration of each young person's clinical, psychological, and social needs. Facilitating this model of care outside of a dedicated adolescent service is experientially more testing however, demanding a shared fervour for the delivery of age-appropriate patient management.

Team working

As individual members of the healthcare team we each contribute to the overall direction and experience of care. Good teamwork recognises this, harnessing each person's knowledge, ability, strengths, and also their limitations. A shared approach to care is not without contention, however, as decisions may sometimes conflict with our own personal beliefs and values. As (Hokkanen *et al.*, 2004) asserted, 'We cannot deny who we are and what we bring to our roles' (p. 10).

We would concur with this: acknowledgement of the influence of our personal life and professional experience informs our work with young people and is imperative if we are to practise with honesty and integrity. Sharing who you are within a multidisciplinary team forum should respect both intrinsic and extrinsic intent, whilst ensuring the patient and their family remain the focus of all our involvement.

As healthcare professionals we instinctively wish to make situations better, and acceptance that we may not achieve this, in its most literal sense, can make us feel a certain degree of inadequacy. It can be hard to allow ourselves space to pause and think about what is really going on when we charge ourselves with the need to actively manage what it feels like in each and every situation. Nursing staff in particular may often 'bridge the gap' (Rosen, 1995; Dixon-Woods *et al.*, 2005) between parents and their son or daughter, fielding questions, facilitating discussion, or acting as a buffer for tension, anger, fear, and distress. Our involvement can easily become all-consuming, and brief disengagement to reflect and refocus is an important activity to foster within the team's approach to supportive care.

Within this chapter we have asserted that family-centred care is integral to the adolescent or young adult with cancer and this, therefore, leads us naturally to question whether staffing young people's services should be the domain of professionals from 'adult' or 'paediatric' training or backgrounds. Published guidance, sensibly, does not prescribe an answer to this debate: instead it suggests an amalgamation of expertise from each professional world (Viner and Keane, 1998; Edwards, 2001; Whelan, 2003). We are in accord with this position and propose that the complexity inherent within the delivery of supportive care to this patient cohort demands, most of all, professionals with a genuine interest and desire to work with young people. We suggest that thoughtful and skilled professionals, irrespective of adult or paediatric backgrounds, will best address the task.

The importance of a working philosophy and physical environment

> It's the times when you are on your own when staff are with you, and they don't need to be . . . I mean they're not giving you an IV or doing anything as such . . . that's really comforting . . . that's what I would call 'supportive care' (Ross, aged 18 years).

It is our belief that addressing each individual's specific and unique needs is the fundamental base of supportive care, and the above quote unequivocally demonstrates the significance of how this care is perceived. Supportive care must be embedded within a philosophy that encompasses emotional and psychological regard for wellbeing. This may be attended to with tangible and deliberate intent yet, as Ross describes, being present, without a task or procedure to complete, can take on particular symbolism and meaning. This resonates with research undertaken by Kelly *et al.* (2003), where healthcare staff appeared to 'know' intuitively when to listen and not ask questions as evidenced in their work. This was perceived as both sensitive and supportive by young cancer patients.

Woodgate (2006) also stressed the importance of a strong perception of support in helping young people to cope with cancer. Her findings portray the significance of 'being there' as a 'psychosocial–emotional presence within a supportive relationship' (Woodgate, 2006, p. 130).

Whilst young people may identify their family and, particularly, their mothers as their most important source of support (Hokkanen *et al.*, 2004), the significance of peer relationships (Coleman and Hendry, 2000) and professional relationships with staff must also be recognised and valued. Being able to be 'present' in this way may be challenging to less experienced professionals however, as it can be difficult to spend time with patients without a physical focus for one's engagement.

Considerable weight has been placed throughout this chapter on describing the philosophy in which supportive care is delivered. However, little emphasis has been placed on the impact of the place of care or its environmental context. The weighting of the importance of these two components of care has been raised for debate (Gibson, 1997). Irrespective of one's views on this, however, there must be 'the provision of highly specialised medical and nursing care needed for cancer treatment' (Whelan, 2003, p. 2573) to coexist with a framework that meets the specific needs of young people (Department of Health, 2004). Meeting a patient's clinical need has ultimately to be one's priority as a key component of the therapeutic context of care.

There is considerable variance in terms of where young people are treated, which is most usually dictated by disease group or a patient's age. In the UK the comprehensive level of care delivered by a Teenage Cancer Trust unit (Geehan, 2003) is not accessible to all and other models of care that meet both cancer- and age-specific needs must, therefore, be explored. A well-resourced ward (for example, with recreational facilities, high-technology equipment, and the right décor) is genuinely important, but a real commitment to a shared working philosophy is needed in order to deliver age-appropriate supportive care. Adopting such a philosophy enables the delivery of good care to young people in less than ideal physical environments. Conversely, a 'good', well-equipped environment cannot replace a cultural way of working that is committed to safe, age-appropriate care.

Clearly neither adult nor paediatric settings provide the optimal physical environment for young people with cancer, yet we acknowledge that the vast majority in the UK still receive their treatment in such facilities. As we have suggested, facilitating good care to a large extent extends beyond physicality, and it is quite possible to meet many young people's needs irrespective of the ward or unit environment. Establishing a philosophy of working that supports the key tasks of adolescence will provide a minimum foundation for the delivery of effective supportive care. In clinical practice this will be delivered by receptive professionals who are open to possibilities, accepting the need to individualise care and not seeking to 'pathologise' the variables of each young person's psychosocial world.

Summary

In this chapter we have explored the dimensions of supportive care in the context of the young person with cancer.

We suggested that providing supportive care requires the team to

'bear all or part of the weight in the provision of what is necessary for the health, welfare, maintenance and protection of the young person with cancer, whilst providing encouragement or emotional help' (Hanvey, 2007, pp. 7–8).

Through the various vignettes and comments in this chapter we have demonstrated that the provision of *what is necessary* requires that significant thought be brought into practise in order to individualise each patient's care and move beyond step-by-step 'interventions'. This locates supportive care in a philosophical rather than interventional context, thus transcending yet including the amelioration of the physical symptoms of cancer. Furthermore, we have demonstrated a necessary relationship between the delivery of supportive care approaches and an understanding of the context in which this care takes place. This understanding requires practitioners to have knowledge of the patient and their world, a high level of self-awareness, and robust professional boundaries. Awareness of the theoretical constructs that enable the team to work through what will be often complex issues is also crucial.

It is clear from our discussion that we believe that these dimensions extend beyond the confines of a unit or ward, or even contact with a particular practitioner. Rather, they extend into the family system and young persons' social world(s), school or work demands, and real or imagined aspirations. Each domain may have emotional, intellectual, temporal, and material elements, such that we must always remind ourselves that there is much that we cannot suppose to know. Correspondingly, we must be prepared to develop supportive care strategies wherever and in whatever way the cancer diagnosis impacts.

In our introduction we argued that it was important to consider how a cancer diagnosis may affect a young person's ability to modify their approach to and development of skills to cope with the biological and psychological and social changes of adolescence. Although we have attempted to focus on one particular task in each vignette, it is apparent that each has relevance to other tasks. For example, John's situation and his inability to make a morally congruent refusal (through the lens of ethical theory at least) also raises questions about his ability to control his behaviour according to social norms, which raises further concerns about his isolated life and how this may have affected his interpersonal skills. This again may have an impact on the development of a coherent identity, and so on. Another example of such linkages is Jack and Pat's relationships with their parents: both needed to acknowledge increased dependence on and the need to negotiate a new role with their parents as a result of their cancer. This impacted on the degree to which they could take responsibility for their behaviour and, as a consequence, on their ability to achieve social independence.

Concluding thoughts

In this chapter we have presented a broad range of complex scenarios demonstrating how young people may require our support as they negotiate cancer and developmental trajectories simultaneously. Readers may make linkages between each vignette and other developmental tasks. One further note is that, as professionals, our world view and approach is informed and influenced by our own discipline. Readers from other disciplines may view each vignette differently and we hope this will stimulate further debate. However, it is our hope that this chapter will encourage healthcare professionals to consider supportive care for young people as a response to their individual needs: bearing witness to their pain, providing a presence as they explore their darkest moments, not just fear of death, but changes to the future, loss of childhood, and returning to childhood; the list goes on. Indeed, if the young person is to live their life during treatment, we must adopt as broad an approach to supportive care as their needs demand.

References

Adams-Greenly, M., Beldock, N., & Moynihan, R. (1986) Helping adolescents whose parents have cancer. *Seminars in Oncology Nursing*, **2**(2), 133–138.

Allen, R. (1997) Adolescent cancer and the family. *Journal of Cancer Nursing*, **1**(2), 86–92.

Armstrong, L. & Jenkins, S. (2000) *It's Not About the Bike: My Journey Back to Life*. Penguin Putnam, New York.

Bahadur, G., Whelan, J., Ralph, D., & Hindmarsh, P. (2001) Gaining consent to freeze spermatozoa from adolescents with cancer: legal, ethical and practical aspects. *Human Reproduction*, **16**(1), 188–193.

Bahadur, G., Ling, K. L. E., Hart, R. *et al.* (2002) Semen quality and cryopreservation in adolescent cancer patients. *Human Reproduction*, **17**(12), 3157–3161.

Barnes, P. (ed.) (1995) *Personal, Social and Emotional Development of Children.* Open University/Blackwell, Oxford.

Barton, C. (2006) The wrong time for cancer! Considerations when caring for a young adult with cancer. *Bone Marrow Transplantation*, **37**(Suppl. 1), S276.

Beauchamp, T. L. & Childress, J. F. (2001) *Principles of Biomedical Ethics*, 5th edn. Oxford University Press, New York, NY.

Bisset, M., Robinson, V., & George, R. (2001) Expanding the remit of palliative care. *Nursing Times*, **97**(21), 38–40.

Burt, K. (1995) The effects of cancer on body image and sexuality. *Nursing Times*, **91**(7), 36–37.

Cancer Research UK (2004) *CancerStats Incidence UK.* Cancer Research UK, London.

Chisholm, L. & Hurrelmann, K. (1995) Adolescence in modern Europe. Pluralized transition patterns and their implications for personal and social risks. *Journal of Adolescence*, **18**, 129–158.

Coleman, J. C. (1993) Understanding adolescence today: a review. *Children and Society*, **7**(2), 137–147.

Coleman, J. C. & Hendry, L. (2000) *The Nature of Adolescence.* Routledge, London.

Conger, J. J. & Galambos, N. L. (1997) *Adolescence and Youth: Psychological Development in a Changing World*, 5th edn. Addison Wesley Longman, New York.

Coscarelli, A. (2000) Treating cancer as a family disease. *Western Journal of Medicine*, **173**, 389–390.

Cutcliffe, J. R. & McKenna, H. P. (2005) *The Essential Concepts of Nursing.* Elsevier Churchill Livingstone, Edinburgh.

Daniels, L. E. (1996) Exploring the physical and psychological implication of central venous devices in cancer patients – interviews with patients. *Journal of Cancer Care*, **3**(1), 45–48.

Department of Health (2001a) *Good Practice in Consent Implementation Guide: Consent to Examination or Treatment.* Department of Health Publications, London.

Department of Health (2001b) *Consent – What You Have a Right to Expect: a Guide for Children and Young People.* Department of Health Publications, London.

Department of Health (2001c) *Consent – What You Have a Right to Expect: a Guide for Parents.* Department of Health Publications, London.

Department of Health (2004) *National Service Framework for Children, Young People and Maternity Services.* Department of Health Publications, London.

Dixon-Woods, M., Young, B., & Heney, D. (2005) *Rethinking Experiences of Childhood Cancer: a Multidisciplinary Approach to Chronic Childhood Illness*, pp. 115–133. Open University Press, Maidenhead.

Djerassi, I. (1967) Methotrexate infusions and intensive supportive care in the management of children with acute lymphocytic leukemia: follow-up report. *Cancer Research*, **27**(12), 2561–2564.

Edge, B., Holmes, D., & Makin, G. (2006) Sperm banking for adolescent cancer patients. *Archives of Diseases in Childhood*, **91**, 149–152.

Edozien, L. (2001) How much information must be given for consent to be valid? The doctrine of informed consent. *Clinical Risk*, **7**, 136–140.

Edwards, J. (2001) A model of palliative care for the adolescent with cancer. *International Journal of Palliative Nursing*, **7**(10), 485–488.

Enskär, K., Carlsson, M., Golsäter, M., & Hamrin, E. (1997) Symptom distress and life situations in adolescents with cancer. *Cancer Nursing*, **20**(1), 23–33.

Erikson, E. H. (1968) *Identity: Youth and Crisis.* Norton, New York.

Evans, M. (1996) Interacting with teenagers with cancer. In: *Cancer and the Adolescent* (eds P. Selby & C. Bailey), pp. 251–263, BMJ Publishing Group, London.

Evans, M. (1997) Altered body image in teenagers with cancer. *Journal of Cancer Nursing*, **1**(4), 177–182.

Fabbri, R., Marsella, T., Diano, C. *et al.* (1999) Ovarian tissue cryopreservation for oncology patients. *International Journal of Gynecological Cancer*, **9**(Suppl. 1), 36–37.

Feiring, C. (1996) Concepts of romance in 15-year-old adolescents. *Journal of Research on Adolescence*, **6**, 181–200.

Finch, A. C. (2003) How do adolescents experience learning about their parent's cancer diagnosis? Unpublished MSc dissertation, King's College London.

Freedman, T. (1994) Social and cultural dimensions of hair loss in women treated for breast cancer. *Cancer Nursing*, **17**(4), 334–341.

Gadow, S. (1989) An ethical case for patient self-determination. *Seminars in Oncology*, **5**(2), 99–101.

Geehan, S. (2003) The benefits and drawbacks of treatment in a specialist teenage unit – a patient's perspective. *European Journal of Cancer*, **39**, 2681–2683.

George, R. (2006) Bioethics: what do we mean by autonomy? In: *Teenage Cancer Trust 4th International Conference on Teenage and Young Adult Cancer Medicine*, pp. 15–16. Teenage Cancer Trust, London (abstract book).

Gibson, F. (1997) Adolescents with cancer: is it the location or philosophy of care which matters? *Journal of Cancer Nursing*, **1**(4), 159.

Gibson, F., Mulhall, A. B., Richardson, A., Edwards, J. L., Ream, E., & Sepion, B. J. (2005) A phenomenologic study of fatigue in adolescents receiving treatment for cancer. *Oncology Nursing Forum*, **32**(3), 651–660.

Gilligan, C. (1982) *In a Different Voice*. Harvard University Press, Cambridge, MA.

Glaser, A. W., Phelan, L., Crawshaw, M., Jagdev, S., & Hale, J. (2004) Fertility preservation in adolescent males with cancer in the United Kingdom: a survey of practice. *Archives of Diseases in Childhood*, **89**, 736–737.

Graber, J. A. & Brooks-Gunn, J. (1996) Transitions and turning points: navigating the passage from childhood through adolescence. *Developmental Psychology*, **32**, 768–776.

Grinyer, A. & Thomas, C. (2001) Young adults with cancer: the effect of the illness on parents and families. *International Journal of Palliative Nursing*, **7**, 162–170.

Gross, R. (2001) *Psychology: the Science of Mind and Behaviour*, 4th edn. Hodder and Stoughton, London.

Gurevich, M., Bishop, S., Bower, J., Malka, M., & Nyhof-Young, J. (2004) (Dis)embodying gender and sexuality in testicular cancer. *Social Science and Medicine*, **58**(9), 1597–1607.

Hall, G. S. (1904) *Adolescence*. Appleton & Co., New York NJ.

Hanvey, J. N. (2007) Maximising personhood: towards a grounded theory of supportive care in adolescent cancer. Unpublished MSc dissertation, City University, London.

Havighurst, R. J. (1952) *Developmental Tasks and Education*. David McKay, New York, NJ.

Hawkins, M. M. & Stevens, M. C. (1996) The long-term survivors. *British Medical Bulletin*, **52**(4), 898–923.

Hilton, B. A. & Gustavson, K. (2002) Shielding and being shielded: children's perspectives on coping with their mother's cancer and chemotherapy. *Canadian Oncology Nursing Journal*, **12**(4), 198–206.

Hinds, P. & Gattuso, J. (1991) Measuring hopefulness in adolescents. *Journal of Pediatric Oncology Nursing*, **8**(2), 92–94.

Hinds, P. S., Quargnenti, A., Fairclough, D., *et al.* (1999) Hopefulness and its characteristics in adolescents with cancer. *Western Journal of Nursing Research*, **21**(5), 600–620.

Hockenberry-Eaton, E. M., Hinds, P., O'Neill, J. B. *et al.* (1999) Developing a conceptual model for fatigue in children. *European Journal of Oncology Nursing*, **3**(1), 5–13.

Hokkanen, H., Eriksson, E., Ahonen, O., & Salantera, S. (2004) Adolescents with cancer: experience of life and how it could be made easier. *Cancer Nursing*, **27**(4), 325–335.

International Council of Nurses (2000) *Code of Ethics for Nurses*. International Council of Nurses, Geneva.

Jones, B. (2000) Legal aspects of consent. *British Journal of Urology International*, **86**(3), 275–279.

Kamm, F. M. (1996) *Morality, Morality*. Oxford University Press, Oxford.

Kelly, D., Mulhall, A., & Pearce, S. (2003) Adolescent cancer – the need to evaluate current service provision in the UK. *European Journal of Oncology Nursing*, **7**(1), 53–58.

Kelly, D., Pearce, S., & Mulhall, A. (2004) 'Being in the same boat': ethnographic insights into an adolescent cancer unit. *International Journal of Nursing Studies*, **41**(8), 847–857.

Kennedy, I. & Grubb, A. (1994) *Medical Law: Text With Materials*, 2nd edn. Butterworths, London.

Koeppel, K. M. (1995) Sperm banking and patients with cancer. *Cancer Nursing*, **18**, 306–312.

Kohlberg, L. (ed.) (1981) *The Philosophy of Moral Development: Vol 1*. Harper & Row, San Francisco, CA.

Koocher, G. & O'Malley, J. (1981) *The Damocles Syndrome*. McGraw-Hill, New York, NJ.

Kuzbit, P. (2004) The psychological effects of chemotherapy induced alopecia following treatment for testicular cancer. *Cancer Nursing Practice*, **3**(8), 10–13.

Lanyado, M. (1999) 'It's just an ordinary pain': thoughts on joy and heartache in puberty and early adolescence. In: *Personality Development: a Psychoanalytic Perspective* (eds D. Hindle & M. Vaciago Smith), pp. 92–115. Brunner-Routledge, New York, NY.

Leonard, R. C. F., Coleman, R. E., O'Regan, J., & Gregor, A. (1996) Special problems of adolescents with cancer. *Journal of Cancer Care*, **5**(3), 117–120.

Lewis, F. M. (1996) The impact of breast cancer on the family: lessons learned from the children and adolescents. In: *Cancer and the Family* (eds L. Baider, C. L. Cooper, & A. Kaplan De-Nour), pp. 271–286, Wiley, Chichester.

Lewis, F. M. (2006) The effects of cancer survivorship on families and caregivers. *American Journal of Nursing*, **106**(3, Suppl.), 20–25.

Lewis, F. M., Zahlis, E. H., Shands, M. E., Sinheimer, J. A., & Hammond, M. A. (1996) The functioning of single women with breast cancer and their school aged children. *Cancer Practice*, **4**, 15–24.

Lore, A. (1973) Adolescents: people not problems. *American Journal of Nursing*, **64**(24), 1232–1234.

Mason, D. L. (2006) Surviving cancer survival. Is the new cancer paradigm good for patients? *American Journal of Nursing*, **106**(3), 11.

Moore, S. & Rosenthal, D. (1998) Adolescent sexual behaviour. In: *Teenage Sexuality: Health, Risk and Education* (eds J. Coleman & D. Roker), pp. 35–58. Harwood Academic Press, London.

Morgan, S. (2003) Supportive and palliative care for patients with COPD. *Nursing Times*, **99**(20), 46–47.

National Council of Hospices and Specialist Palliative Care Services (2002) *Briefing Paper 11: Definitions of Supportive and Palliative Care*. National Council of Hospices and Specialist Palliative Care Services, London.

National Institute for Health and Clinical Excellence (2004) *Improving Supportive and Palliative Care for Adults with Cancer – The Manual*. National Institute for Health and Clinical Excellence, London.

National Institute for Health and Clinical Excellence (2005a) *Guidance on Cancer Services: Improving Outcomes in Children and Young People With Cancer – The Manual*. Department of Health, London.

National Institute for Health and Clinical Excellence (2005b) *Guidance on Cancer Services: Improving Outcomes in Children and Young People With Cancer – The Evidence Review*. Department of Health, London.

Neven, R. S. (1997) *Emotional Milestones from Birth to Adulthood: a Psychodynamic Approach*. Jessica Kingsley, London.

Newby, N. M. (1996) Chronic illness and the family life cycle. *Journal of Advanced Nursing*, **23**, 786–791.

Northouse, L. L. (1992) Psychological impact of the diagnosis of breast cancer on the patient and her family. *Journal of the American Medical Women's Association*, **47**(5), 161–164.

Novakovic, B., Fears, T. R., Horowitz, M. E. *et al.* (1996) Experiences of cancer in children and adolescents. *Cancer Nursing*, **19**(1), 54–59.

Nursing and Midwifery Council (2002) *Code of Professional Conduct*. Nursing and Midwifery Council, London.

Papadatou, D. (1989) Caring for dying adolescents. *Nursing Times*, **85**(18), 28–31.

Pape, T. (1997) Legal and ethical considerations of informed consent. *AORN Journal*, **65**(6), 1122–1127.

Parry, C. (2003) Embracing uncertainty: an exploration of the experience of childhood cancer survivors. *Qualitative Health Research*, **13**(2), 227–246.

Patenaude, A. F. (2000) A different normal: reactions of children and adolescents to the diagnosis of cancer in a parent. In: *Cancer and the Family*, 2nd edn (eds L. Baider, C. L. Cooper, & Kaplan De-Nour, A.), pp. 239–254. Wiley, Chichester.

Pearsal, J. & Hanks, P. (eds) (1998) *The New Oxford Dictionary of English*. Oxford University Press, Oxford.

Piaget, J. (1932) *The Moral Judgement of the Child*. Routledge and Kegan Paul, London.

Poirot, C., Vacher-Lavenu, M., Helardot, P., Guibert, J., Brugieres, L., & Jouannet, P. (2003) Human ovarian tissue cryopreservation: indications and feasibility. *Obstetrical & Gynecological Survey*, **58**(2), 119–120.

Popay, J., Rodgers, A., & Williams, G. (1998) Rationale and standards for the systematic review of qualitative literature in health services research. *Qualitative Health Research*, **8**(3), 341–351.

Quinn, B. & Kelly, D. (2000) Sperm banking and fertility concerns: enhancing practice and the support available to men with cancer. *European Journal of Oncology Nursing*, **4**(1), 55–58.

Redmond, K. (1996) Advances in supportive care. *European Journal of Cancer Care*, **5**(Suppl. 2), 1–7.

Regnard, C. & Kindlen, M. (2002) *Supportive and Palliative Care in Cancer: an Introduction*. Radcliffe Medical Press, Abingdon.

Richardson, A. (2004) Creating a culture of compassion: developing supportive care for people with cancer. *European Journal of Oncology Nursing*, **8**(4), 293–305.

Richer, M. C. & Ezer, H. (2002) Living it, living with it and moving on: dimensions of meaning during chemotherapy. *Oncology Nursing Forum*, **29**(1), 113–119.

Richie, M. (2001) Self-esteem and hopefulness in adolescents with cancer. *Journal of Pediatric Nursing*, **16**(1), 35–42.

Robinson, C. & Janes, K. (2001) 'Is my Mom going to die?' Answering questions when a family member has cancer: the 2000 Shering Lecture. *Canadian Oncology Nursing Journal*, **11**(2), 62–66.

Rolfe, G. (2000) *Research, Truth & Authority: Postmodern Perspectives on Nursing*. Macmillan Press, Basingstoke.

Rosen, D. (1995) Between two worlds: bridging the cultures of child health and adult medicine. *Journal of Adolescent Health*, **12**, 10–16.

Rosen, J. C., Srebnik, D., & Saltzberg, E. (1991) Development of a body image avoidance questionnaire. *Journal of Consultant Clinical Psychology*, **3**(1), 32–37.

Rotter, J. B. (1966) Generalized expectancies for internal versus external control of reinforcement. *Psychological Monographs*, **80**, 1–28.

Russell-Johnson, H. (2000) Adolescent survey. *Paediatric Nursing*, **12**(6), 15–19.

Sainio, C. & Lauri, S. (2003) Cancer patients' decision making regarding treatment and nursing care. *Journal of Advanced Nursing*, **41**(3), 250–260.

Schenker, J. G. & Fatum, M. (2004) Should ovarian tissue cryopreservation be recommended for cancer patients? *Journal of Assisted Reproduction & Genetics*, **21**(11), 375–376.

Schover, L. R., Brey, K., Lichtin, A., Lipshultz, L. I., & Jeha, S. (2002a) Knowledge and experience regarding cancer, infertility, and sperm banking in younger male survivors. *Journal of Clinical Oncology*, **20**(7), 1880–1889.

Schover, L. R., Brey, K., Lichtin, A., Lipshultz, L. I., & Jeha, S. (2002b) Oncologists' attitudes and practices regarding banking sperm before cancer treatment. *Journal of Clinical Oncology*, **20**(7), 1890–1897.

Shaw, M. C. & Halliday, P. H. (1992) The family, crisis and chronic illness: an evolutionary model. *Journal of Advanced Nursing*, **17**(5), 537–543.

Shell, J. A. & Miller, M. E. (1999) The cancer amputee and sexuality. *Orthopaedic Nursing*, **18**(5), 53–64.

Siegelman, M. H. (1964) Advances in the supportive care of children with acute leukaemia. *Medical Record and Annals*, **57**, 439–441.

Sontag, S. (1979) *Illness as Metaphor*. Allen Lane, London.

Souhami, R., Whelan, J., McCarthy, J., & Kilby, A. (1996) Benefits and problems of an adolescent oncology unit. In: *Cancer and the Adolescent* (eds P. Selby & C. Bailey), pp. 276–283. BMJ Publishing Group, London.

Stattin, H. & Magnusson, D. (1996) Anti-social development: a holistic approach. *Development and Psychopathology*, **8**, 617–645.

Steefel, L. (2000) Adolescent cancer survivors are mature beyond their years. *Nursing Spectrum* (New York/New Jersey Metro Edition), **12a**(24), 6–7.

Stotland, E. (1969) *The Psychology of Hope*. Josey-Bass, San Francisco, CA.

Taylor, J. & Müller, D. J. (1995) *Nursing Adolescents: Research and Psychological Perspectives*. Blackwell Science, Oxford.

Thompson, I. E., Melia, K. M., & Boyd, K. M. (2000) *Nursing Ethics*, 4th edn. Churchill Livingstone, Edinburgh.

Thompson, J. K. (1990) *Body Image Disturbance: Assessment and Treatment*. Pergamon Press, New York, NY.

Tschudin, V. (2003) *Ethics in Nursing: the Caring Relationship*, 3rd edn. Butterworth-Heinemann, London.

US Department of Health, Education and Welfare (1979) *Nursing Adolescents: Research and Psychological Perspectives*. Blackwell, London.

Viner, R. & Keane, M. (1998) *Youth Matters. Evidence-based Best Practice for the Care of Young People in Hospital. Caring for Children in the Health Services*. Action for Sick Children, London.

Wahlstrom, K. (2002) Changing times: findings from the first longitudinal study of later high school start times. *NASSP Bulletin*, **86**, 633.

Wallace, W. H. B. & Thomson, A. B. (2003) Preservation of fertility in children treated for cancer. *Archives of Diseases in Childhood*, **88**, 493–496.

Wells, M. (2001) The impact of cancer. In: *Cancer Nursing Care in Context* (eds J. Corner & C. Bailey), pp. 63–85. Blackwell Science, Oxford.

Whelan, J. (2003) Where should teenagers with cancer be treated? *European Journal of Cancer Care*, **39**, 2573–2578.

White, C. (2000) Body image dimensions and cancer: a heuristic cognitive behavioural model. *Psycho-Oncology*, **9**(3), 183–192.

Whiteson, M. (2003) The Teenage Cancer Trust – advocating a model for teenage cancer services. *European Journal of Cancer*, **39**, 2688–2693.

Wilkinson, S. (2002) Is honesty the best policy? *International Journal of Palliative Nursing*, **8**(1), 4.

Woodgate, R. (2005) A different way of being: adolescents' experiences with cancer. *Cancer Nursing*, **28**(1), 8–15.

Woodgate, R. L. (2006) The importance of being there: perspectives of social support by adolescents with cancer. *Journal of Pediatric Oncology Nursing*, **23**(3), 122–134.

Zani, B. (1993) Dating and interpersonal relationships in adolescence. In: *Adolescence and Its Social Worlds* (eds S. Jackson & H. Rodriguez-Tome), pp. 95–116. Lawrence Erlbaum, Hove.

Zeltzer, L. (1993) Cancer in adolescents and young adults: psychosocial aspects. *Cancer*, **71**, 3463–3468.

Chapter 6

Getting on with Life During Treatment

Roberta Woodgate

Introduction

Adolescence is famously a time of momentous growth and development. Developmental changes are characterised by significant physical, psychological, social, and maturational processes. These processes may be extremely challenging for adolescents. However, for those with a cancer diagnosis, coping with the normative developmental processes may be additionally daunting. The challenges arising from these developmental changes, a cancer diagnosis, and subsequent treatment may cause a dual crisis (Zevon *et al.*, 1987; Kyngäs *et al.*, 2001).

Situated in the words and lived experiences of a group of adolescents receiving cancer treatment, the aim of this chapter is to consider the complexities of 'getting on with life' (Woodgate, 2001). Foundationally, the chapter will include key research findings specific to adolescents' cancer experiences. The findings are part of a larger longitudinal qualitative interpretative study that sought to describe how childhood cancer and its symptom course were experienced by 39 families of children with cancer (Woodgate, 2001). The study took place in a city in western Canada between the period of July 1998 and December 2000. Fifteen of the 39 families had an adolescent child diagnosed with cancer. They ranged from 12 to 18 years of age and eight were male and seven were female. The majority were diagnosed with either leukaemia or lymphoma (*n* = 12) and three were diagnosed with a solid tumour. Data were collected through qualitative open-ended individual and focus group interviews with the adolescents and by observing them during various periods and at different points in time. The findings will be grounded in the literature in order to explicate further the challenges faced and key coping strategies used by adolescents.

Challenges facing adolescents with cancer

A diagnosis of cancer causes uncertainty, disruption, restrictions in daily life, increased psychological and physical work, lengthy and rigorous treatment regimens, and multiple losses. As such, cancer in adolescence can be viewed as a major life transition, complete with a wide range of negative and positive experiences (Hedstrom *et al.*, 2004).

At times, the challenging nature of cancer has been described as extremely over-whelming, as one 16-year-old female adolescent with leukaemia expressed:

> I've never been in the hospital before now. And then all of a sudden, it's just like crazy and I can't go to parties with my friends. And then I'm 16 and I can't drive . . . I have too much on my plate, you know? So it just kind of sucks that I'm 16 and I have all this . . .

Research reveals that adolescents consistently identify the aspects of cancer treatment as one of the most stressful aspects about having cancer (Enskär *et al.*, 1997). In fact, childhood cancer survivors report feeling more affected by the painful and visible side effects of treatment than by the more abstract threat of their illness (Di Gallo *et al.*, 2003). Cancer treatment may restrict an adolescent's ability to lead a normal life as they struggle with the many challenges related to body image and sense of self, peer relations, family relations, sexual health, education, and employment.

Body image and sense of self challenges

Research shows that adolescents with cancer experience feelings of being differ-ent, while having a dynamic sense of self throughout the cancer trajectory (Hinds and Martin, 1988; Rechner, 1990; Weekes and Kagan, 1994; Enskär *et al.*, 1997; Hockenberry-Eaton *et al.*, 1998). The cancer and subsequent bodily changes experi-enced require individuals to renegotiate their identity and interaction with others, and may affect them developing a positive sense of self (Mathieson and Stam, 1995; Ritchie, 2001a; Kameny and Bearison, 1999; Hedstrom *et al.*, 2004; Skolin and Von Essen, 2004). The subsequent impact of these changes on their sense of self was reinforced by a female adolescent's words:

> Um, losing my hair is hard . . . Because it makes me feel really depressed . . . It's one of the things that like totally derails you (14-year-old with leukaemia).

The young person's altered sense of self is closely tied to their changing body as a result of the cancer- and treatment-related symptoms (Woodgate, 2005). The bodily changes and changing self-perceptions were experienced by adolescents in six ways of being in the world: (1) life as a ' klutz' due to an unruly and unreliable body, (2) life as a 'prisoner' due to a dependent body, (3) life as an invalid due to a 'really sick' body, (4) life as an 'alien' due to a distorted and foreign body, (5) life as a 'zombie' due to a tired body, and (6) life as a kid in a renewed body. In addi-tion to feeling betrayed by their bodies, they also report bodily changes to have a profound impact on their sense of identity and may also have greater difficulty in rediscovering themselves within the new confines of cancer (Palmer *et al.*, 2000).

Peer relation challenges

Friends have an important role to play in the lives of young people (Hokkanen *et al.*, 2004). Adolescents with cancer need to maintain strong peer relationships and the knowledge that friends care for them is especially vital to them, as one participant reinforced:

> Yeah, knowing that my friends care is important. Well, at school I remember sometimes when I was in the hospital and my best friends came up and they brought a huge poster that most of the school had signed (13-year-old male with non-Hodgkin's lymphoma).

For adolescents with cancer, loss of friends is a primary fear (Hedstrom *et al.*, 2004). The maintenance of peer relationships may be a difficult task for young people, who must deal with the many challenges of undergoing treatment (Heiney, 1989; Palmer *et al.*, 2000; Kameny and Bearison, 1999). Undergoing treatment makes it difficult for them to engage in those activities that encourage interactions with their peers. For example, one 16-year-old girl expressed that she was afraid that she was not going to have a 'normal teenage life like most of her friends'. She reinforced this:

> They'll be partying or hanging out while I'm getting sick from my treatment. Leukaemia sucks!

Adolescents also express concern about the challenges of being treated differently by their friends. Even during those times when they really do feel different or unlike themselves or 'abnormal' they want their friends to respond to them like they were the same person. They 'do not want to be singled out as being different' or to be labelled as 'special' by their friends (Woodgate, 2005).

Family relation challenges

The onset of cancer always changes the dynamics and relationships of family members (Kyngäs *et al.*, 2001; Woodgate, 2006a). Adolescents with cancer face a change of focus within their family, whereby family life becomes more centred on their cancer treatments. This change of focus is at times hard for them to accept, as evidenced by the following comment:

> Sometimes I feel sorry you know my family always has to run around and do this stuff and I'm just sitting here like a queen (12-year-old female with leukaemia).

Specific challenges within the family also include the struggles young people have with their parents. Autonomy and independence from parents is quite difficult to attain for young people, who by the nature of their illness and treatment require increased parental support and care (Hokkanen *et al.*, 2004). Although they value support from their parents, it can also be a source of a great deal of stress, as noted in the following comment:

> At times it kind of got overwhelming. When I just wanted everyone to leave me alone, it was like 'Go away!' (18-year-old female with Wilm's tumour with relapse).

They also experience a sense of helplessness and guilt in not always being able to be with their siblings. The time required for cancer treatments impacts on the amount of time they wish they could spend with their siblings.

Sexual health challenges

Having cancer does not preclude young people from facing sexual and reproductive challenges. In fact, cancer and the effects of treatment may impact on their self-image, peer relationships, psychosexual development, and sexual activity, which in turn can heighten sexual and reproductive challenges (Heiney, 1989). In addition to the general challenges faced by adolescents (e.g. ambivalent feelings regarding their sexuality, sexual orientation, and the lack of knowledge of normal sexual development, birth control, or sex acts), those with cancer are at risk of problems that may be synergistic (Heiney, 1989; Roberts *et al.*, 1998). For example, the bodily changes experienced by young people due to treatment may lead to self-doubt about his/her femininity or masculinity, lowered self-concept, and isolation from peers, all of which may become an obstacle to developing intimate relationships (Heiney, 1989). The lack of any type of intimate relationship with their peers whilst undergoing treatment was a subject of discussion during research interviews (Woodgate, 2001). One participant, while talking about the losses experienced as a result of cancer, frequently expressed 'Here I am, sweet 16, and I have never been kissed!'

Education and employment challenges

In addition to acquiring academic and vocational skills, the school setting helps to promote developmental tasks that include dealing with successes and failures, acquiring social skills, and promoting peer relationships (Glasson, 1995). However, young people with cancer may not experience the full benefits of school due to the potential disruptions associated with treatment regimes (Roberts *et al.*, 1998). Trying to keep up with their studies becomes a struggle for them, especially when they experience increased symptom distress, particularly in relation to extreme fatigue (Woodgate, 2001). Besides missing their friends by not being at school, they expressed fears of getting behind in school, as this 15-year-old female with leukaemia noted:

> Now that I am in high school it is not even fun to miss a day of school because I had sat at home and it was not like I could have fun relaxing and watching television and you know I would think 'people are sitting in my English honour class right now and I am going to have to catch up on everything they did.'

Concerns about part-time employment and future employment in the adult years are also common concerns of adolescents with cancer. The diagnosis, subsequent treatment, and associated symptoms may prevent them from experiencing specific developmental tasks such as part-time employment and making career plans (Hedstrom *et al.*, 2004). In addition, there is evidence to suggest that young people make changes in their vocational goals as a result of the cancer diagnosis (Roberts *et al.*, 1998). One 17-year-old male with leukaemia noted that:

> One of my dreams that I wanted to be was a fire pilot and that was kind of taken away because you need good science and good math. And you need to be very physically fit which I'm not . . . I have to say maybe the roughest part (treatment) is over but it is still, it is still there, it is so there.

Getting on with life

Despite the challenges faced, research shows that adolescents have dual goals. They endeavour to deal with their cancer diagnosis and treatment, while at the same time resume their daily lives (Rechner, 1990; Woodgate, 2001; Hinds, 2004). In order to get on with life, it is important to face the challenges posed by cancer or as they put it, to 'get through' all the 'rough spots' (Woodgate, 2001). Adolescents have expressed that 'getting through' as opposed to 'getting over' the difficult aspects of cancer is necessary in order for them to be able to regain some sense of life and freedom from the cancer, as one 14-year-old female with leukaemia reinforced:

> It is getting through it, NOT OVER IT! It is getting through in two ways. I guess getting over it makes it seem like you are always there and you are always trying to get over it. I don't know, I have weird little visions in my mind of things, it is like a barricade. And for me it is not going over it and getting past it, it is going through it ripping it all down and tearing it into pieces. Like I don't want it to be something whole that is just behind me but is something that I destroyed and ripped down and is just not there any more. Getting over it, it is still there, it would just always bother me . . .

By defining cancer as something to get through, young people are able to move forward. In moving forward, they reported that they used seven main strategies: (1) hoping for the best, (2) having the right attitude, (3) knowing what to expect, (4) making some sense out of a bad situation, (5) taking one day at a time, (6) taking time for yourself, and (7) staying connected (Woodgate, 2001). Their use of various coping strategies is situated and supported in the literature.

Hoping for the best

Hoping for the best is a coping strategy that refers to adolescents remaining hopeful and believing that, no matter how bad things are or become during treatment, there is a light at the end of the dark tunnel. Holding on to the belief that one will get through all the difficult aspects of the cancer treatment and ultimately survive the cancer became a common strategy used soon after diagnosis, as one 17-year-old male with a Ewing's sarcoma reinforced:

Like I never really looked at it like I could die, you know? Except for that one time when I first got diagnosed. But after that I just decided to throw away that thought and really believed I would be alright.

Maintaining a sense of hopefulness has been identified as a key coping strategy by adolescents at all stages of the illness trajectory while dealing with cancer and other chronic illnesses (Hinds and Martin, 1988; Woodgate, 1998; Hinds, 2004). However, at times the maintenance of hope becomes difficult, especially when the fears and challenges associated with cancer (e.g. increased symptom distress) are more evident. There is evidence to suggest that certain important conditions come into play to sustain hope. Firstly, the knowledge that others, especially their parents, believe and express to them that they will get through the cancer trajectory. Hinds and Martin (1988) noted that reflecting on and finding comfort in the expressed certainty others have for their health recovery helped young people to sustain a sense of hopefulness. Hokkanen *et al.* (2004) also noted that adolescents with cancer want professional caregivers to show more encouragement and a positive attitude. Indeed, the participants reinforced to the author how important it is to have others tell them that 'you're going to be okay' and 'you can make it.' Secondly, making plans for future goals (short- and long-term goals). Short-term goals are more immediate and smaller and may include plans to spend an hour at school even when not feeling well. Long-term goals are larger goals, such as graduating from high school with one's peers. A faith in God also engenders a feeling of hope that everything will turn out for the best and provides a basis for meaning and hope for some.

Having the right attitude

The participants reinforced that having the right attitude and/or a fighting attitude is very important to getting through the cancer trajectory. They viewed having the right attitude as something that goes hand-in-hand with being hopeful, as this 17-year-old male with a Ewing's sarcoma noted:

Hope and faith go with having a good attitude, having a good attitude to know that sometime you'll get through it. It is like having faith it will sometime be over and having the hope that everything will turn out all right it goes with having a positive attitude.

In having the right attitude, they stressed that a strong sense of tenacity or perseverance is key to not giving up during treatment, as reinforced by the following comment:

See a lot of ways people say stubbornness and bull-headedness isn't good but when you have cancer it is what I think one of the best assets you could ever have (17-year-old male with a Ewing's sarcoma).

More importantly, having a negative attitude and feeling sorry for oneself only makes the treatments harder to get through, as this participant expressed:

> Yeah, you cannot start feeling sorry for yourself because people who start feeling sorry for themselves and will just sit there and go 'oh, this sucks you know, I didn't deserve to have this happen to me, why is this happening to me, this all sucks!' And they become kind of bitter and get down on everything and then it is really hard to go through it . . . it is just kind of keeping higher spirits . . . (15-year-old female with leukaemia).

They also gained a sense of accomplishment in fighting hard during each course of their cancer régime and, in turn, this made them even more determined to get through their treatment, as noted by the following:

> Knowing I haven't given up helps me . . . I mean when I looked at the road map [treatment regimen] the first time, you know the first time they ever showed it to me, it was like 'I am never going to get through this. It is like each page is 2 months; I am never going to get through this.' Then I finished the first page and it was like 'wow I get to flip the page.' . . . Like once I am done all that, that to me will be such an accomplishment, you know like it is all going to be like I have finished it all, I have gone through it! (14-year-old female with leukaemia).

Having a positive life atitude and willingness to fight the illness as main coping resources for young people with cancer is supported in the paediatric oncology literature (Kyngäs *et al.*, 2001). In addition, the participants also pointed out that, during the times when they did feel negative, it was important 'not to get down on your self' (Woodgate, 2001). More importantly, they felt that, once in a while, it was alright 'to have a bad attitude' and, in fact, it was their right, considering all the challenges that they had to face. In effect, they stressed the importance of not being too critical of oneself when they felt like not always fighting or when things did not go as smoothly. The participants stressed that 'doing whatever it takes' is what gets one through the treatment.

Knowing what to expect

With a diagnosis of cancer, adolescents express feeling lost and that their sense of understanding of their self or their world was shaken. Accordingly, they need to know what to expect with respect to what they will go through and experience during their cancer treatment or, as some would refer, to the 'new routine' (Woodgate, 2001). Knowing what to expect helps them to get on with their daily lives, as well as prepare them for the rough times. In order to be successful at knowing what to expect, they become attentive to the world around them as framed within the context of the cancer trajectory. Young people watch and listen, as well as seek out and receive information. They reinforce that it is very important that health professionals tell them exactly what to expect, and to be told the 'whole picture':

> My doctor thinks that you should know everything that is going to happen and I agree because I think it's important that you understand what is going on

because it is your life and it's important for you to know (17-year-old male with a Ewing's sarcoma).

The need to know the 'whole picture' is consistent with previous research that has shown that young people with cancer desire a wide array of information related to their cancer experience. The need to know requires information about adjusting to their diagnosis, dealing with procedures, relationships with friends, relationships with family, finishing treatment, and getting back to school (Decker *et al.*, 2004). It appears that they consider it extremely important that they know about their illness and how it will impact on their future (Hokkanen *et al.*, 2004). Although they acknowledge the importance of health professionals informing them of all aspects of their cancer and cancer treatment, they feel it is important for health professionals to recognise that each person is an individual. Hence, young people suggest that how the information is delivered (e.g. the timing and amount) should be based on each person's unique needs and situation. They also expressed it was important that health professionals convey a sense of hope and are positive when talking to them.

Among the most important information pieces that they want to know in order to plan ahead are about what to expect with their treatment regimens, the type of symptoms that they will experience (Woodgate, 2001), what they are allowed to do in relation to treatment, and how to cope in socially embarrassing situations (Hokkanen *et al.*, 2004). Understandably, they become more attentive to their bodies and aware of the changes that are taking place. Just as young people have to find out and understand about their new way of living or changes within their life, they also have to discover and understand more about their sense of self and the changes their bodies experience because of the many side effects from treatment. They also want to know about the long-term impacts of medication and treatments (Hokkanen *et al.*, 2004).

An integral part of knowing what to expect is coming to terms with the fact that, despite how well informed one may be, it is important to expect the unexpected or to be prepared for all those unexpected events, such as treatment being postponed due to low blood counts (Woodgate, 2001). The participants noted that, by sometimes expecting the unexpected, they were less disappointed by situations or events that did not transpire the way they were supposed to. They reinforced that it is unrealistic to be prepared for everything and that it is important to live with some degree of 'not knowing' or uncertainty whilst undergoing treatment.

Making some sense out of a bad situation

Making some sense out of a bad situation is a strategy that refers to young people coming to terms with the cancer and its treatment by trying to make some sense out of a bad situation. Basically it involves them finding meaning behind the question 'because of cancer I. . . .'. Only by reflecting on and assigning meaning to their experience with cancer are they able to put the cancer in its proper place while they continue with their daily lives. A sense of normalcy is created in two ways. Firstly, through the reinterpretation of the cancer experience and, secondly, through personal reflection on what cancer means and how it affects their personal lives; which helps them maintain a sense of balance (Rechner, 1990; Weekes and Kagan, 1994).

Adolescents express needing to find meaning not so much with respect to why they were the ones that were diagnosed with cancer, but why it is important for them to fight and get through the cancer trajectory. They reason that they need to get through the cancer trajectory because of their families. They reason that if they gave up and stopped going to treatment that this would only cause more suffering for their families, as one 16-year-old female with leukaemia reinforced:

> I will keep on fighting. I am my mom and dad combined. Dad and mom are my total role models or idols because they have been through so much in their lives but they are still as strong and probably stronger then anyone else! If I was to die I could see it would hurt them.

Adolescents also tried to make sense out of their cancer by reflecting on how it affected their sense of being within their family. Most expressed that, because of cancer, they became closer to their family. The participants reinforced that, because of having cancer, they came to realise just how much their family really cared and loved them:

> Well, you kind of knew that your family cared, but it is just that they never really had a chance to show you. It kind of gives them a chance to show you (14-year-old female with leukaemia).

Making some sense out of a bad situation also involves reasoning that cancer had helped to strengthen certain relationships involving friends, as well as leading to the development of new relationships. Although adolescents experienced weakened relationships with certain friends, they also experienced strengthened relationships with others. In fact, they reasoned that cancer helped them to discover who their 'true friends' really were, based on who was there for them during the more difficult treatment times.

They made sense of their cancer situation by reinforcing that their particular circumstances could always be worse. The participants always expressed that there were always others who had experienced a lot more pain or suffering than they did, as one 16-year-old female with leukaemia said:

> . . . so treatment for me at the beginning was never really that bad (pause) . . . But for someone who catches it really, really late like 'Eve' did, like she was in the hospital for a long time and was getting a feeding tube.

In addition, they made sense of their cancer treatment by believing that the cancer gave them an excuse not to partake in certain undesirable activities, such as the consumption of alcohol at parties or becoming sexually active.

Lastly, they made sense of their cancer by reflecting upon how it changed them as individuals. Adolescents reinforced the positive self-changes that emerged, such as becoming a more mature person who is more sensitive and caring to others, which is consistent with the research literature (Bearison, 1991; Haase and Rostad, 1994; Enskär *et al.*, 1997).

Taking one day at a time

The strategy 'taking one day at a time' refers to young people learning to live life more in the present or in the very moment. Adolescents needed to concentrate and direct all their energies in getting though the treatment by focusing on what needed to be accomplished on a day-to-day basis. They found that taking one day at time helped them from becoming too overwhelmed in having to deal with all the roughness associated with cancer and its treatment. Taking one day at a time helped them to 'hang in' and not give up during the more difficult periods when they were seriously ill and/or experiencing a lot of symptoms. In fact, during the more difficult times they further described living moment-by-moment instead of day-by-day.

While taking one day at time helped them to focus on the treatment and its related symptom trajectory, it also gave them a break in some respect from the hectic life of things not directly related to the cancer world. They did not have to worry about every single problem or issue that they normally would have worried about prior to their cancer diagnosis. In learning to take one day at a time they still nonetheless needed to maintain connections to the past and future. Talking about the past and planning for the future were important to the extent that it helped them to focus on why it was important to take one day at a time:

> Yes, it is important to take one day at a time, but it is also important to look ahead! To know that someday it is going to be done and someday you are working towards something. So it is taking one day at a time, but each day is one day less going towards August 10, the last day of my treatment (15-year-old female with leukaemia).

Whilst undergoing cancer treatment it was also important to enjoy the good times as they occur and not to think of cancer in terms as something that overall is a good or bad thing. It was important not to label each day as good or bad but instead to take each day as it comes and enjoy the good times when they occur, as one 14-year-old female with leukaemia said:

> I don't like to think of it that way, good and bad times, because then you think of it as the majority being bad times and it is like saying you have to cling on to the few good times you can get so you just live it when the good times come . . . When you are enjoying it, enjoy it, and when you can't, you just go through it.

Taking one day at a time also involved them becoming more patient, as now they had to wait for many things that prior to the cancer experience was not required. Waiting involved learning to put certain life and daily plans on hold. This included the 'big plans of life' like planning a vacation to visit relatives.

However, the most important waiting was waiting for the treatment to be over, as well as waiting for news that the treatment was successful. By taking one day at a time this strategy helped young people to celebrate the smaller successes of the cancer treatment such as completing one course of chemotherapy.

Taking time for yourself

This strategy of 'taking time for yourself' involves finding time for oneself during or between cancer treatments. In effect it involves taking some sort of break from cancer and focusing on finding time and personal space for a sense of self. Adolescents viewed taking a break as necessary, considering how hard the cancer trajectory could be for them. Often, taking time involved them trying to do 'fun' things that they liked doing best, in spite of not feeling so well, as one 15-year female with leukaemia told us:

> I always wanted to go shopping but I was too tired. I couldn't go and walk around the mall and like after a while I didn't want to go to the mall because I knew I would see somebody I knew. My cheeks would be all puffy from the medication and I was all bald and stuff. So in the middle of the day when all of my friends were in school, my sister used to drive me down to the shopping centre and borrow a wheelchair and then she'd drive me around the centre and we would go shopping. We used to go into the stores and there would be such small spaces and we would end up knocking things over (laughs)!

Adolescents stress the importance of remaining connected to those events or activities that they always appreciated doing prior to their cancer diagnosis. The importance of maintaining certain activities like sports across the cancer experience has been shown to have a positive impact on the psychosocial well-being of adolescents with cancer (Keats *et al.*, 1999). The participants also emphasised that it is important not to make cancer their only priority or their number 1 priority in life, but to have a balanced life:

> You kind of have to have a balance. Kind of like an equilibrium thing there, so you can kind of have it where you have to plan things around the cancer because you have these important treatments but at the same time you shouldn't let it run your life, because then you will pretty much have no life (17-year-old male with leukaemia).

In making time for a life other than cancer, they said it is important to try live a life that was as normal as possible:

> I think the best way of dealing with a lot of things is to try and make your life as normal to other regular, I guess regular kids as possible, you know? I have my band. I jam with them. I play drums and in 5 years we kick ass! (17-year-old male with a Ewing's sarcoma).

Sometimes getting away from the cancer experience also meant taking breaks away from individuals that they cared for the most, including family members:

But then sometimes I just want to get lost, you know? . . . because there are a lot of people in this house and I don't know, sometimes it just drives me nuts (15-year female with leukaemia).

Whilst they recognised the importance of taking time to do things that they liked to do, often the amount of time they could take was dictated or controlled by the timing of the treatment course and subsequent symptom distress. Most distressing to them was having to go into hospital for treatment during the times when they are feeling fairly well. For some, this was like throwing away valuable time or days in which they could be doing things they liked doing because they were feeling fairly well physically. One 15-year male with lymphoma noted that:

Oh, I'm feeling great like I was before I had to go in [the hospital] and then I start to feel like crap after this [after treatment]. God you put this stuff through me just to make me feel like crap! And I know it is helping and everything but still it is like I want to wait until at least until I get the flu or something and then put me in a hospital and give the stuff. If I'm feeling sick it won't be so bad.

Although for the most part they described having to wait to do things in their lives because of their cancer and treatment regime, there are times when they made the cancer wait for them. Some, with the support of their families, acknowledged it was important, regardless of the treatment regimen, to take time to do certain things that they needed or wanted to do. 'Taking time' allowed them or gave them permission at times to keep the cancer waiting, as this 17-year-old male with leukaemia expressed:

I found that I could have said that the cancer waits for me, type thing because we went on trips and stuff . . . We kind of said this is our date. It [cancer] sort of had to wait for me. Um, like we'd go on vacations and stuff and like we would reschedule appointments. When we came back you'd have to go but it [cancer] kind of held for us. We did what we needed to do and sort of came back and did the treatment.

Staying connected

Staying connected is a strategy that involves the maintenance of a sense of presence around those individuals important to young people in spite of having to undergo cancer treatment. Staying connected was important as it helped them to maintain a sense of belonging as opposed to feeling alone or abandoned in the world. They stayed connected by being with others, by others being there for them, and by them being there for others (Woodgate, 2006b).

'Being with others' referred to adolescents being around those individuals whom they liked and cared about the most, such as good friends and family. It involved spending time with friends and families in activities that brought pleasure to them as well as their friends and family. One of the most important 'being with' activities that they cherished was going out for lunch or supper with their parents after they attended the cancer clinic for a scheduled treatment. For many it became a ritual to go out after their clinic appointment. Another important 'being with' activity was to attend school because it afforded them the opportunity to be with their friends, as one 16-year-old female with leukaemia reinforced:

> I like school cause I like being with my friend. Even though I am still young and I know you go there to learn or whatever but school is more of the sociable place to me.

Another example of 'being there for them' refers to family, friends, and other significant individuals (e.g. clinic nurse) standing by and being there for them throughout the cancer trajectory and especially during those times when the symptom distress was more intense. 'Being there' involved more than just a physical presence, but also a psychosocial–emotional presence that further helped them feel accepted and connected to individuals identified as important to them. Sometimes it involved others doing something physically to the adolescent, while other times it just involved the simple act of a family member or friend sitting beside them. The latter was preferred when their bodies became really sensitive as a result of their symptoms. It was during those times that the participants would express to others to 'be there, but don't touch me!'.

Adolescents identified a number of ways that others could be there for them, including (1) to comfort them, (2) to hold their hand, (3) to keep them from feeling less lonely, (4) to help them maintain a life other than the life that evolved around the cancer and its treatment, (5) to help them maintain a positive attitude, and (6) to help them feel loved and wanted despite those times when they feel or act differently (Woodgate, 2006b). These six options were viewed to be important sources of social support and may offer practical assistance, as a strong support system has been found to help adolescents cope with cancer (Neville, 1998; Ishibashi, 2001; Kyngäs *et al.*, 2001; Ritchie, 2001b; Haluska *et al.*, 2002).

The third way that helped to maintain a sense of presence involved adolescents 'being there for others'. This involved supporting their friends and family when they needed help in dealing with some type of concern or problem. They stressed the importance of a reciprocal relationship with friends and families who provided steadfast support. Having family and friends stand by them during their cancer treatments made them not only appreciate the importance of supportive relationships, but resulted in them feeling more responsible and caring to their family and friends, as is made evident by the following comment:

> But with like my friends, I am very careful when it comes to my friends and stuff. Then again, they are really careful when it comes to me (13-year-old male with non-Hodgkin's lymphoma).

Implications for health professionals

Despite the many challenges, research suggests that adolescents wish to get on with life whilst undergoing treatment. The resilient nature of adolescents with cancer reinforces the need to approach them not from a deficit-centred model, but from a resilient-centred one that focuses on coping, competence, adjustment, and adaptation (Woodgate, 1999a,b). While caring for adolescents with cancer, health professionals, including practitioners and service providers, need to be not only aware of adolescents' personal coping strategies, but also when it may be deemed appropriate to encourage or support their use of additional sources of coping. Accordingly, a list of supportive behaviours has been developed that health professionals can use as a guide to promote coping in adolescents with cancer (refer to Box 6.1). Acknowledging the value that young people with cancer place on others being there for them, health professionals can also help them cope by implementing supportive acts that indicate 'being there' and 'standing by' them throughout the cancer trajectory (refer to Fig. 6.1).

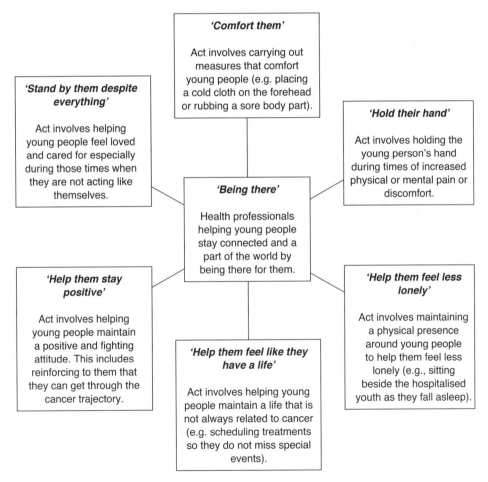

Fig. 6.1 'Being there': health professionals' supportive acts that help young people with cancer stay connected.

Box 6.1   Supportive behaviours that promote coping strategies in adolescents with cancer

Coping strategy 1: hoping for the best
    Refers to the adolescent sustaining a sense of hope.
    Supportive behaviours

- Convey a sense of hope to the adolescent that he/she will get through the cancer trajectory.
- Try to maintain a positive attitude.
- Work with the adolescent in developing short- and long-term goals.

Coping strategy 2: having the right attitude
    Refers to the adolescent maintaining a positive and fighting attitude.
    Supportive behaviours

- Praise the adolescent for all his/her successes (minor and major).
- Support and comfort the adolescent when they are 'feeling down'.
- Help the adolescent deal with any negative feelings about how he/she is coping.

Coping strategy 3: knowing what to expect
    Refers to the adolescent needing to know what to expect with respect to the 'whole' cancer course.
    Supportive behaviours

- Educate the adolescent about all aspects of cancer and the cancer treatment.
- Deliver the information in a manner that recognises the adolescent's unique needs.
- Balance hope with honesty when delivering information.

Coping strategy 4: making some sense out of a bad situation
    Refers to the adolescent coming to terms with the cancer.
    Supportive behaviours

- Provide opportunities for the adolescent to reflect on his/her cancer experience (e.g. 'talk time' and daily journaling).
- Offer specialised supportive services (e.g. individualised counselling and art therapy).
- Accept whatever meanings that the adolescent assigns to his/her cancer experience.

Coping strategy 5: taking one day at a time
    Refers to the adolescent learning to live life more in the present or in the very moment.
    Supportive behaviours

- Help the adolescent maintain connections to the past and future.
- Encourage the adolescent to celebrate and enjoy the 'good' moments in life.
- Help the adolescent to deal with having to put certain life and daily plans on hold.

Coping strategy 6: taking time for yourself
    Refers to the adolescent finding time for him-/herself amongst or in between going through the cancer treatment.
    Supportive behaviours

- Help the adolescent to carry on with activities that he/she likes doing.
- Acknowledge to the adolescent that cancer is only one part of his/her life.
- Arrange appointments so that they do not to conflict with the adolescent's favourite activities (when possible).

Coping strategy 7: staying connected
    Refers to the adolescent maintaining a sense of presence around family and friends.
    Supportive behaviours

- Ensure that the adolescent is able to spend time with his/her family and friends.
- Educate family and friends how they can be there for the adolescent.
- Educate the adolescent how he/she can be there for family and friends.

Conclusion

This chapter has provided insight into some of the challenges faced by young people undergoing cancer treatment and some of the coping strategies used to 'get on with life'. Supportive behaviours that help to sustain adolescents' coping strategies were also presented. Whilst research is growing in this area, more work needs to be done that will further advance our understanding of how adolescents both experience and cope with cancer and how health professionals can best sustain young people's coping strategies. Both research and practice needs to be directed at helping adolescents to get through cancer treatment and, in so doing, ensure they will 'succeed' no matter what the eventual outcome of treatment. As one 14-year-old with leukaemia told us:

> For me it was not like a race like you had to win because no matter what, if you get through, you have won. I just see it if you get through it, you have won!

References

Bearison, D. (1991) *'They Never Want to Tell You': Children Talk About Cancer.* Harvard University Press, Cambridge, MA.

Decker, C., Phillips, C., & Haase, J. (2004) Information needs of adolescents with cancer. *Journal of Pediatric Oncology Nursing*, **21**(6), 327–334.

Di Gallo, A., Amsler, F., Gwerder, C., & Bürgin, D. (2003) The years after: a concept of the psychological integration of childhood cancer. *Supportive Care in Cancer*, **11**, 666–673.

Enskär, K., Carlson, M., Golsäter, M., & Hamrin, E. (1997) Symptom distress and life situation in adolescents with cancer. *Cancer Nursing*, **20**(1), 23–33.

Glasson, J. (1995) A descriptive and exploratory pilot study into school re-entrance for adolescents who have received treatment for cancer. *Journal of Advanced Nursing*, **22**, 753–758.

Haase, J. & Rostad, M. (1994) Experience of completing cancer therapy: children's perspectives. *Oncology Nursing Forum*, **21**(9), 1483–1492.

Haluska, H., Jessee, P., & Nagy, C. (2002) Sources of social support: adolescents with cancer. *Oncology Nursing Forum*, **29**(9), 1317–1324.

Hedstrom, M., Skolin, I., & Von Essen, L. (2004) Distressing and positive experiences and important aspects of care for adolescents treated for cancer. Adolescent and nurse perceptions. *European Journal of Oncology Nursing*, **8**(1), 6–17.

Heiney, S. (1989) Adolescents with cancer: sexual and reproductive issues. *Cancer Nursing*, **12**(2), 95–101.

Hinds, P. (2004) Adolescent-focused oncology nursing research. *Oncology Nursing Forum*, **31**(2), 281–287.

Hinds, P. & Martin, J. (1988) Hopefulness and the self-sustaining process in adolescents with cancer. *Nursing Research*, **37**(6), 336–340.

Hockenberry-Eaton, M., Hinds, P., Alcoser, P. *et al.* (1998) Fatigue in children and adolescents with cancer. *Journal of Pediatric Oncology Nursing*, **15**(3), 171–182.

Hokkanen, H., Eriksson, E., Ahonen, O., & Salantera, S. (2004) Adolescents with cancer: experience of life and how it could be made easier. *Cancer Nursing*, **27**(4), 325–335.

Ishibashi, A. (2001) The needs of children and adolescents with cancer for information and social support. *Cancer Nursing*, **24**(1), 61–67.

Kameny, R. & Bearison, D. (1999) Illness narratives: discursive constructions of self in pediatric oncology. *Journal of Pediatric Nursing*, **14**(2), 73–79.

Keats, M., Courneya, K., Danielsen, S., & Whitsett, S. (1999) Leisure-time physical activity and psychosocial well-being in adolescents after cancer diagnosis. *Journal of Pediatric Oncology Nursing*, **16**(4), 180–188.

Kyngäs, H., Mikkonen, R., Nousiainen, E. *et al.* (2001) Coping with the onset of cancer: coping strategies and resources of young people with cancer. *European Journal of Cancer Care*, **10**, 6–11.

Mathieson, C. & Stam, H. (1995) Renegotiating identity: cancer narratives. *Sociology of Health and Illness*, **17**(3), 283–306.

Neville, K. (1998) The relationships among uncertainty, social support, and psychological distress in adolescents recently diagnosed with cancer. *Journal of Pediatric Oncology Nursing*, **15**(1), 37–46.

Palmer, L., Erickson, S., Shaffer, T., Koopman, C., Amylon, M., & Steiner, H. (2000) Themes arising in group therapy for adolescents with cancer and their parents. *International Journal of Rehabilitation and Health*, **5**(1), 43–54.

Rechner, M. (1990) Adolescents with cancer: getting on with life. *Journal of Pediatric Oncology Nursing*, **7**, 139–144.

Ritchie, M. (2001a) Self-esteem and hopefulness in adolescents with cancer. *Journal of Pediatric Nursing*, **16**(1), 35–42.

Ritchie, M. (2001b) Sources of emotional support for adolescents with cancer. *Journal of Pediatric Oncology Nursing*, **18**(3), 105–110.

Roberts, C., Turney, M., & Knowles, A. (1998) Psychosocial issues of adolescents with cancer. *Social Work in Health Care*, **27**(4), 3–18.

Weekes, D. & Kagan, S. (1994) Adolescents completing cancer therapy: meaning, perception, and coping. *Oncology Nursing Forum*, **21**(4), 663–670.

Woodgate, R. (1998) Adolescents' perspectives of chronic illness: 'it's hard'. *Journal of Pediatric Nursing*, **13**(4), 210–223.

Woodgate, R. (1999a) A review of the literature of resilience in the adolescent with cancer: part II. *Journal of Pediatric Oncology Nursing*, **16**(2), 78–89.

Woodgate, R. (1999b) Conceptual understanding of resilience in the adolescent with cancer: part I. *Journal of Pediatric Oncology Nursing*, **16**(1), 35–43.

Woodgate, R. L. (2001) Symptom experiences in the illness trajectory of children with cancer and their families. Doctoral dissertation, University of Manitoba, Winnipeg, MB.

Woodgate, R. L. (2005) A different way of being: adolescents' experiences with cancer. *Cancer Nursing*, **28**(1), 8–15.

Woodgate, R. L. (2006a) Life is never the same: childhood cancer narratives. *European Journal of Cancer Care*, **15**(1), 8–18.

Woodgate, R. L. (2006b) The importance of 'being there': perspectives of supportive relationships by adolescents. *Journal of Pediatric Oncology Nursing*, **23**(3), 122–134.

Zevon, M., Tebbi, C., & Stern, M. (1987) Psychological and familial factors in adolescent oncology. In: *Major Topics in Adolescent Oncology* (ed. C. Tebbi), pp. 325–349. Futura Publishing Company, Inc., New York, NY.

Chapter 7
End of Treatment Issues: Looking to the Future

Nelia Langeveld and Julia Arbuckle

Introduction

Completion of therapy is a milestone in the life of any young cancer patient. The final day of the patient's therapy will offer emotional and psychosocial relief to the whole family, as well as the promise of resolution of many of the physical problems that occur during treatment, including low blood counts, hair loss, mouth sores, and nausea and vomiting. Now everyone can move on and truly get back to a normal way of life. However, long-term survivors of childhood cancer face an uncertain future. The clinical success achieved with this patient population has come at some cost in terms of patients' level of functioning and sense of wellbeing. Studies have documented that two-thirds of survivors suffer at least one chronic or late-occurring complication (late effect) of their cancer therapy, with about one-third having serious or life-threatening complications (Stevens *et al.*, 1998; Oeffinger *et al.*, 2000). In addition, some survivors will encounter job discrimination, difficulties obtaining insurance, and emotional or social problems (Kelaghan *et al.*, 1988; Hays *et al.*, 1992; Zeltzer, 1993; Haupt *et al.*, 1994; Evans and Radford, 1995; Rauck *et al.*, 1999; Langeveld *et al.*, 2002).

One of the growing challenges in medicine today is providing appropriate health care for survivors of childhood and adolescent cancer. In the past survivors were often on their own after treatment ended. When it became apparent that these young people often faced complex medical and psychosocial effects from their years of treatment, late-effects clinics, using a multidisciplinary team to monitor and support survivors, were established. These follow-up clinics not only provide comprehensive care for survivors, but also participate in research projects that may improve the quality of life for current and future long-term survivors.

This chapter will discuss the ongoing support needs of those young people finishing cancer treatment, and addresses the planning for this phase of care. Some considerations for long-term follow-up will be given and potential models of care will be presented.

The ongoing support needs of young people finishing cancer treatment

Stopping active treatment is a phase that young people and parents often describe as an experience fraught with conflicting emotions (Wiard and Jogal, 2000). The protocol schedules and frequent appointments served to provide reassurance and structure. Many young people and parents feel 'safe' during treatment and assume that the therapy is keeping the cancer away. The end of treatment often leaves families feeling exposed and vulnerable. Concerns about relapse are an almost universal response since the cancer is no longer being actively treated (Keene *et al.*, 2000). Healthcare professionals can help smooth the transition from the acute phase of treatment to the 'off treatment' period by having a meeting with the young person and their parents near the end of treatment. Factual information should include a discussion about the disease, the treatment, and possible late effects, suspicious symptoms to be aware of, a schedule of the follow-up visits and screening tests yet to come, and a discussion of any concerns. The young person and their parents should receive written information that includes the most important facts about the disease and treatment, such as name of their disease, date of diagnosis, place of treatment, total dosages of drugs, amounts of radiation, and necessary follow-up (Keene *et al.*, 2000). This will also help the survivor provide all future physicians with comprehensive information on their medical history. Furthermore, they should be prepared for the fact that the process of reintegration and adjustment takes time. This insight might help to set more realistic expectations for the process of recovery after treatment. Ideally, teaching about all of these issues should begin several months before the young person is to complete therapy. Counselling and anticipatory guidance about reactions, feelings, and other issues to expect after the end of active treatment can help them and their families prepare for this time.

The guidance provided by the National Institute for Health and Clinical Excellence (2005), entitled *Improving Outcomes in Children and Young People with Cancer*, stresses that

> 'Psychological support needs are highly individual and will change as individuals and families move through the different stages of the patient pathway' (p. 85).

Therefore, an assessment of young people's psychological support needs is just as vital at the end of treatment as at the beginning. Eiser *et al.* (2000) noted that survival is actually a 'separate and ongoing phase' of care in itself.

Trajectory of need

Although physical recovery from the illness and treatment has started, emotional recovery may only just be beginning, and many may need time and support to achieve this. There is an assumption that moving off treatment means that anxieties disappear. Instead, many young people and parents experience this phase as a time of increased anxiety. Once the focus has shifted from the day-to-day grind of treatment, often the reality of their situation hits them and they then start to face other worries they may not have had the time or energy to process during treatment – such as infertility and mortality.

Some young people will feel very emotionally drained after treatment has finished. They are often expected to be happy that they have been given the 'all clear' and, although many do feel very relieved, they can also experience a range of feelings, including guilt, anger, anxiety, blame, sadness, loss, and fear, which can be quite overwhelming. It can be very difficult for these survivors to feel positive about the future again, and the pressure of other people's expectations to 'get on with life' and plan ahead can make them feel isolated and frustrated. Young people can often feel abandoned by the medical systems that once enveloped them and occupied and determined their whole life and routine, but which are now reduced to sporadic follow-up clinic appointments. Of course, some young people are able to move on quickly and can use their experiences to reassess their lives in a positive way. Facing up to and beating a life-threatening illness can inspire people to live in a different way and can provide clarification about what and who is truly important to them (Zebrack and Chesler, 2001).

Although every individual has different experiences and needs, there are certain common adjustments, issues, and areas of support that are experienced by this client group and should be expected to be addressed. These are (1) re-establishing an individual, social, and sexual identity as a cancer survivor, (2) renegotiating relationships with families and friends, (3) re-engaging with life after treatment by occupying their time with meaningful activity, and (4) coping with the after-effects of treatment.

Each of these areas will be discussed in the following sections and a case report (referred to as D) will be used to illustrate them. It should be noted that not all survivors and family members suffer from psychological consequences and maladaptive behaviour that requires professional input. In clinical practice the consequences of treatment may result in a wide variety of reactions. However, childhood cancer can affect the whole family, as illustrated by the case of D.

> D was diagnosed with leukaemia when she was 16 years old and still at school. She lived with her parents and an older sibling (who has since left home) and underwent 2 years of treatment for her disease before going into remission nearly 3 years ago. A Cancer and Leukaemia in Children social worker for young people met her halfway through her first treatment and has been working with her for 4 years, supporting her through the various stages of her cancer journey.

Re-establishing an individual, social, and sexual identity

Evans (1996) suggested that a diagnosis of cancer puts young people at risk of psychological disturbance, since the developmental tasks of this age group focus on identity formation and independence: therefore, a cancer diagnosis may disrupt this developmental process. At the very time that young people are seeking independence, cancer increases their dependence and alters their identity, singling them out from their peers as different. This was certainly the case for D, who had to leave school when she began treatment and spent her time in hospital or at home.

Establishing a new identity

In the transition from 'patient' to 'survivor' young people must establish a new identity that incorporates their cancer experience, but does not let it define who they are. They must also re-establish their independence and find a comfortable way of defining themselves, deciding what 'their story' is and preparing themselves for when and how they want to tell it. Hollen and Hobbie (1995) wrote that we must help young people to define their own 'wellness role'. This is a difficult task because long and complicated treatment processes may mean that, for many years, their disease has defined them. They now have to redefine themselves as an individual, not as a patient who is part of a medical team and treatment system, but as a person who is now part of a different society. They must rejoin a whole new world of 'well' people, despite having missed out on time spent in this society and with their peers. Their challenge now is to reintegrate and find a place again. They may have lost a lot of their social confidence and need to build this up at their own pace by going out in public, to shops, and so on and so increase interactions with peer groups. However, some young people will have found cancer an isolating experience and may need a great deal of support to do this. They may look different if their hair has grown back a different colour or their weight has changed or they have scars or have had an amputation, and this may constantly remind them of the illness. A changed body image can make them feel 'not like themselves' and so less attractive. Lozowski's (1993) survivors study reported that young people had negative concerns and perceptions of 'being different', as well as more social anxieties compared to their non-cancer peers.

> In D's case, when she went into remission, the transition from patient to survivor was quite difficult and she needed time and support with this process. This was partly due to the age and stage she was when she became ill, as she had only just begun to seek more independence from her parents. However, it was also due to her and her family's coping mechanisms, which were to place themselves fully under the care and guidance of the hospital and follow every instruction to the letter. D and her mother became 'a team' and went through everything together, to the exclusion of other family members, who were also involved, but not as closely. In fact, her mother referred to every procedure D had as 'we', for example 'we had a bone marrow test today' and D felt that this was comforting and made her feel that she did not have to cope with painful procedures alone. This strategy helped D feel less frightened in the treatment process, but also helped her mother feel less anxious, as she had a role in her daughter's care. However, as a result, D only felt safe within the hospital environment or at home if her mother was with her and was doing everything for or with her. When she went into remission, it took a lot of time for D to feel safe

again in the outside world – and without her mother. Gradually she had to build up her trust and self-confidence to do everyday things, such as making a telephone call, taking a bus, or seeing her friends on her own. It took over 6 months of gradual support for D to feel able to come into town on a bus to meet the social worker for a coffee alone. For a long time, even after her hair had grown back (although it was finer and not the same as before), she believed that people would know she had had cancer just by looking at her, as she still felt so different from her peers and looked so different than before she was ill. D had lost all of her social confidence and felt exposed and vulnerable, but gradually, through re-engaging with her old friends and going on outings and trips with someone outside of the family that she felt safe with, and together with other young people who had survived cancer, she began to build up her confidence and felt able to take part in life again.

Sexual identity

In terms of sexuality, this subject is often avoided during young people's cancer treatment. It is as if it is put 'on hold' and is often an ignored part of young people's identities. However sexuality can no longer remain a neglected area of patient care (Coughlan, 1987).

Young people need to be supported with their emerging sexuality during and after their cancer treatment, as it may also have been affected by their cancer experience. Young people can experience issues such as a loss of sexual confidence and feelings of unattractiveness due to a changed body image, and some of their treatment may also have affected their sex drive and sexual function.

D was just starting to explore her sexuality and relationships when she was diagnosed with cancer. The relationship she was in did not survive once her treatment started. This was very upsetting for her and made her feel that she had been rejected because of the cancer. When her treatment finished and she began to think about relationships again, the fear of rejection, along with the effect of treatment on her body image, made her very apprehensive about having a sexual relationship, although she wanted this and saw it as a way of helping her to feel 'normal' again. Her body was not the same as it had been before treatment and she had been left with scars and a feeling of physical fragility from the fear that her body would let her down again. In time, she did embark on a relationship, which later became sexual, but she needed time and support to feel able do this.

Renegotiating relationships with family and friends

Family

Relationships are affected by and often change during cancer treatment. If young people are not already living at home then they often return to live in their family home during treatment. Even if they were still living at home, the dynamic of the relationship will change because of their increased dependence when they are ill. Both parties may find this difficult to accept or adjust to (Stam *et al.*, 2005). Often, just when they have adjusted, the situation changes again and both parties can find it hard to cope with a relationship that needs to be renegotiated through the different stages of cancer. Established family roles are difficult to change, and the balance between young people feeling overprotected and abandoned is often a very difficult one for family members to predict. As a patient their needs will have changed at various stages of their treatment and what made them feel safe when they were ill can make them feel smothered when they are well. Some young people will need to reclaim their independence very slowly in order to feel safe with this process, whereas others want to claim it back quickly and feel frustrated if they feel they are being held back. Some continue to live independently or with friends or partners during their treatment; however, this does not mean that relationships are unaffected, and they may need to be renegotiated in the same way as by those living at home.

Cancer affects the whole family and can impact on all of the roles and dynamics within it (Van Dongen-Melman, 2000). Differing coping mechanisms can isolate family members if they are not understood or respected. A major illness places a family under a great deal of strain, and this includes siblings and friends. Siblings can experience their own feelings of fear, anxiety, resentment, guilt, and isolation within the family and with their peers (Houtzager, 2004).

Friends

Young people feel very different to their 'well' peers during and after their treatment – and vice versa – and some friendships do not survive because of this. The loss of young people's time with their friends needs to be acknowledged, as well as the particular losses when they did not feel able to keep up with certain friends and missed out on important social outings, such as birthdays. Some may refer to and separate out their 'cancer' and 'non-cancer' friends, and it is often very difficult after treatment for them to catch up with peers whose lives have moved on. These friends may not even begin to understand what has happened unless the young person felt able to share it with them by including them as visitors or keeping in touch in some way, such as explaining experiences. However, this is often very hard to do. It can be very frustrating and irritating for young people when they do not feel understood or feel pressure because of expectations from friends that they will simply return 'to their old selves'. Encouraging young people to keep in touch with and include their friends, as well as joining or attending groups and clubs, may help them to establish new networks whilst keeping and renegotiating existing ones.

Illustration of negotiating relationships

When D became ill, her family relationships changed as her mother stopped working and became her primary carer, whilst her father and older sibling continued with their jobs. As a result D and her mother became a 'closed unit' and 'the experts' on her disease and treatment and her father and older sibling were excluded from being involved in her care.

Throughout her treatment, D slept in her mother's bed with her and her father slept in D's room, as neither D nor her mother felt safe when they were apart. D's mother also slept over with her whenever she was in hospital. This changed the dynamic of all of the relationships within the family and, even when D was in remission, it took a long time for her to feel safe enough to return to her own bedroom. This was also difficult for her mother to adjust to. However, D was actually ready before her and, as a result, would often wake in the night to the sight of her mother standing over her to check that she was breathing normally. D redecorated and then gradually reclaimed her room back as well as her own private space and some of her previous independence. However, she still remains much closer to her mother, to the exclusion of other family members and does not feel that they fully understand her illness/treatment or trust them to 'look after' her.

Re-engaging with life after treatment by occupying time with meaningful activity

Re-engaging with life after treatment involves young people making decisions about how to use their time. These are highly individual decisions that will depend on their physical and emotional energy levels. Therefore, it is vital to move at the young person's pace, whilst providing them with a variety of ideas and options to stimulate motivation. Young people can feel drained for some time after treatment has finished. It can be quite daunting for them to begin life after treatment with a big blank canvas, which is often the case if they were not on an education or employment path before treatment or now reassess and seek new opportunities. Sudden interaction after isolation is difficult for some young people, and confusing, since their role/job was to get better. Their new role may now be unclear and, again, what is their new story? They need to find a new sense of 'normal' in their lives.

Young people often need support with education (such as restarting school, college, or university) to look for or restart work, as well as thinking creatively about other options such as open learning/home study or voluntary work. It can be very hard to resume studies and/or work after such a life-changing experience – compounded by a significant gap in education or employment. Occupying time in a meaningful way can itself be a major step on the road to their recovery, but can offer a sense of structure and security and a distraction from thinking about their illness/health. However, this also has to happen at their pace and some young people need considerable time, space, and support to rethink their lives.

The Scottish Intercollegiate Guidelines Network (2004) publication *Long Term Follow Up of Survivors of Childhood Cancer: a National Clinical Guideline* suggests that treatment for childhood cancer 'may have an impact on educational and social function later in life' (p. 19).

Adjustment to life after cancer may include low mood/anxiety, low self-esteem, and some evidence of post-traumatic stress disorder. Therefore, it is vital to acknowledge that young people may need support with the process of seeking and maintaining meaningful activity.

> By the time that D had finished her 2 years of treatment, she had missed the last 2 years of her education and all of her friends had left school and were starting work or further education. However, D did not feel able to do either (or want to return to school) as she still felt very fatigued and physically fragile and had lost her social confidence. Although she had previously been a successful student, she was worried that she had forgotten how to study and was particularly anxious about her ability to concentrate and retain information. She needed a variety of options to consider and time to consider them whilst doing something with her time as she had started to become well enough to feel bored. Having previously enjoyed art at school, she began making her own greeting cards and this helped her to occupy her time and build up her confidence with no pressure. She then felt able to do some home study courses through a local college, and the social worker supported her by invigilating her tests at her home, and, once she had completed these, she felt able to attend college on a full time basis.

Coping with the after-effects of treatment

As already described, a cancer diagnosis and treatment affects a young person's identity and relationships, and they can also be left with numerous physical after-effects, such as fatigue, changes to their body, and infertility, all of which can seriously affect their quality of life and ability to move on. Infertility, in particular, is often an effect that has not been discussed in great depth during treatment. It may not be apparent straight away, and can be extremely distressing in terms of a loss of identity and hopes for the future.

> Infertility is an issue that D has to live with. Infertility at any age is a loss, but D also sees this as yet another part of her life that has been damaged by her cancer and a part of the future that she expected that has been taken from her because of it.

In terms of psychosocial after-effects, fear of relapse is a major cause of anxiety for some young people for a long time after their treatment has finished (Lozowski, 1993; Langeveld *et al.*, 2004). Returning for outpatient appointments can be an extremely stressful reminder, although, for some, their anxieties may lessen as time goes on. At the end of treatment young people are told that they are better, but having to return for follow-up appointments seems to contradict that, so they often do not feel 'better'. The first cold or flu after treatment can be traumatic for them, and aches or pains that they previously shrugged off now contribute to a fear of cancer returning. For some young cancer survivors 'that fear' is made all the more real when relapse does occur after the completion of treatment.

Albritton and Bleyer (2003) stated that:

> 'Even after treatment, adolescents can maintain persistently abnormal perceptions of their body and/or their health, manifested as counter phobic or reckless behaviour or hypochondria' (p. 2596).

Facing mortality

Young people can be left with altered perceptions about their mortality after they have survived cancer. Some feel invincible at having won, whilst others feel convinced the disease will return and that they will not survive it this time when it does. Whilst they were ill they had a very uncertain future, and they may continue to feel uncertain about the future for some time. Planning for a future can be difficult and feel like a very strange process.

Mortality is not something that 'well' young people generally consider until much later in life. Once it has been faced, however, there is no way back to a time when it was not an issue. Young people are usually able to take life for granted, but this is difficult to do when trust in the future has been taken from them as a result of cancer. Wasserman *et al.* (1987) noted higher risk-taking behaviour among survivors of Hodgkin's disease during childhood or adolescence. Their theories on why this should occur included survivors experiencing feelings of invincibility having beaten cancer or feelings of inferiority for having had it. Their life has been 'saved', but they still take life-threatening risks, leading Wasserman *et al.* (1987) to hypothesise that some could only feel alive by cheating death again and again.

Some young people may also experience survivor's guilt in relation to the fact that they survived when others did not. This can lead to feelings of pressure to live life to the full or, alternatively, to prove that they are worthy of surviving.

> Two of the young cancer survivors D knew well died and she attended both of their funerals. Whilst D understood that one person's survival did not necessarily affect that of another, she still experienced feelings of guilt at having survived when they did not.

Other practical issues that young cancer survivors encounter are difficulties with travel and life insurance (Hobbie *et al.*, 1993). These can cause a great deal of distress, especially if blunt questions are asked that they find difficult to answer. They often need support at such times in terms of advice on where to go or what to say about their illness and health status as a cancer survivor.

Being a cancer survivor

Many young people may need support to explore all of these issues, at their own pace, by skilled and experienced support staff with an awareness of the issues and the ability to listen and to really hear the often painful feelings which accompany them. Professionals need to acknowledge and not minimise young cancer survivors' losses and life changes, but at the same time remain flexible and respond to windows of opportunity when young people want to talk and have the energy to consider different options (such as social interaction or study).

It needs to be acknowledged that there is no 'return to normal' for young people after cancer treatment, because normal was hospital and now normal will be something else, a 'something' they will need to define. The ability to motivate, as well as the sensitivity to create a safe environment without pushing, is essential. Throughout and beyond treatment, young people need to have a space where they can say whatever they feel and be heard and supported.

The need for aftercare

From this case study it is clear that the transition from patient to survivor can be a powerful experience, not only for the patient, but also for those closely involved with him or her. D's case shows that, although she is the most seriously affected family member, childhood cancer has also psychosocial effects for her parents and her sibling. This indicates the need for medical and psychosocial aftercare, not only for the survivor, but also for his or her family. It is evident that the care of the young person does not end with the last dose of chemotherapy. Nor can it end 3 or 5 years later when the chance of recurrent disease declines.

The need for comprehensive survivorship care has been gaining international attention and recognition. Support for the development of specialised programmes, guidelines, and educational initiatives are taking place at local, national, and federal levels. The Institute of Medicine published a report entitled *Childhood Cancer Survivorship: Improving Care and Quality of Life* (Hewitt *et al.*, 2003): this report emphasises the importance of establishing follow-up programmes, developing healthcare guidelines, and educating both cancer survivors and related healthcare professionals. The publication *A National Action Plan for Cancer Survivorship: Advancing Public Health Strategies* (Lance Armstrong Foundation, 2004) set as a goal 'access to high-quality care throughout every stage of cancer survivorship' for all survivors (p. 2). Similarly, in the UK the National Institute for Health and Clinical Excellence's (2005) *Guidance on Cancer Services: Improving Outcomes in Children and Young People with Cancer* includes specific recommendations on the management of long-term sequelae.

The requirement for long-term surveillance is quite clear; what is less clear, however, is how surveillance should be designed. To date, there are no evidence-based or uniformly effective long-term models of follow-up care for young cancer survivors. Although various national groups have addressed the problem with the development of long-term follow-up guidelines, which provide a foundation for what elements of follow-up care need to be delivered, the recommendations may not be completely consistent (Friedman *et al.*, 2006). Furthermore, there are several barriers to the delivery of 'survivor healthcare'. Oeffinger and

Wallace (2006) recently assessed the current status of follow-up care in the USA and UK. They found that the majority of survivors, including those at highest risk, were not receiving recommended healthcare in the US or the UK, partly due to survivor-related, physician-related, or healthcare system-related barriers. These included a general lack of awareness of late effects by survivors, a lack of capacity for survivor care within cancer institutions, primary care physicians being unfamiliar with the health needs of survivors, and a general lack of communication between survivors, cancer centres, and primary physicians. At the present time, potential strategies for overcoming these barriers are being tested in the USA and the UK, such as the development of a 'passport for care', an Internet-based tool that provides an individualised summary of the *Children's Oncology Group Long-term Follow-up Guidelines* (Children's Oncology Group, 2006) based on the patient's cancer treatment history. Medical colleagues from the USA and the UK are also testing the feasibility of using a virtual information centre, which is accessible through the Internet or a free telephone number, to link high-risk Hodgkin's disease survivors, their primary care physicians, and cancer centres (Oeffinger and Wallace, 2006). In the UK, the production of an information booklet, treatment summary, and separate information sheets has been evaluated in the clinical setting (Blacklay *et al.*, 1998). The purpose of this was to improve access to follow-up care and raise awareness of possible vulnerability to future health issues among survivors of younger cancer. The results of the evaluation suggest that the intervention enhanced awareness among survivors about the importance of follow-up and the need for vigilance in their health care (Eiser *et al.*, 2000).

Models of follow-up care

The perspective of healthcare professionals has dominated most models of follow-up care. However, the success of any long-term follow-up programme is also dependent on participation by the survivors themselves. All patients, from childhood through adolescence to adulthood, will have views on their continuing care needs. It is important to listen to the survivors themselves and to find out which models are preferred by them and why. Because of the current lack of knowledge about the opinions of survivors on follow-up care, research is clearly warranted. Chapter 10 explores this issue in greater depth.

Ideally, models of care for long-term survivors of childhood cancer should be flexible enough to meet the needs of both adolescents and young adults and be sensitive to change throughout the life cycle. Evaluations should be individualised based on the survivor's treatment history and may include screening for potential somatic and psychosocial complications. At the same time, it will be important to maintain a balance between over-screening, which might induce unnecessary fear of unlikely but remotely plausible complications, and under-screening for potential life-threatening complications that could be missed at an early phase and, thus, require more aggressive intervention when the complication becomes clinically apparent (Landier *et al.*, 2006).

Friedman *et al.* (2006) described a variety of models that can be proposed for long-term follow-up clinical care. The model most commonly employed at the moment is a cancer centre-based model, where the follow-up is coordinated by the primary oncology team in the oncology clinic by a dedicated late effects team in the oncology clinic – or by a dedicated late effects team outside of the oncology clinic. The late effects team can vary widely, involving some or all of the following members: paediatric oncologist, medical oncologist, advanced practice nurse, psychologist, social worker, radiation oncologist, and paediatric and medical sub-specialists. Some paediatric oncology centres have also established formalised transition programmes with specialised long-term follow-up programmes for adult survivors of childhood cancer.

A second model is the community-based model, where health professionals in typical practices, such as paediatricians, family medicine specialists, internists, medical/paediatric specialists, advanced practice nurses, or physician assistants, carry out the follow-up of the survivor. The advantage of a community-based model is that there may be coordination between the risk-adapted follow-up that the survivor requires and the general primary care that promotes independence on the part of the survivor and their families.

A third model is the combined cancer centre and community model. This appears to be the most ideal. An example would be follow-up in the cancer centre model for a specified time period with the transfer of follow-up care to a community-based primary care practice with variable levels of continued involvement from the late effects team. The time of transfer should be dependent on several factors, such as the risk for developing adverse late effects, the complexity of those late effects, psychosocial and developmental issues, and the knowledge demonstrated by the survivor or their family.

It is probably unrealistic to assume, as Friedman *et al.* (2006) also reflected in their article, that consensus will be reached for a unified model across all centres and countries. This is due to the heterogeneity within the survivor population, the variety of healthcare systems that exist, and the resources that are available – both nationally and locally. In establishing a formal follow-up programme, there is a need to examine local needs and resources and to determine how best to apply them so that the basic elements can be provided in a manner that is age appropriate, culturally sensitive, and clinically and cost-effective.

The transition process

As survivors of childhood and adolescent cancer increase both in number and in age, their health requirements will demand expertise and resources from the adult healthcare system. Most paediatric oncology centres have an upper age limit for care, and there is also the recognition that older survivors cannot receive appropriate care in a paediatric institution. In most circumstances survivors cannot avoid the transition from the 'sheltered' environment of paediatrics to the independent environment of adult medicine. Specialist adolescent services may or may not be available as an option. Therefore, paediatric centres should prepare survivors for this transition by allowing time for this process to occur relatively seamlessly. The optimal transition process occurs gradually, is organised in advance, and should begin years before the actual transition takes place. As more and more chronically ill young people survive into their third decade and beyond, researchers working with these groups have generated the majority of existing guidelines and principles for the transitional process (Bowes *et al.*, 1995). Although cancer survivors do not display active disease, as do patients with cystic fibrosis and other chronic disorders, the basic principles of transition can be applied legitimately to this population. The principles of successful transition from a Society for Adolescent Medicine position study (Blum, 2002) are outlined below and include the following.

1. The healthcare setting must be chronologically and developmentally appropriate.
2. Common concerns of young adulthood must be addressed to speciality care needs.
3. Transition should promote autonomy, personal responsibility, and self-reliance in young adults.
4. Transition programmes must be flexible enough to meet the needs of young adults.
5. A designated professional must take responsibility for the transition process in conjunction with the young adult and their family.

A factor that facilitates a smooth transition from a paediatric or adolescent cancer centre to an adult centre is a comprehensive medical summary, which should be provided to the new members of the healthcare team as well to the survivor and their family. Furthermore, the survivors themselves must also possess knowledge obvious to their disease and the treatment they received, and should be encouraged and feel able to question and speak for themselves in medical situations.

Conclusion

The case study described in this chapter shows that cancer affects many aspects of life for survivors and his or her family. The complexity, seriousness, and persistence of the late consequences of cancer underscore the need for medical and psychosocial aftercare when treatment ends. The obvious goal of follow-up care is to maximise the survivors' health and quality of life, while minimising the morbidity associated with cancer treatment exposure. This goal has been achieved to date through survivorship programmes in paediatric or adolescent cancer centres where a multidisciplinary team provides comprehensive surveillance of medical and psychosocial late effects, including early identification, intervention, education, and health promotion. As survivors of cancer grow in number and age, it is essential to develop a systematic plan for healthcare that extends not just through childhood and adolescence, but also through the lifetime of the survivor. Since the majority of young adult cancer survivors receive care outside of a cancer centre, educating survivors about their disease, treatment, and lifelong follow up care needs will remain imperative. Likewise, paediatricians, internists, family practitioners, nurses, and psychologists will require ongoing education regarding the potential long-term physiological and psychological effects of adolescent cancer. This is a real challenge that faces oncology healthcare providers, and will be the impetus for finding optimal mechanisms for providing care for young adult cancer survivors as they achieve independence (Ginsberg *et al.*, 2006).

> At the present time D has been 'off treatment' for more than 3 years and has been transitioned to a longitudinal programme focused on her long-term healthcare needs. She has a boyfriend who comes to the appointments with her instead of her mother. She also uses the word 'I' instead of 'we' again, thereby separating herself from her mother and asserting her individuality. A year ago the support of the CLIC Sargent social worker came to an end. Although D still appreciated the contact with the social worker, she did not need her assistance anymore. D is doing really well.

References

Albritton, K. & Bleyer, W. A. (2003) The management of cancer in the older adolescent. *European Journal of Cancer*, **39**(18), 2584–2599.

Blacklay, A., Eiser, C., & Ellis, A. (1998) Development and evaluation of an information booklet for adult survivors of cancer in childhood. The United Kingdom Children's Cancer Study Group Late Effects Group. *Archives of Diseases in Childhood*, **78**, 340–344.

Blum, R. W. (2002) Introduction. Improving transition for adolescents with special health care needs from pediatric to adult-centered health care. *Pediatrics*, **110**, 1301–1303.

Bowes, G., Sinnema, G., Suris, J. C., & Buhlmann, U. (1995) Transition health services for youth with disabilities: a global perspective. *Journal of Adolescent Health*, **17**, 23–31.

Children's Oncology Group (2006) *Children's Oncology Group Long-term Follow-up Guidelines*. Children's Oncology Group.

Coughlan, U. (1987) Dear nurse. *Nursing Times*, **83**(42), 32–34.

Eiser, C., Hill, J. J., & Blacklay, A. (2000) Surviving cancer: what does it mean for you? An evaluation of a clinic based intervention for survivors of childhood cancer. *Psycho-Oncology*, **9**, 214–220.

Evans, M. (1996) Interacting with teenagers with cancer. In: *Cancer and the Adolescent* (eds P. Selby & C. Bailey), pp. 251–263, BMJ Publishing Group, London.

Evans, S. E. & Radford, M. (1995) Current lifestyle of young adults treated for cancer in childhood. *Archives of Disease in Childhood*, **72**, 423–426.

Friedman, D. L., Freyer, D. R., & Levitt, G. A. (2006) Models of care for survivors of childhood cancer. *Pediatric Blood & Cancer*, **46**, 159–168.

Ginsberg, J. P., Hobbie, W. L., Carlson, C. A., & Meadows, A. T. (2006) Delivering long-term follow-up care to pediatric cancer survivors: transitional care issues. *Pediatric Blood & Cancer*, **46**, 169–173.

Haupt, R., Fears, T. R., Robison, L. L. *et al.* (1994) Educational attainment in long-term survivors of childhood acute lymphoblastic leukemia. *JAMA*, **272**, 1427–1432.

Hays, D. M., Landsverk, J., Sallan, S. E. *et al.* (1992) Educational, occupational, and insurance status of childhood cancer survivors in their fourth and fifth decades of life. *Journal of Clinical Oncology*, **10**, 1397–1406.

Hewitt, M., Weiner, S. L., & Simone, J. V. (eds) (2003) *Childhood Cancer Survivorship: Improving Care and Quality of Life*. National Cancer Policy Board, Institute of Medicine. The National Academies Press, Washington, DC.

Hobbie, W., Ruccione, K., Moore, I. K., & Truesdell, S. (1993) Late effects in long-term survivors. In: *Nursing Care of the Child with Cancer* (eds G. V. Foley, D. Fochtman, & K. H. Mooney), pp. 466–496, W.B. Saunders Company, Orlando, FL.

Hollen, P. J. & Hobbie, W. L. (1995) Establishing comprehensive specialty follow up clinics for long-term survivors of cancer. Providing systematic physiological and psychosocial support. *Supportive Care in Cancer*, **3**(1), 40–44.

Houtzager, B. (2004) Siblings of pediatric cancer patients. Coping, risk factors and psychological health. Unpublished thesis, University of Amsterdam.

Keene, N., Hobbie, W., & Ruccione, K. (2000) *Childhood Cancer Survivors. A Practical Guide to your Future*, 1st edn, pp. 1–29, O'Reilly & Associates, Sebastopol, CA.

Kelaghan, J., Myers, M. H., Mulvihill, J. J. *et al.* (1988) Educational achievement of long-term survivors of childhood and adolescent cancer. *Medical & Pediatric Oncology*, **16**, 320–326.

Lance Armstrong Foundation (2004) *A National Action Plan for Cancer Survivorship: Advancing Public Health Strategies*. Centers for Disease Control and Prevention, Department of Health and Human Services, Atlanta.

Landier, W., Wallace, W. H. B., & Hudson, M. M. (2006) Long-term follow-up of pediatric cancer survivors: education, surveillance, and screening. *Pediatric Blood & Cancer*, **46**, 149–158.

Langeveld, N. E., Ubbink, M. C., Last, B. F., Grootenhuis, M. A., Voûte, P. A., & De Haan, R. J. (2002) Educational achievement, employment and living situation in long-term young adult survivors of childhood cancer in The Netherlands. *Psycho-Oncology*, **11**, 1–13

Langeveld, N. E., Grootenhuis, M. A., Voûte, P. A., De Haan, R. J., & Van den Bos, C. (2004) Quality of life, self-esteem and worries in young adult survivors of childhood cancer. *Psycho-Oncology*, **13**(12), 867–881.

Lozowski, S. (1993) Views of childhood cancer survivors. *Cancer*, **71**, 3354–3357.

National Institute for Health and Clinical Excellence (2005) *Guidance on Cancer Services: Improving Outcomes in Children and Young People with Cancer*. National Institute for Health and Clinical Excellence, London.

Oeffinger, K. C. & Wallace, W. H. B. (2006) Barriers to follow-up care of survivors in the United States and the United Kingdom. *Pediatric Blood & Cancer*, **46**, 135–142.

Oeffinger, K. C., Eshelman, D. A., Tomlinson, G. E., Buchanan, G.R., & Foster, B.M. (2000) Grading of late effects in young adult survivors of childhood cancer followed in an ambulatory adult setting. *Cancer*, **88**, 1687–1695.

Rauck, A. M., Green, D. M., Yasui, Y., Mertens, A., & Robison, L. L. (1999) Marriage in the survivors of childhood cancer: a preliminary description from the Childhood Cancer Survivor Study. *Medical & Pediatric Oncology*, **33**, 60–63.

Scottish Intercollegiate Guidelines Network (2004) *Long Term Follow Up of Survivors of Childhood Cancer: a National Clinical Guideline*. Scottish Intercollegiate Guidelines Network, Edinburgh.

Stam, H., Grootenhuis, M. A., & Last, B. F. (2005) The course of life of survivors of childhood cancer. *Psycho-Oncology*, **14**(3), 227–238.

Stevens, M. C., Mahler, H., & Parkes, S. (1998) The health status of adult survivors of cancer in childhood. *European Journal of Cancer*, **34**, 694–698.

Van Dongen-Melman, J. E. W. M. (2000) Developing psychosocial aftercare for children surviving cancer and their families. *Acta Oncologica*, **39**(1), 23–31.

Wasserman, A. L., Thompson, E. I., Wilimas, J. A., & Fairclough, D. L. (1987) The psychological status of survivors of childhood/adolescent Hodgkin disease. *American Journal of Diseases of Children*, **141**(6), 626–631.

Wiard, S. & Jogal, S. (2000) The psychosocial impact of cancer. In: *Childhood Cancer. A Handbook from St Jude Childrens's Research Hospital* (eds G. Steen & J. Mirro), pp. 461–469. Perseus Publishing, Cambridge, MA.

Zebrack, B. J. & Chesler, M. (2001) Health-related worries, self-image, and life outlooks of long-term survivors of childhood cancer. *Health & Social Work*, **26**(4), 245–256.

Zeltzer, L. K. (1993) Cancer in adolescents and young adults: psychosocial aspects. Long-term survivors. *Cancer*, **71**, 3463–3468.

A Young Person's Experience 3

Life After Treatment or Chemotherapy Saves the Lost Boy

Alan Pitcairn

I began my cancer treatment with an almost spiritual belief that it would cure me. I was 16 years old. Now I am aged 31. Before medical intervention, cancer consumed my pelvis, my strength, and my spirit for over 2 years. Scans then a biopsy revealed the cause of this decline. An orthopaedic consultant delivered my diagnosis. He told me I had a Ewing's sarcoma in my right iliac crest. When he and his entourage had departed, I asked a nurse if this was cancer. Then I cried. I was devastated but relieved. I had suffered for years because my general practitioner (GP) could not comprehend the intensity or the implications of my pain. Now 'they' knew what was wrong with me. Now my fight back could begin.

On diagnosis day a registrar, who had been part of the consultant's circle, returned. He said that, of the 200 types of cancer, mine was not among the most lethal. More importantly, he told me there were drugs that could kill my tumour, but that they did not work on everybody so I would have to fight with the chemotherapy, to fight for my life. The registrar's rallying words lessened the impact of my diagnosis: not all cancers were equal, not all cancers meant death. No, I would fight and I would live. I imagined the cancer as a black mass at the tip of my pelvis. Treatment and willpower would transform the black into white healthy bone. Later my parents had to absorb the consultant's grimmer assessment of my condition, a sub-10% chance of survival. Neither they nor the doctors thought I could deal with this dark prediction. I think they were right.

For my treatment I was moved to an oncology ward across town. Again the staff did not tell me anything I might find traumatic, while my parents maintained an air of positive strength. Mum and dad censored clinical information before it reached me. In many ways it was more difficult for my younger brother than it was for my parents or me. They had each other and I became the focus of their devotion and my relatives' attention. As a result, Neil grew more independent of us, living a tribal existence with his friends, while I receded still further from my contemporaries. Perhaps he felt neglected: I am not sure if anyone asked him.

My initial time in the oncology ward was spent in a daze that prevented me from comprehending the reality of my situation. Years of struggle against undiagnosed cancer had crushed me into a permanent state of collapse. After this period of disjointed and detached GP cover, I revelled in the high-level medical attention I was now receiving. Doctors were finally taking me seriously. It did not occur to me that the oncologists' full-on intervention might have come too late, even when they could not conceal their alarm at my months of continual coughing. Later I realised they suspected the tumour had spread to my lungs, which is common with established bone cancer. Such potential consequences of my late diagnosis were not discussed with me. I was spared sinister projections. My calmness would have given way to abject panic had the medics' suspicion of spread been disclosed.

My oncology consultant, said chemotherapy would be our key anticancer weapon. In the ward, over the course of a year, I would receive as many treatment sessions as my body could withstand. There would be sufficient home leave between sessions for my white blood count to recover, typically 3–4 weeks. A Hickman line was fitted to ease the chemotherapy into me. This plastic vein linked me to a volumetric infusion pump that bore various bags of liquid across its shoulders. The biggest bag, a 3-litre beast, was swathed in a sinister black cloak. It would take 72 hours for the Mesna it contained to drain into my bloodstream, which set the duration of each treatment at 3 days. Vincristine hung in a smaller, transparent bag and, at some point during the 72 hours, a syringe-full of Adriamycin was administered. A discussion about the toxicity of my chemotherapy prepared me for the inevitability of side effects, although I anticipated only hair loss plus a hint of unpleasantness. What occurred was more like gastric Armageddon.

Initially, I tried mixing food with the treatment. This failed no matter how much anti-emetic I swallowed. As I fasted through further chemotherapy sessions, they became almost routine, but no more bearable. I dreamed of a drug that would knock me out for days, thereby rendering me oblivious to the rigours of treatment. Distractions could never eclipse the horror of it all: the ceaseless retching of an achingly empty stomach, bowels that screamed to be emptied, but locked when I tried, the constant nausea, and the toxic fatigue. However, my parents' visits made each 3-day therapy more palatable, as did brief but frequent encounters with staff whose continuity allowed relationships to be established. Health service workloads did not allow it but, even if they had, chemotherapy's side effects would have prevented me from enjoying sustained dialogue with the professionals on my ward. There was no need to rise to the occasion when my parents sat at my bedside: I was free to be passively wretched while they made all the effort.

Yes, chemotherapy put me in an unsociable mood. Feeling as rough as I did, I appreciated the privacy of a single room whenever one was available. In the wider ward, beyond the sanctuary of my isolation, dwelled too many hauntingly ill souls, the ghosts of cancer. It was an adult ward where most patients were older and sicker than I was. Any exposure to the decline evident in their hollowed, hanging faces traumatised me. It threatened the security of my belief. I did not want to see the disease that I had destroying the lives of others. Conversely, meeting 'cancer survivors' might have given me tangible hope. Sharing experiences with teenage cancer patients might have helped me gain insight and perspective. However, for selfish reasons, I could not have faced anyone who was gravely ill.

On home leave between treatments I felt relatively well. In these periods I would have been more receptive to although not necessarily enthusiastic about organised 'cancer contact', had it been offered. Beyond the sphere of my disease I yearned for greater contact with my peer group. Cancer had relentlessly reduced the scope of my existence since I was 14 years old: its prison of pain had shut me away from the excitement and exploits of my generation for too long.

In the 2+ years of my illness pre-diagnosis I diminished and withdrew from aspects of life beyond schoolwork, eating, and sleeping. My social spirit waned and I became a forgotten, invisible outsider. I was a lost boy, lost to cancer. I maintained friendship with only a couple of guys who lived nearby. Once they knew I had cancer, they did not treat me as more fragile or with any reverence because I was afflicted by this potentially fatal condition. There was no syrupy sympathy or melodramatic compassion. Our socialising became sporadic and structured, but those friends saw me as the 'me' from before. Whereas in their eyes I was unchanged, I saw them mature and grow. Disease denied me advancement through regular interaction with peers and it took many years post-treatment before I was comfortable with new people my own age. However, in many other ways I did make personal headway, learning much from my cancer odyssey.

After the first treatment session I was composed enough to consider fragments of life beyond cancer. Addressing my schooling took precedence over social and personal progress. The prospect of immersing myself in the 1000-pupil frenzy of my school was too daunting. I remained shy and did not want to stray from the cocoon of my restricted but cushioned life as a patient. Furthermore, educational institutions abound with germs and I imagined plague stalking the corridors waiting to ambush my chemotherapy-suppressed immune system. Home schooling was to help me keep pace with my former classmates. I did not want to be left behind. Naively, I considered that it was only in the academic arena this might happen. I lacked the foresight to realise other aspects of a teenager's development might be arrested by cancer. Growing up is an experience shared with one's peers, and my separation from them would curtail this process. Ideally, my treatment plan would have tackled this, somehow.

Opting for a scholarly focus was natural for me. I had always been diligent. Lack of rebellious spirit meant this was inevitable, given that my mother and father were teachers. In partnership with my parents, teachers from school provided generous support. My maths teacher, even gave me tutoring at her home twice weekly before cooking her husband's dinner. I gained most of my university entrance qualifications on schedule, but kept English for the next year because of an unassailable literature backlog. Thus, with my magnificent teachers, educational parentage, and studious nature, I was ideally placed to keep abreast academically at a time when illness and treatment dominated my life. Perhaps an agency could support teenage patients with less favourable circumstances.

Four treatments into my protocol I underwent numerous scans and X-rays to assess the status of my tumour. I was not aware that 'they' were also searching for secondary tumours. The spectre of metastasis did not enter my consciousness until the next clinic appointment, when I learned the cancer had not spread. Until that day, when I was told a cure was within reach, I had been shielded from the possibility of cancer colonising more of me. The scanners may have peered deep, but only a biopsy could provide definitive proof of my chemotherapy's efficacy and so I found myself in an orthopaedic ward again. Before the operation I knew there was an outside chance that, when the surgeon confronted my tumour in the flesh, he would feel confident enough to excise the whole thing. If this best-case scenario proved elusive, a radiotherapy broadside would be unleashed against my cancer. Either way, several chemotherapy sessions lay ahead. When I woke after surgery, my father was standing over me. I whispered 'Did they take it out?' He nodded and I felt such relief the bed cradled me like loving arms. My cancerous bone was pink because of the rich blood supply it demanded. The bone doctor could therefore cut safely around the margins of my tumour. I wanted to see my cancer's corpse, but it was already buried in pathology where studies revealed only a few living cells lingering. Chemotherapy had done for the rest. So there would be no radiotherapy and the chemotherapy ahead would be to mop up any rogue elements, invisible to the scanners, that might be lurking inside me. My tumour was located where a leg muscle joins the pelvis. With the cancerous bone gone, some biological engineering was required to give the newly detached end of my muscle a new point of anchor. This reconfiguration of my musculature meant I had to learn to walk again and, although my body remains 'funny' down there, it is a battle scar rather than a restrictive handicap.

During cancer treatment I was stronger than I could have imagined myself being before those days. Positive thought saw me through, but there was no negative clinical reality to dent my certainty. I was told I had cancer. I was told I could be cured. And I was. My cancer did not spread. It did not resist treatment. After diagnosis, there was no bad news. My situation was never so desperate that I felt a need for extra-familial support. Anyway, had it been offered, my mindset probably would have prevented me from 'engaging'. I was holding myself together with strong yet brittle cords of belief. Professional probing of my psyche might have fractured these bands of hope. No, it was post-treatment, after I had removed my psychological armour, that I was in need of help my family could not provide. Re-establishing a 'normal' existence floored me. Cancer had stifled my life when I was 14–17 years old: it had hijacked what should have been formative years. I could not go back to the life I led before cancer: life had moved on. Neither was I equipped to build a contemporary life as if cancer had never happened. How would I fill the vacuum left by those desolate years? I could not instantly grant myself the growth, wisdom, and peer group experiences they would have endowed. In short, I needed help to bridge the gap between my pre- and post-cancer worlds. I am not sure how this could have been achieved but, for me, it would have made a world of difference. I was a lost boy, lost to cancer. Chemotherapy saved me but, in the life it granted, I still had to find myself.

Chapter 8

Long-term Effects of Cancer Treatment

Gill Levitt and Debra Eshelman

Introduction

A cancer survivor's journey does not end after curative treatment. Successful multi-modality treatment is not tumour specific and, as a result, normal tissue is damaged. In addition, there is psychological trauma to the patient and family when given the diagnosis of a life-threatening illness. After cure, when the risk of relapse is receding, is a time when this damage requires assessment and management. Encouragingly, the number of young adult, childhood, and adolescent survivors continues to increase. It has been projected that, by the year 2010, one in 715 young people will be survivors of cancer. Therefore, it is vital we understand the consequences of treatments and have specific pathways of how to manage this increasing population (Campbell *et al.*, 2005).

The needs of adolescents change over time, different issues being paramount at various ages and time points from diagnosis (Jenney and Levitt, 2002). A young person who was treated as a baby will have different fears, needs, and information requirements from a person diagnosed when an adolescent, who has had little time to acclimatise to the label. In addition, they will have had their normal adolescent life experience disrupted by treatment. This chapter will review the main issues affecting cancer survivors in both categories.

Information on treatment-related toxicities is increasingly reported: much of this is through *childhood* cancer survivor studies, but care must be taken in extrapolating these results directly to *adolescent* cancer survivors. In addition, late effects studies suffer from many methodological pitfalls, which should be acknowledged when reviewing them, such as self-reported data and selection bias (hospital-based versus population-based studies), small single institution studies, differing control groups, measurement variances, and many others. Quality of life research in particular suffers from inconsistencies in addition to those problems listed above: evaluation of the research requires an appreciation of the outcome in relation to differing cultural norms and society expectations, which are largely dependent on the country of origin.

Long-term survival

The most critical period is the first 5 years after the cancer diagnosis, but even though the long-term outcome for our patients is excellent, we are aware that, compared with their peers, there is an increased risk of early death.

Long-term survival data have been extensively reported for childhood cancer survivors and, to a degree, can be used to inform deficiencies in our knowledge for adolescents with cancer. Long-term survival data only include patients who have survived 5 years from diagnosis. Mertens *et al.* (2001) reported an 11-fold increased risk of death compared with the normal population. Both hospital- and population-based studies found that 10% of 5-year survivors died 5–35 years post-treatment (Robertson *et al.*, 1994; Hudson *et al.*, 1997; Mertens *et al.*, 2001; Moller *et al.*, 2001). Survival after treatment is dependent on the risk of late recurrence of the primary tumour and treatment-related organ damage. The highest risk of tumour recurrence occurs most commonly in the first 5 years after completing therapy, but remains the commonest cause of late mortality up to 10 years. Studies have suggested that 61–75% of late deaths are due to tumour recurrence (Robertson *et al.*, 1994; Mertens *et al.*, 2001). Childhood-type embryonal cancers, with the exception of certain brain tumours, tend to relapse early, compared with adult-type cancers. The range of cancers seen in adolescents and young adults differs from that in childhood, with an increased percentage of adult-type cancers (10–20%): thus it may be that this group is more at risk of later relapses (Birch *et al.*, 2003; Desandes *et al.*, 2004). Hodgkin's disease, for example, a disease primarily of adolescents and young adults, can cause death as late as 15 years from diagnosis due to multiple recurrences (Aleman *et al.*, 2003). This is an important consideration when planning long-term follow-up clinics, which tend to concentrate on late sequelae surveillance. About 20% of deaths are due to treatment-related organ damage, with second malignant tumours and cardiovascular and pulmonary toxicity the main problems reported. However, this figure may be reduced in the future with improved surveillance and treatment modification. The treatment of Hodgkin's disease highlights this, with a marked reduction in cardiac deaths after mediastinal radiation doses were reduced, accompanied by increased shielding of the heart with no increase in relapse rates (Hancock and Donaldson, 1993).

It is important to appreciate that late mortality studies usually relate to treatments given decades before, which may differ markedly from present day regimes in their intensity, chemotherapy combinations, and radiation sources, doses, and fields. Therefore, these reports can only act as a guide to long-term outcomes for the present era.

Long-term sequelae

Cancer treatment can cause problems with both physical and psychosocial health, which in turn reduces the quality of life of our survivors, and therefore both aspects will be addressed. In this section we have not attempted to give a comprehensive overview of late sequelae, but have tried to identify the problems that are most relevant to the adolescent and young adult population. There are other texts (Wallace and Green, 2004) for more detailed information on other sequelae not covered here, as well as newly released comprehensive screening guidelines for late effects from the Children's Oncology Group (2004) in the USA, the Scottish Intercollegiate Guidelines Network (2005), and the United Kingdom Children's Study Group (Skinner *et al.*, 2005).

Late effects are defined as the physical, psychological, social, and/or economic chronic or late occurring consequences of cancer treatment persisting or occurring at least 5 years from diagnosis. The type and severity of late effects are dependent on the age and gender of the patient, total doses of treatment, and other host variables. This will govern the follow-up management depending on whether organ function requires to be monitored or damage requires active treatment. Certain groups, such as young people with a brain tumour and those requiring bone marrow or peripheral stem cell transplantation, may require sequelae management before the risk of recurrence recedes.

The appearance of clinically relevant morbidity can vary, with some being manifest at the end of treatment or many years from diagnosis, with the possibility of progression as the survivor matures and the follow-up interval lengthens. Our knowledge of the problems has improved over the last decade and many sequelae are now predictable, which can inform our management.

Physical late effects

The issues that we felt required consideration were fertility, cardiac sequelae, second malignant neoplasms (SMNs), obesity, osteopenia, and neurocognitive disorders, but patients may not be exempt from dysfunction of other endocrine organs, the kidneys, the lungs, special senses, and growth.

Much of our information comes from childhood cancer survivors studied in single centres, although recently a large epidemiological study from the USA (the Childhood Cancer Survivors Study) has provided volumes of data on late effects, their incidence, and risk factors (Robison *et al.*, 2002). In addition, a population-based study is under way on British survivors (British Childhood Cancer Study), and this will expand our knowledge further (Taylor *et al.*, 2004). Data from these childhood studies can be extrapolated in some circumstances to include the adolescent population, although there is a need for more data on adolescent cancer survivors. The majority of studies are in agreement that at least 50% of survivors have medical problems as a result of their treatment, although care must be taken in interpreting these reports, as patient selection and the methods of reporting may differ (Stevens *et al.*, 1998; Lackner *et al.*, 2000; Humpl *et al.*, 2001).

Pubertal development and fertility

Pubertal development and normal sexual function with assurance of fertility are important milestones in adolescence and may affect future quality of life. Unfortunately, cancer treatment may impact on all these aspects, with infertility being the most difficult to resolve (Aubier *et al.*, 1989; Chiarelli *et al.*, 1999; Relander *et al.*, 2000).

Normal pubertal progression and fertility are dependent on functional gonads and an intact pituitary–hypothalmic axis. Pubertal maturation occurs over years, and the onset can vary enormously in the general population. The majority of survivors will progress through puberty, albeit that some may deviate from the normal range. An early onset of puberty can occur in females who have undergone low-dose cranial radiation, as in the older leukaemia regimes (pre-1990s), and in both sexes with higher doses (25–50 Gy) (Leiper *et al.*, 1988; Ogilvy-Stuart *et al.*, 1994; Darzy *et al.*, 2004). This may well cause emotional problems as well as physical change and a reduction in final height due to early fusion of the epiphysis, particularly when combined with a reduced growth velocity. Delayed or absent pubertal progression can occur as a result of ongoing cancer treatment during adolescence, gonadal/cranial radiation including total body radiation (Sanders *et al.*, 1983; Leiper *et al.*, 1986), and high-dose alkylating agents (Leiper *et al.*, 1986). These patients need prompt referral to an endocrinologist for assessment and initiation of hormone replacement therapy where appropriate. The timing is important from a psychological viewpoint in patients who may already feel at a disadvantage compared to their peers, and also to maximise bone density (Bonjour *et al.*, 1994).

Fertility is primarily dependent on normal sperm production in the male and the presence of oocytes in the female, in addition to sufficient hormone production, which can sometimes be artificially supplemented if necessary. In males germ cell production occurs for the first time at puberty and continues throughout adult life. This is different from females, where the full complement of eggs is present at birth and attrition occurs normally throughout life. Menopause occurs when the oocytes are depleted. It is vital to be able to give accurate information on the possibility of subfertility and, conversely, reassurance if the risk of infertility is minimal. There are many studies on the risk factors, but accurate information for individuals is not always available because of the cumulative effect of multimodality treatment and the heterogeneity of patient groups. Gonadal radiation usually causes irreversible damage to germ cell production (Sanders *et al.*, 1983; Leiper *et al.*, 1986) and cranial radiation affects hormonal secretion from the hypothalamic–pituitary axis. Many different chemotherapy agents are implicated in gonadal damage, but the most important group are the alkylating agents (Bramswig *et al.*, 1990; Wallace *et al.*, 2005). Other risk factors include gender, age at treatment (Wallace *et al.*, 2005), and cancer diagnosis. Males are at greatest risk, and for them progression through puberty is not an assurance of fertility. This is due to the differential susceptibility to damage of the cells in the testes. The sertoli cells (sperm-producing cells) of the testes are much more sensitive to radiation and gonadotoxic drugs then the Leydig cells, which produce testosterone. In females the divergence in sensitivity of the ovarian follicular components is less and it is unusual to be infertile if post-pubertal with a normal menstrual cycle, but treatment may have reduced the reproductive lifespan, thereby leading to an early menopause.

In males alkylating agents, such as single-agent moderate doses of cyclophos-phamide (>7.5 g/m^2), ifosfamide, and combinations of chemotherapy, have been reported to cause oligospermia or azoospermia (Mackie *et al.*, 1996; Kenney *et al.*, 2001; Williams *et al.*, 2005). In females ovarian damage may result in an early menopause, except in high-dose schedules such as those used in bone marrow transplant regimes where primary ovarian failure may occur (Sanders *et al.*, 1983). The older the female is at the time of treatment the greater the risk of a premature menopause. To date this has been very difficult to predict, but there are some interesting hormone assays being developed, which may give valuable warning of ovarian failure (Wallace *et al.*, 2005).

Assessment of the risk of infertility is important at the time of diagnosis, when the treatment plan is formulated, so that consideration of fertility preservation techniques can be discussed. In mature males sperm can be cryopreserved and used with successful outcomes at a later date (Agarwal *et al.*, 2004). This needs to be sensitively handled in pubertal boys who are also coping with a diagnosis of cancer (Bahadur *et al.*, 2002). Some patients, particularly those with a diagnosis of Hodgkin's disease, may have impaired spermatogenesis prior to treatment: nevertheless, sperm preservation should be attempted (Rueffer *et al.*, 2001).

In females the preservation of fertility is a more complex problem. Cryopreser-vation of embryos and later implantation into a receptive uterus can expect a favourable outcome of a live birth. This technique can be used for females of reproductive age who have a stable partner, where time allows for hormonal manipulation and the procurement of mature oocytes for *in vitro* fertilisation. Currently, the preservation of mature oocytes is being evaluated for *in vitro* fertil-isation, but the chance of a successful outcome is less assured. For immature boys and girls there is at present no optimal method of preserving fertility, although many groups are pursuing this objective. It will nevertheless be many years before this can be offered routinely (Wallace *et al.*, 2005). There are obviously ethical issues to address in the under-age child. They can take part if it can be shown they have sufficient understanding to make an informed decision (Gillick competence) (Great Britain England. Court of Appeal, Civil Division, 1985). Females who have had pelvic radiation may have perinatal problems related to a reduced uterine function, resulting in poor implantation rates, increased miscarriage rates, and small for date and premature babies. On a positive note, various studies have found no increased incidence of congenital abnormalities or cancer in the offspring of both male and female survivors (Hawkins *et al.*, 1989; Winther *et al.*, 2004).

It is rare for pathways involved in potency and normal sexual activity to be damaged, but patients with pelvic tumours requiring surgery or high-dose radi-ation involving the genital tract and attendant nerve supply may be at risk. In particular, in survivors of prostatic/base of bladder rhabdomyosarcoma, where disruption of the autonomic nervous system and vascular supply occurs, this can cause erectile and ejaculation dysfunction. These patients need early informa-tion, sensitive counselling, and referral to an andrology department for males and a gynaecologist for females (Hendry, 1995; Sklar and La Quaglia, 1998; Spunt *et al.*, 2005).

Cardiac effects

Morbidity and mortality as a result of cardiac damage from anthracyclines and chest radiation are well recognised (Green *et al.*, 1999; Hinkle *et al.*, 2004; Levitt and Saran, 2004). Our patient population is particularly at risk, as more than 50% will receive anthracyclines as part of their first-line treatment, and treatment of Hodgkin's disease may include mediastinal radiation. Anthracyclines cause cardiomyocyte damage at the time of administration, but the onset of clinical symptoms or subclinical abnormalities can vary. Symptoms can rarely present acutely within 12 months of the end of therapy or over many years from treatment. Clinically, patients present with heart failure, arrhythmias, or, unusually, sudden death (Hinkle *et al.*, 2004). The true clinical incidence is unknown. Reports differ depending on the diagnostic group, total anthracycline doses (Nysom *et al.*, 1998b), and follow-up interval. Kremer *et al.* (2002a) reported an incidence of early cardiac decompensation of 1.6% in a childhood cancer cohort, whereas other studies have failed to identify cases. Subclinical damage occurs in 0–57% and can progress to clinical status (Nysom *et al.*, 1998a; Kremer *et al.*, 2002b). The major risk factor is the cumulative dose of anthracyclines linked to the increasing duration from the end of treatment (Nysom *et al.*, 1998b; Kremer *et al.*, 2002b; Sorensen *et al.*, 2003). Although all dose levels have been implicated, long-term studies have suggested that a threshold below 250 mg/m^2 may represent a lower risk of deterioration in cardiac damage over 10–15 years (Sorensen *et al.*, 2003; Pein *et al.*, 2004; Lipshultz *et al.*, 2005).

Adolescents are at particular risk for two reasons. Firstly, cardiac dysfunction is progressive and childhood cancer survivors may have been off treatment for many years by the time they reach adolescence. Secondly, adolescent cancer survivors are in the age group more commonly diagnosed with tumours such as osteosarcoma and peripheral primitive neuroectodermal tumours, which are tumour types that usually require higher doses of anthracyclines (>300 mg/m^2) for cure. Other risk factors are their age at treatment, cardiac radiation, female gender, and use of other cardiotoxic agents (Kremer *et al.*, 2002b). At present it is not possible to predict whether a patient is at risk of cardiac morbidity at the end of treatment, and no plateau has been identified at which cardiac function stabilises.

Cardiac radiation can affect all layers of the heart, from the outer pericardium, myocardium, valves, and the endothelium of the capillaries and coronary vessels. The majority of publications have been reports on survivors of Hodgkin's disease receiving mediastinal radiation. The radiation damage is primarily caused by vascular damage resulting in tissue ischaemia, cell death, and replacement fibrosis. The incidence of cardiac disease varies according to the era of treatment, the dose to the heart, and the age at diagnosis. Early onset coronary artery disease was highlighted as a worrying cause of late deaths in the Hodgkin's population in the early 1990s. Analysis determined that those most at risk were patients at each end of the age spectrum receiving radiation doses in excess of 40 Gy. The majority of studies include mixed ages, but an American study reported the cumulative risk of coronary artery disease in patients treated under the age of 21 years to be 8% at 22 years post-treatment (Hancock and Donaldson, 1993).

Pericardial disease also occurs post-radiation, but, reassuringly, a study on childhood and adolescent survivors found no patients with clinical symptoms at a median of 90 months follow-up, although 43% had evidence of pericardial thickening on scanning (Green *et al.*, 1987). Valvular disease has been identified in 16–42% of patients treated with doses >35 Gy, with no cases having been reported in patients receiving <35 Gy (Adams *et al.*, 2004). Conduction defects are also more common when higher doses are required. Myocardial dysfunction is rare with radiotherapy alone, but an in-depth study did show evidence of diastolic dysfunction but no systolic abnormalities. Diastolic decompensation is thought to herald the onset of heart failure at a later date, although there were no reports from this study (Adams *et al.*, 2004).

Screening programmes suggest that all patients exposed to anthracyclines should have regular cardiac monitoring, usually using non-invasive techniques such as echocardiography (Children's Oncology Group, 2004; Scottish Intercollegiate Guidelines Network, 2005; Skinner *et al.*, 2005). There is debate as to whether drug intervention with medication aimed at reducing the after-load should be used for preventing the progression of damage, as there is little evidence of long-term gain (Silber *et al.*, 2001; Lipshultz *et al.*, 2002; Van Dalen *et al.*, 2003). Echocardiography and electrocardiography should be offered to those who receive significant cardiac radiation.

For our adolescent population cardiac damage adds further anxiety regarding their long-term future. The consequences for those with subclinical abnormalities can be far-reaching, affecting physical activities and employment choices (Evans and Cooke, 2003). Fitness training involving isometric exercises (weight training) is not encouraged, as this causes an increased workload on the damaged heart and may worsen the situation. All females need to be warned that cardiac surveillance during pregnancy is important, as the increased workload during the third trimester, labour, and early postnatal period may unmask cardiac dysfunction (Levitt and Jenney, 1998; Bar *et al.*, 2003). For those with symptomatic heart failure there is a significant risk that progression will lead to consideration of heart transplantation (Levitt *et al.*, 1996).

SMNs

Although adolescents may worry about a relapse of their original cancer, they may also be concerned about the development of another cancer in their lifetime. It is known that survivors of childhood cancer are at an increased risk of the development of second cancers compared to the population at large, but the risk is generally low and should be considered in relation to the overall success in the cure rates of childhood cancer. Epidemiological studies on childhood and adolescent cancer survivors from different countries have identified a 1.5–7-fold increased risk compared with the general population. The risk is highest during the first 10 years, but the increased risk extends throughout life (Olsen *et al.*, 1993).

Clinicians should focus their attention on identifying those adolescents who may be at risk of another cancer, teaching them preventive healthcare practices whenever possible and intervening early in order to optimise treatment.

The types of SMNs that develop may be primarily influenced by the type of treatment modalities and combinations employed for curing the initial cancer. The primary cancer diagnosis, time from initial treatment, age at treatment, gender, and genetic predisposition may also influence the development of SMNs (Meadows *et al.*, 1985; Pui *et al.*, 1991; Bhatia *et al.*, 1996; Wong *et al.*, 1997; Hisada *et al.*, 1998; Neglia *et al.*, 2001; Jenkinson *et al.*, 2004). What has not yet been identified is the interaction between specific cancer treatment modalities, the ageing process, and the risk of SMNs. It is beyond the scope of this chapter to discuss each SMN in detail, but a general overview is provided to briefly review the findings in the literature.

Radiation and SMNs

Numerous studies have reported on the incidence of SMN development in previously irradiated tissues or near irradiated fields from presumed 'scatter' radiation. Two-thirds of SMNs occur in association with radiation. Patients who received higher doses of radiation and/or those who were treated during the era when different energy sources and radiation techniques were used, which allowed for an increased absorption of radiation into nearby tissues, i.e. cobalt radiation, seem to be most at risk. Second neoplasms that have been reported in association with radiation include breast carcinoma in females at a young age, particularly in association with Hodgkin's disease, thyroid neoplasms, bone sarcomas, soft tissue sarcomas, central nervous system (CNS) tumours (both benign and malignant), carcinomas of the oral cavity, and skin cancers (melanoma, basal cell carcinoma, and atypical nevi) (Rimm *et al.*, 1987; Bhatia *et al.*, 1996; Neglia *et al.*, 2001; Travis *et al.*, 2003; Kenney *et al.*, 2004; Cohen *et al.*, 2005; Guibout *et al.*, 2005). The increased risk of developing a radiation-induced SMN is lifelong. Tumours may present a few years after treatment or many decades later. Surveillance therefore has to be long-term and effective screening, such as for breast cancer in those who received chest radiation, is vital.

Chemotherapy and SMNs

Therapy-related acute leukaemias have been associated with several chemotherapy agents, including alkylating agents (Meadows *et al.*, 1985; Boivan *et al.*, 1995), topoisomerase II inhibitors (epipodophyllotoxins) (Sandler *et al.*, 1997; Le Deley *et al.*, 2003), anthracyclines (Breslow *et al.*, 1995), and platinum medications (Travis *et al.*, 1999). Alkylating agents and anthracyclines have also been associated with the development of secondary bone cancers and soft tissue sarcomas (Tucker *et al.*, 1987; Neglia *et al.*, 2001; Cohen *et al.*, 2005). Some studies have reported no increased risk for the development of secondary leukaemias after exposure to the above agents (Neglia *et al.*, 2001). This calls attention to the fact that reports of

SMNs must be interpreted in light of the methodologies reported in studies, including the characteristics of the cohort being studied, total drug doses, and length of time since treatment.

Genetic factors and SMNs

Certain genetic conditions have been associated with an increased risk for the development of SMNs, including hereditary retinoblastoma, Li–Fraumeni syndrome, neurofibromatosis, hereditary non-polyposis colorectal cancer, multiple endocrine neoplasm, Gorlin's, and familial adenomatous polyposis (Li and Fraumeni, 1969; Kingston *et al.*, 1987; Friedman *et al.*, 1999). Repeated enquiry into family histories is vital to forewarn families that they maybe at risk of familial cancer syndromes and may need to see a geneticist for additional information.

Medical knowledge about the incidence of SMNs has been enhanced because of increased survival rates and growing interest in late effects research, but stands in jeopardy if adolescent cancer survivors who are reaching adulthood are not given relevant information or followed clinically in a systematic fashion across their lifespan. As yet there are no fully effective screening programmes for early diagnosis of second tumours. Breast screening by magnetic resonance imaging in the young female exposed to chest radiation is the only screening systematically performed in the UK. Evaluation of the programme in the UK for female Hodgkin's survivors is ongoing.

Osteopenia/osteoporosis

Osteopenia and osteoporosis are diseases primarily of adulthood that originate during childhood and the adolescent years (Kaste, 2004). Bone mineral accumulation normally occurs during the same timeframe as the onset of a diagnosis of a paediatric or adolescent malignancy and reaches a peak in the third decade. The risk factors for impaired mineral density, in addition to cancer treatment protocols, include gonadal failure with inadequate replacement, physical inactivity (Prince *et al.*, 1991; Mora *et al.*, 1994; Tillmann *et al.*, 2002), nutritional deficits (Prince *et al.*, 1991; Sentipal *et al.*, 1991), genetic factors (Ferrari *et al.*, 1995; Tokita *et al.*, 1996), age at onset of puberty (Mora *et al.*, 1994), and lifestyle choices such as smoking and carbonated beverage consumption (Krall and Dawson-Hughes, 1999; Wyshak, 2000). The incidence and onset of bone mineral density changes, extent of the contribution of cancer treatment protocols, and the degree of recovery after treatment ends is not yet conclusively delineated in the adolescent cancer literature.

The most studied groups at risk for bone mineral density changes have been children treated for acute lymphoblastic leukaemia, brain tumours, allogeneic bone marrow transplant patients, and, more recently, patients with solid tumours (Aisenberg *et al.*, 1998; Kaste *et al.*, 1999; Tillmann *et al.*, 2002; Kelly *et al.*, 2005). It is well proven that children who receive chronic steroid therapy are at risk for bone mineral deficits (Halton *et al.*, 1996; Kaste *et al.*, 2001). Other cancer therapies also contribute to bone mineral density changes. Anti-metabolites (methotrexate) appear to alter bone metabolism directly by reducing bone metabolism during treatment, thereby inhibiting full development of the peak bone mass (Nysom *et al.*, 1998c). Cranial radiation may cause hypothalamic–pituitary dysfunction, resulting in low levels of growth hormone secretion or hypogonadotropic hypogonadism (Gilsanz *et al.*, 1990; Hyer *et al.*, 1992). Cyclophosphamide and ifosfamide may affect gonadal function leading to premature ovarian failure or Leydig cell dysfunction, thereby promoting bone loss (Hyer *et al.*, 1992).

Whatever the causative factor, the implication for early detection in adolescent cancer survivors is clear. The aim should be to maximise the peak bone mass in early adulthood and identify a low bone mineral density before fracture occurs when prevention measures, such as appropriate growth hormone and sex hormone replacement, calcium, exercise, biphosphonates, and modification of lifestyles choices (smoking, drinking carbonated beverages, and a sedentary lifestyle), may be beneficial. Longitudinal evaluations are clearly needed in order to understand better the multifactorial relationships between cancer-related treatment factors, genetic influences, lifestyle choices, physical inactivity, and nutritional deficits and the development of osteopenia or osteoporosis in at-risk adolescent cancer survivors.

Obesity

Being overweight and obesity, as defined by a body mass index of 25–29 kg/m^2 and in excess of 30 kg/m^2, respectively, are becoming more prevalent in the developed world among both adults and children (Rogers *et al.*, 2005; Stamatakis *et al.*, 2005). Unfortunately, studies are reporting an increased incidence of obesity in cancer survivor groups compared with the normal population, leading to a rise in long-term health risks.

Obesity is known to be associated with an increased cardiovascular morbidity, breast, colorectal, and prostatic cancer, depression, and low self-esteem (Gortmaker *et al.*, 1993). It is an important pointer to the development of a collection of metabolic abnormalities, namely glucose intolerance, diabetes mellitus, dyslipidaemia, and hypertension, which in turn affects cardiovascular wellbeing (Talvensaari *et al.*, 1996). Obesity is caused by an imbalance of calorie intake versus energy expenditure, but a multitude of factors impact on this equation, such as hormonal dysfunction. A number of studies have identified risk groups, namely acute lymphoblastic leukaemia survivors, particularly females who were young at diagnosis and received cranial radiation, and, similarly, young people with brain tumours treated with radiation (Craig *et al.*, 1999; Lustig *et al.*, 2003; Oeffinger *et al.*, 2004). The theory for radiation-related obesity is that there is an effect on the hypothalamus–pituitary axis affecting leptin sensitivity (Ross *et al.*, 2004). Leptin is a hormone, the production of which is governed by negative feedback of the adipose tissue. In addition, reduced physical activity, growth hormone insufficiency, and development of the metabolic syndrome contribute to the problem (Warner *et al.*, 1998). There is debate whether chemotherapy contributes in the long term, but steroid treatment certainly causes obesity in the short term. Encouragement of healthy lifestyles may help in reducing increases in weight gain and body fat.

Neurocognitive effects

Adolescents may be cognitively impaired as a direct result of intrathecal or systemic chemotherapy (e.g. methotrexate) or as a result of radiation treatment to the CNS. Cognitive deficits may become more evident as educational goals increase. Generally, the neurotoxic effects of chemotherapy and radiation are more pronounced in certain subgroups of patients, including those who have been treated for leukaemia, lymphoma, and brain tumours, in children treated at a younger age, and in those with radiation to the whole brain, head, and neck. Cognitive dysfunction may result in a plethora of problems, such as memory deficits, spatial processing problems, a decline in overall intelligence quotient points, alterations in reading comprehension, decreased mathematical skill, a decline in executive functioning abilities, or slower processing of the learning of new skills (Ris and Noll, 1994; Zeltzer *et al.*, 1997; Rodgers *et al.*, 1999; Mulhern and Palmer, 2001). Learning difficulties impact on the psychosocial wellbeing of young people and may prevent them from functioning as independent, self-supporting adults. In order to obtain their maximum potential, early identification of problems, with good support pathways, should be established.

Psychosocial late effects

Just as certain exposures to cancer treatments may affect the physical structure and functioning of an adolescent body, so too may they affect the psychological and social functioning of this vulnerable group. The normal psychological development of adolescents is complex and involves obtaining a personal identity, an increasing independence, the development of a body image, and peer approval. Normal adolescents find this period disturbing and difficult, so how much more complicated must it be for survivors who may have had disruption to their education, received treatments that may have had detrimental effects on their neurocognitive progress and body image, and fewer opportunities for independence.

Studies suffering from methodological weaknesses as described earlier make it difficult to come to definitive conclusions about psychosocial functioning for adolescent cancer survivors. Historically a number of studies have suggested that a fair proportion of childhood cancer survivors are troubled psychologically (Stuber *et al.*, 1996; Hobbie *et al.*, 2000). In a study of 5736 adult survivors of childhood leukaemia and Hodgkin's and non-Hodgkin's lymphoma Zebrack *et al.* (2002) found a significantly increased risk for reporting symptoms of depression and somatic distress, and that intensive chemotherapy added to this risk. In a childhood cancer survivor study of 9535 young adult survivors Hudson *et al.* (2003) reported moderate to severe impairment in some aspect of mental health across all diagnostic groups studied, and patients diagnosed with Hodgkin's disease, sarcomas, and bone tumours had significantly higher levels of self-reported cancer-related anxiety and fears, which adversely affected their perception of their health status.

Other researchers have reported conflicting results. In a comprehensive review of 30 studies Langeveld *et al.* (2002) reported that most young adult survivors of childhood cancer functioned well psychologically and did not have significantly more emotional problems than controls. The subgroup of survivors who reported problems mentioned depression, mood disturbances, tension, anger, confusion, and anxiety. Female gender, an older age at follow-up, a greater number of relapses, the presence of impaired physical functioning, cranial radiation, and minority survivors were associated with an increased risk of emotional problems.

Significantly, there appear to be no reports of an increased risk of depression in childhood cancer survivors, although young people with brain tumours may exhibit more depressive symptoms. Unfortunately we have only limited information regarding the survivors of adolescent cancer who may be at increased risk of psychological effects (Pemberger *et al.*, 2005). Other work has highlighted the possibility that some of our survivors may suffer other psychosocial difficulties due to a change in their body image, sexuality, and the effects of fatigue and post-traumatic stress syndrome. Although the evidence is sparse, when assessing patients it is worth considering these possibilities. Therefore we will discuss them briefly below.

Body image

Body image becomes an important issue for survivors, and the reason for an abnormal body image is probably multifactorial, involving physical looks and an altered perception of body appearances. Alopecia, abnormal growth patterns with face and body asymmetry, limb amputations, and obesity can contribute to the problems related to body image, which then impact on the quality of life. It is important that more good studies are performed in order to inform healthcare professionals about the best treatment options and not to assume that modern techniques are best. This has been demonstrated in studies on young people with bone tumours who may have the option of amputation or limb salvage surgery. On the surface it may seem better to have limb salvage surgery with an improved mobility and body image, but studies have shown that repeated hospital admissions for revisions, treatment of infections, and chronic pain have overshadowed the advantages. Overall, studies have shown very similar results regarding body image and quality of life (Eiser, 2004).

Sexuality

Few studies have considered the effect of treatment and diagnosis on sexuality. It may be assumed that a life-threatening illness and the experience of treatment may cause an effect on sexual behaviour, sexual attitudes, and behaviour. A small study performed in Finland suggested that female survivors of childhood- and adolescent-onset leukaemia had similar sexual behaviour when compared with their peers. However, their sexual attitudes were immature and sexual images were restrictive in nature (Puukko *et al.*, 1997). The literature concerning male survivors is restricted to adult cancer survivors with genitourinary cancer, but psychologists accept the need for support in this area although the prevalence of the problem has not been ascertained. The males at most risk are those treated for pelvic tumours, who may have both physical and emotional causes for their sexual dysfunction that require multidisciplinary management, but the knowledge of infertility *per se* may well affect sexuality.

Fatigue

Cancer-related fatigue has been defined in the oncology literature as a persistent, subjective sense of tiredness related to cancer or cancer treatment that interferes with usual functioning (National Comprehensive Cancer Network and the American Cancer Society, 2005). Multiple studies have suggested that cancer-related fatigue may exist months to years after treatment involving adult patients (Andrykowski *et al.*, 1998; Broeckel *et al.*, 1998; Fossa *et al.*, 2003). Little is known about adolescents, but they may be more at risk than childhood cancer survivors, who have been noted to have similar rates as compared to their peer group. The important message is the observed two-way interaction between depression and fatigue (Langeveld *et al.*, 2003; Meeske *et al.*, 2005).

Post-traumatic stress

The model of post-traumatic stress has gained attention in recent years for its usefulness in trying to understand the long-term psychological effects of a cancer experience (Kazak *et al.*, 2004). Post-traumatic stress disorder refers to the development of symptoms following exposure to a particularly severe stressor, and that stressor must involve either experiencing or witnessing an event capable of causing death, injury, or threat to physical integrity to oneself or another person. A review of the literature from 1991 to 2001 estimated the prevalence of post-traumatic stress in childhood cancer survivors and/or their parents to be between 2% and 30% in survivors and between 10% and 30% in parents. In some studies survivors seemed to be no different from controls in their levels of post-traumatic stress (Kazak *et al.*, 1997). This evolving literature about the impact of the cancer experience as a stressor or traumatic event is also leading to work on 'resilience' or 'thriving', enhanced quality of life, and post-traumatic growth (Zebrack and Zeltzer, 2003).

Health behaviours

Health behaviours in survivors can be thought of in either a positive fashion, such as those that are likely to promote future health, or in a negative fashion, commonly referred to as risk-taking behaviours, namely behaviours that could compromise a person's wellbeing. Given the risks for adverse sequelae of treatment, it would seem that risk-taking behaviours might be particularly health-compromising for the cancer survivor. Tyc *et al.* (2001) found that, in a small cohort of survivors, they generally appreciated that they were more at risk of health problems and therefore had a greater need to protect their health by avoidance of risky health behaviours. Whether this translates to health-promoting activities such as cancer prevention screening, exercise, the use of sunscreen, or safe sex practices have not been addressed in the literature.

It should be recognised then that assessing the psychosocial concerns of adolescents during the long-term follow-up period should be viewed with equal importance to assessing the physical late effects of treatment. Clinicians should be cognisant of the psychological impact of surviving cancer during adolescence and, consequently, should strive to keep the psychological and emotional wellbeing of the patient in mind during clinical evaluation. Risk-taking behaviours should be identified and a strong emphasis placed on health-promoting behaviours. The remainder of this section will address risk-taking behaviours, bearing in mind that the data presented are self-reported.

Smoking

Early US studies of the smoking rates in survivors of childhood cancer suggested that the smoking rates were comparable with the age-matched population (Corkery *et al.*, 1979; Haupt *et al.*, 1992): however, more contemporary studies have reported that survivors seemed to be smoking at rates below the general population (Emmons *et al.*, 2002). In a British study comparing the risk behaviours of survivors with age- and sex-matched controls and a group of siblings Larcombe *et al.* (2002) reported that the survivors were significantly less likely than the controls to have ever smoked or to be current smokers. These results support similar findings in the American literature (Mulhern *et al.*, 1995; Tao *et al.*, 1998). Butterfield *et al.* (2004) demonstrated that childhood cancer survivors who smoked had a number of other risk factors for the development of preventable disease. An Australian study (Bauld *et al.*, 2005) investigated smoking among adolescent survivors of childhood cancer and found that 13–17 year olds were at a lower risk of tobacco use when compared to their healthy peers. They concluded that, although the risks were reduced, a substantial proportion of survivors engaged in risky behaviours.

Alcohol use

Several American and Canadian studies (Gray *et al.*, 1992; Hollen and Hobbie, 1993; Mulhern *et al.*, 1995) have found that survivors were less likely than their peers to drink, and that the incidence of 'problem' drinking was low. Mulhern *et al.* (1995) reported that fewer survivors were current drinkers than controls or siblings and fewer survivors regularly exceeded the limit of five units of alcohol at a single sitting (binge drinking).

Illicit drug use

Data regarding illicit drug use are scarce in the survivor population and are confounded by self-report bias. Hollen and Hobbie (1993) found that 17% of survivors aged 12–19 years had tried marijuana. In a British study (Larcombe *et al.*, 2002) comparisons showed that significantly fewer survivors of either sex than controls had ever used recreational drugs or were users at the time of the study. In a recent Australian study, investigators found that 13–17 year olds were at an increased risk of reporting pain reliever use for non-medical purposes, but at lower risk of cannabis use or illicit drug use when compared to their healthy peers (Bauld *et al.*, 2005).

Occupational and insurance status

There is very little literature available that describes educational achievements, frequency of problems in the workplace, current employment status, or the ability to obtain affordable healthcare insurance in the survivor population. A study carried out over a decade ago by Hays *et al.* (1992) in the USA concluded that, with the exception of individuals with CNS tumours, childhood cancer survivors treated in the era 1945–1975 had few economic sequelae. Anecdotally, in more recent American literature there are numerous accounts of discrimination in the workplace, in the armed services, and in the receipt of affordable health and life insurance, suggesting that, in fact, these discriminatory practices are happening. The insurance industry is very quick in interpreting long-term follow-up data for informing their decisions, but the key is for workers to try and support the survivor if the insurer is being unreasonable. Educational attainment is an important positive predictor of employment, as seen in lower limb amputees and in the poor employment record of brain tumour survivors (Nagarajan *et al.*, 2003). In the UK the armed forces rarely accept cancer survivors, unless a cancer specialist contests a strong case (Children's Cancer and Leukaemia Group, 2005). Further research is necessary in order to delineate the prevalence of unfair discrimination.

Delivery of care

The delivery of longitudinal health care to ageing adolescent cancer survivors has historically been guided by treatment exposures. It is universally accepted that adolescent cancer survivors need risk-based follow-up by providers knowledgeable about chemotherapy and radiation exposures (Wallace *et al.*, 2001). How this is best accomplished is variable and dependent on multiple factors (Friedman *et al.*, 2005).

In the USA risk-based health is often influenced by factors such as the age limitations of the treating institution, insurance barriers, lack of insurance, or inaccessibility due to geographical location. In Europe the limitations have not been in association with health insurance, but more associated with the background of the proponent of the follow-up service and their ability to provide care in an age-appropriate setting. As a result, several models of cancer survivor care are emerging.

Many agencies have looked at the attributes required for a successful service, including the Institute of Medicine's report *Childhood Cancer Survivorship: Improving Care and Quality of Life* (Hewitt *et al.*, 2003) and, in the UK, the National Institute for Health and Clinical Excellence's (2005) document on improving outcomes in children and young people with cancer, which contains recommendations for the management of long-term follow-up. Unfortunately there are barriers to providing high-quality care on both sides of the Atlantic (Oeffinger and Wallace, 2006), such as the patient's knowledge of the risks of adverse health outcomes, which may affect their attitude to follow-up and the ability of the agencies to provide informed healthcare professionals in the clinical settings preferred by the survivors. A few studies are now appearing that provide information about how informed survivors wish the service to develop, which may differ from the views of the healthcare professionals and will require increased input from governmental organisations (Earle *et al.*, 2005; F. Gibson, A. Richardson, H. Haslett, and G. Levitt, unpublished report).

One of the biggest issues is the effective transition of survivors from the cosy setting of the paediatric cancer centre to the more appropriate adolescent/adult arena, whether it be the adult cancer centre, adult hospital being reviewed by paediatric oncologists or adult physicians, or family practitioner (Viner, 2003; Ginsberg *et al.*, 2006). Other specialities, such as respiratory medicine for the transition of patients with cystic fibrosis, or endocrinology and diabetes, have successfully achieved good transition to their adult colleagues, but unfortunately cancer patients have multiple needs addressed by a variety of medical/psychological experts, so one model does not fit all.

The key is that each survivor has a coordinator of care, who is assigned depending on the future requirements of the survivor and that there is flexibility in the service to change the type of care if required. For patients with a low risk of sequelae it maybe appropriate to keep only telephone/e-mail contact with a follow-up administrator, who can give information for assisting with employment and insurance issues and direct patients where to obtain further help. In others, such as brain tumour or transplant survivors, more complicated pathways are necessary. In addition, all patients should have detailed, accurate information about their diagnosis, treatment, risks of sequelae, and suggested follow-up plan.

Patient education

Various studies have evaluated the knowledge that survivors have about their diagnosis and treatment (Kadan-Lottick, N., *et al.*, 2002; Earle *et al.*, 2005; Landier *et al.*, 2006). Invariably they have misinformation, and they are often unaware of the risks of adverse health outcomes. To an extent this is the fault of the paediatric oncologist, often in association with parents, in trying to shield survivors from any further bad news, but in the long run this is counterproductive: the more informed patients are, the more able they are to be in control of their future.

We have already alluded to the importance of providing adequate information for our survivors in order to empower them to understand their future risks and to have an informed input into their follow-up management. There are now a number of publications providing excellent levels of information, although for those with educational problems the information may not be readily comprehensible and will require additional input from their follow-up clinician and family. The public can access the majority via the Internet (Children's Oncology Group, 2004; Scottish Intercollegiate Guidelines Network, 2005; Skinner *et al.*, 2005; Children's Cancer and Leukaemia Group, 2005).

This chapter has also highlighted the need for further research applicable to adolescent cancer survivors in terms of incidence, risk factors, and the severity of late sequelae. Accurate information can help protocol designers in reducing late sequelae where possible and provide an evidence base for long-term follow-up. Entwined in this research is the need to engage the adolescent and young adult so as to be able to provide for their needs in a more acceptable, cost-effective manner.

Conclusion

The objective of care after cure is to maximise the potential of the patient affected by the physical and emotional burden of a diagnosis of cancer and its treatment, and obtain the best possible quality of life across the many domains involved. Included in this is the hope that the adolescent and young adult will feel they are in control of their destiny and, wherever possible, we must try to 'demedicalise' our survivors. When discussing adolescents and young adults we must not ignore other family members, who may also have issues that need addressing.

References

Adams, M. J., Lipsitz, S. R., Colan, S. D. *et al.* (2004) Cardiovascular status in long term survivors of Hodgkin's disease treated with chest radiotherapy. *Journal of Clinical Oncology*, **22**, 3139–3148.

Agarwal, A., Ranganathan, P., Kattal, N. *et al.* (2004) Fertility after cancer: a prospective review of assisted reproductive outcome with banked semen specimens. *Fertility & Sterility*, **81**, 342–348.

Aisenberg, J., Hsieh, K., Kalaitzoglou, G. *et al.* (1998) Bone mineral density in young adult survivors of childhood cancer. *Journal of Pediatric Hematology/Oncology*, **20**(3), 241–245.

Aleman, B. M. P., Van den Belt-Dusebout, A. W., Klokman, W. J., Van't Veer, M. B., Bartelink, H., & Van Leeuwen, F. E. (2003) Long-term cause-specific mortality of patients treated for Hodgkin's disease. *Journal of Clinical Oncology*, **21**, 3431–3439.

Andrykowski, M. A., Curran, S. L., & Lightner, R. (1998) Off-treatment fatigue in breast cancer survivors: a controlled comparison. *Journal of Behavioral Medicine*, **21**, 1–18.

Aubier, F., Flamant, F., Brauner, R., Caillaud, J. M., Chaussain, J. M., & Lemerle, J. (1989) Male gonadal function after chemotherapy for solid tumors in childhood. *Journal of Clinical Oncology*, **7**, 304–309.

Bahadur, G., Ling, K. L., Hart, R. *et al.* (2002) Semen production in adolescent cancer patients. *Human Reproduction*, **17**, 2654–2656.

Bar, J., Davidi, O., Goshen, Y., Hod, M., Yaniv, I., & Hirsch, R. (2003) Pregnancy outcome in women treated with doxorubicin for childhood cancer. *American Journal of Obstetrics & Gynecology*, **189**, 853–857.

Bauld, C., Toumbourou, J., Anderson, V., Coffey, C., & Ollson, C. (2005) Health risk behaviours among adolescent survivors of childhood cancer. *Pediatric Blood & Cancer*, **45**, 706–715.

Bhatia, S., Robison, L., Oberlin, O. *et al.* (1996) Breast cancer and other second malignant neoplasms after childhood Hodgkin's disease. *New England Journal of Medicine*, **334**, 745–751.

Birch, J. M., Alston, R. D., Quinn, M., & Kelsey, A. M. (2003) Incidence of malignant disease by morphological type, in young persons aged 12–24 years in England, 1979–1997. *European Journal of Cancer*, **39**, 2622–2631.

Boivan, J., Hutchinson, G., Zauber, A. *et al.* (1995) Incidence of second cancers in patients treated for Hodgkin's disease. *Journal of the National Cancer Institute*, **87**, 732–741.

Bonjour, J. P., Theintz, G., & Law, F. (1994) Peak bone mass. *Oesteoporosis International*, **1**, 7–13.

Bramswig, J. H., Heimes, U., Heiermann, E., Schlegel, W., Nieschlag, E., & Schellong, G. (1990) The effects of different cumulative doses of chemotherapy on testicular function. Results in 75 patients treated for Hodgkin's disease during childhood or adolescence. *Cancer*, **65**, 1298–1302.

Breslow, N., Takashima, J., Whitton, J., Moksness, J., D'Angio, G., & Green, D. (1995) Second malignant neoplasms following treatment for Wilms' tumor: a report from the National Wilms' Tumor Study Group. *Journal of Clinical Oncology*, **13**, 1851–1859.

Broeckel, J. A., Jacobsen, P., Horton, J., Balducci, L., & Lyman, G. (1998) Characteristics and correlates of fatigue after adjuvant chemotherapy for breast cancer. *Journal of Clinical Oncology*, **16**, 1689–1696.

Butterfield, R., Park, E., Puleo, E. *et al.* (2004) Multiple risk behaviors among smokers in the Childhood Cancer Survivors Study cohort. *Psycho-Oncology*, **13**, 619–629.

Campbell, J., Wallace, W. H., Bhatti, L. A., & Brewster, D. H. (2005) *Cancer in Scotland: Trends in Incidence, Mortality and Survival 1975–1999*. Information and Statistics Division, Edinburgh (www.isdscotland.org/cancer information).

Chiarelli, A. M., Marrett, L. D., & Darligton, G. (1999) Early menopause and infertility after treatment for childhood cancer diagnosed in 1994–1988 in Ontario Canada. *American Journal of Epidemiology*, **150**, 245–354.

Children's Cancer and Leukaemia Group (2005) *After Cure Booklet*. Children's Cancer and Leukaemia Group, Leicester (www.aftercure.org).

Children's Oncology Group (2004) *Long-term Follow-up Guidelines for Survivors of Childhood, Adolescent, and Young Adult Cancers* (www.survivorshipguidelines.org).

Cohen, R., Curtis, R., Inskip, P., & Fraumeni, J. (2005) The risk of developing second cancers among survivors of childhood soft tissue sarcoma. *Cancer*, **103**(11), 2391–2396.

Corkery, J., Li, F., McDonald, J. *et al.* (1979) Kids who really shouldn't smoke. *New England Journal of Medicine*, **300**, 1279.

Craig, F., Leiper, A. D., Stanhope, R., Brain, C., Meller, S. T., & Nussey, S. S. (1999) Sexually dimorphic and radiation dose dependent effect of cranial irradiation on body mass index. *Archives of Disease in Childhood*, **81**, 500–504.

Darzy, K. H., Gleeson, H. K., & Shalet, S. M. (2004) Growth and neuroendocrine consequences In: *Late Effects of Childhood Cancer* (eds D. Green & H. Wallace), pp. 189–211. Arnold, London.

Desandes, E., Lacour, B., Sommelet, D. *et al.* (2004) Cancer incidence among adolescents in France. *Pediatric Blood & Cancer*, **43**, 742–748.

Earle, E. A., Davies, H., Greenfield, D., Ross, R., & Eiser, C. (2005) Follow-up care for childhood cancer survivors: a focus group analysis. *European Journal of Cancer*, **41**, 2882–2886.

Eiser, C. (2004) Quality of life and body image. In: *Late Effects of Childhood Cancer* (eds D. Green & H. Wallace), pp. 338–339. Arnold, London.

Emmons, K., Li, F., Whitton, J. *et al.* (2002) Predictors of smoking initiation and cessation among childhood cancer survivors: a report from the Childhood Cancer Survivor Study. *Journal of Clinical Oncology*, **20**, 1608–1616.

Evans, S. A. & Cooke, J. N. C. (2003) Cardiac effects of anthracycline treatment and their implications for aeromedical certification. *Aviation, Space, & Environmental Medicine*, **74**, 1003–1008.

Ferrari, S., Rizzoli, R., Chevalley, T., Slosman, D., Eisman, J. A., & Bonjour, J.-P. (1995) Vitamin-D-receptor-gene polymorphisms and change in lumbar-spine bone mineral density. *Lancet*, **345**, 423–424.

Fossa, S. D., Dahl, A., & Loge, J. (2003) Fatigue, anxiety, and depression in long-term survivors of testicular cancer. *Journal of Clinical Oncology*, **21**, 1249–1254.

Friedman, D. & Meadows, A. (1999) Pediatric tumors. In: *Multiple Primary Cancers* (eds A. I. Neugent, A. T. Meadows, & L. Robison), pp. 235–256. Lippincott Williams & Williams, Philadelphia, PA.

Friedman, D. L., Freyer, D. R., & Levitt, G. A. (2005) Models of care for survivors of childhood cancer. *Pediatric Blood & Cancer*, **46**, 159–168.

Gilsanz, V., Carlson, M. E., Roe, T. F., & Ortega, J. A. (1990) Osteoporosis after cranial irradiation for acute lymphoblastic leukemia. *Journal of Pediatrics*, **117**, 238–244.

Ginsberg, J. P., Hobbie, W. L., Carlson, C. A., & Meadows, A. T. (2006) Delivering long-term follow-up care to pediatric cancer survivors: transitional care issues. *Pediatric Blood & Cancer*, **46**, 169–173.

Gortmaker, S. L., Must, A., Perrin, J. M., Sobel, A. M., & Dietz, W. H. (1993) Social and economic consequences of overweight in adolescence and young adults. *New England Journal of Medicine*, **329**, 1008–1012.

Gray, R., Doan, B., Shermer, P. *et al.* (1992) Psychological adaptation of survivors of childhood cancer. *Cancer*, **70**, 2713–2721.

Great Britain England. Court of Appeal, Civil Division (1985) Gillick v Weat Norfolk and Wisbech Area Authority. *All England Law Reg*, 533–539.

Green, D. M., Gingell, R. L., Pearce, J., Panahon, A. M., & Ghoorah, J. (1987) The effect of mediastinal irradiation on cardiac function of patients treated during childhood and adolescence for Hodgkin's disease. *Journal of Clinical Oncology*, **5**, 239–245.

Green, D. M., Hyland, A., Chung, C. S., Zevon, M. A., & Hall, B. C. (1999) Cancer and cardiac mortality among 15-year survivors of cancer diagnosed during childhood or adolescence. *Journal of Clinical Oncology*, **17**, 3207–3215.

Guibout, C., Adjadj, E., Rubino, C. *et al.* (2005) Malignant breast tumors after radiotherapy for a first cancer during childhood. *Journal of Clinical Oncology*, **23**, 197–204.

Halton, J. M., Atkinson, S. A., Fraher, L. *et al.* (1996) Altered mineral metabolism and bone mass in children during treatment for acute lymphoblastic leukemia. *Journal of Bone & Mineral Research*, **11**, 1774–1783.

Hancock, S. L. & Donaldson, S. S. (1993) Radiation-related heart disease: risks after treatment of Hodgkin's disease during childhood and adolescence. In: *Cardiac Toxicity After*

Treatment for Childhood Cancer (eds J. T. Bricker, D. M. Green, & G. D'Angio), pp. 35–43. Wiley-Liss, New York, NY.

Haupt, R., Byrne, J., Connelly, R. *et al.* (1992) Smoking habits in survivors of childhood and adolescent cancer. *Medical & Pediatric Oncology*, **20**, 301–306.

Hawkins, M. M., Draper, G. J., & Smith, R. A. (1989) Cancer among 1348 offspring of survivors of childhood cancer. *International Journal of Cancer*, **43**, 975–978.

Hays, D., Landsverk, J., Sallan, S. *et al.* (1992) Educational, occupational and insurance status of childhood cancer survivors in their fourth and fifth decades of life. *Journal of Clinical Oncology*, **10**, 1397–1406.

Hendry, W. F. (1995) Iatrogenic damage to male reproductive function. *Journal of the Royal Society of Medicine*, **88**, 579–584.

Hewitt, M., Weiner, S., & Simone, J. V. (eds) (2003) *Childhood Cancer Survivorship: Improving Care and Quality of Life*. National Cancer Policy Board; Institute of Medicine and National Research Council. The National Academies Press, Washington, DC.

Hinkle, A. S., Proukou, C. B., Deshpande, S. S. *et al.* (2004) Cardiovascular complications: cardiotoxicity caused by chemotherapy. In: *Late Effects of Childhood Cancer* (eds D. Green & H. Wallace), pp. 85–100. Arnold, London.

Hisada, M., Garber, J., Fung, C., Fraumeni, J., & Li, F. (1998) Multiple primary cancers in families with Li–Fraumeni syndrome. *Journal of the National Cancer Institute*, **15**, 606–611.

Hobbie, W. L., Stuber, M., Meeske, K. *et al.* (2000) Symptoms of posttraumatic stress in young adult survivors of childhood cancer. *Journal of Clinical Oncology*, **18**, 4060–4066.

Hollen, P. & Hobbie, W. (1993) Risk taking and decision making of adolescent long term survivors of cancer. *Oncology Nursing Forum*, **20**, 769–776.

Hudson, M. M., Jones, D., Boyett, J., Sharp, G. B., & Pui, C. H. (1997) Late mortality of long term survivors of childhood cancer. *Journal of Clinical Oncology*, **15**, 2205–2213.

Hudson, M. M., Mertens, A. C., Yasui, Y. *et al.* (2003) Health status of adult long term survivors of childhood cancer. *JAMA*, **290**(12), 1583–1592.

Humpl, T., Fritsche, M., Bartels, U., & Gutjahr, P. (2001) Survivors of childhood cancer for more than twenty years. *Acta Oncologica*, **40**, 44–49.

Hyer, S. L., Rodin, D. A., Tobias, J. H., Leiper, A., & Nussey, S. S. (1992) Growth hormone deficiency during puberty reduces adult bone mineral density. *Archives of Disease in Childhood*, **67**, 1472–1474.

Jenkinson, H. C., Hawkins, M. M., Stiller, C. A., Winter, D. L., Marsden, H. B., & Stevens, M. C. (2004) Long-term population-based risks of second malignant neoplasms after childhood cancer in Britain. *British Journal of Cancer*, **91**, 1905–1910.

Jenney, M. E. & Levitt, G. A. (2002) The quality of survival after childhood cancer. *European Journal of Cancer*, **38**, 1241–1250.

Kaste, S. (2004) Bone-mineral density deficits from childhood cancer and its therapy. *Pediatric Radiology*, **34**, 373–378.

Kaste, S. C., Chesney, R. W., Hudson, M. M., Lustig, R. H., Rose, S. R., & Carbone, L. D. (1999) Bone mineral status during and after therapy of childhood cancer: an increasing population with multiple risk factors for impaired bone health. *Journal of Bone & Mineral Research*, **14**(12), 2010–2014.

Kaste, S. C., Jones-Wallace, D., Rose, S. R. *et al.* (2001) Bone mineral decrements in survivors of childhood acute lymphoblastic leukemia: frequency of occurrence and risk factors for their development. *Leukemia*, **5**, 728–734.

Kazak, A. E., Barakat, L. P., Meeske, K. *et al.* (1997) Posttraumatic stress, family functioning, and social support in survivors of childhood leukemia and their mothers and fathers. *Journal of Consulting and Clinical Psychology*, **65**, 120–129.

Kazak, A. E., Alderfer, M., Rourke, M. T., Simms, S., Streisand, R., & Grossman, J. R. (2004) Posttraumatic stress disorder (PTSD) and posttraumatic stress symptoms (PTSS) in families of adolescent cancer survivors. *Journal of Pediatric Psychology*, **29**(3), 211–219.

Kelly, J., Damron, T., Grant, W. *et al.* (2005) Cross-sectional study of bone mineral density in adult survivors of solid pediatric cancers. *Journal of Pediatric Hematology/Oncology*, **27**(5), 248–253.

Kenney, L. B., Laufer, M. R., Grant, F. D., Grier, H., & Diller, L. (2001) High risk of infertility and long term gonadal damage in males treated with high dose cyclophosphamide for sarcoma during childhood. *Cancer*, **91**, 613–621.

Kenney, L. B., Yasui, Y., Inskip, P. D. *et al.* (2004) Breast cancer after childhood cancer: a report from the Childhood Cancer Survivor Study. *Annals of Internal Medicine*, **141**(8), 590–597.

Kingston, J., Hawkins, M., Draper, G., Marsden, H., & Kinnier Wilson, L. (1987) Patterns of multiple primary tumours in patients treated for cancer during childhood. *British Journal of Cancer*, **56**, 331–338.

Krall, E. & Dawson-Hughes, B. (1999) Smoking increases bone loss and decreases intestinal calcium absorption. *Journal of Bone & Mineral Research*, **14**, 215–220.

Kremer, L. C., Van Dalen, E. C., Offringa, M., & Voute, P. A. (2002a) Frequency and risk factors for anthracycline-induced clinical heart failure in children: a systematic review. *Annals of Oncology*, **13**, 503–512.

Kremer, L. C. M., Van der Pal, H. J. H., Offringa, M., Van Dalen, E. C., & Voute, P. A. (2002b) Frequency and risk factors of subclinical cardiotoxicity after anthracycline therapy in children: a systematic review. *Annals of Oncology*, **13**, 819–829.

Lackner, H., Benesch, M., Schagerl, S., Kerbl, R., Schwinger, W., & Urban, C. (2000) Prospective evaluation of late effects after childhood cancer therapy with a follow-up over 9 years. *European Journal of Pediatrics*, **159**, 750–758.

Landier, W., Wallace, W. H. B., & Hudson, M. M. (2006) Long term follow-up of pediatric cancer survivors: education, surveillance, and screening. *Pediatric Blood Cancer*, **46**, 149–158.

Langeveld, N. E., Stam, H., Groottenhuis, M. A., & Last, B. F. (2002) Quality of life in young adult survivors of childhood cancer. *Supportive Care in Cancer*, **10**, 579–600.

Langeveld, N. E., Grootenhuis, M. A., Voute, P. A., De Haan, R. J., & Van den Bos, C. (2003) No excess fatigue in young adult survivors of childhood cancer. *European Journal of Cancer*, **39**, 204–214.

Larcombe, I., Mott, M., & Hunt, L. (2002) Lifestyle behaviours of young adult survivors of childhood cancer. *British Journal of Cancer*, **87**, 1204–1209.

Le Deley, M. C., Leblanc, T., Shamsaldin, A. *et al.*; Société Française d'Oncologie Pediatrique (2003) Risk of secondary leukemia after a solid tumor in childhood according to the dose of epipodophyllotoxins and anthracyclines: a case–control study by the Société Française d'Oncologie Pédiatrique. *Journal of Clinical Oncology*, **21**, 1074–1081.

Leiper, A. D., Grant, D. B., & Chessells, J. M. (1986) Gonadal function after testicular radiation for acute lymphoblastic leukaemia. *Archives of Disease in Childhood*, **61**, 53–56.

Leiper, A. D., Stanhope, R., Preece, M. A., Grant, D. B., & Chessells, J. M. (1988) Precocious or early puberty and growth failure in girls treated for acute lymphoblastic leukaemia. *Hormone Research*, **30**, 72–76.

Levitt, G. A. & Jenney, E. M. (1998) The reproductive system after childhood cancer. *British Journal of Obstetrics & Gynaecology*, **105**, 946–953.

Levitt, G. A. & Saran, F. H. (2004) Cardiovascular complications: radiation damage. In: *Late Effects of Childhood Cancer* (eds D. Green & H. Wallace), pp. 101–113. Arnold, London.

Levitt, G. A., Bunch, K., Rogers, C. A., & Whitehead, B. (1996) Cardiac transplantation in childhood cancer survivors in Great Britain. *European Journal of Cancer*, **32A**(5), P826–P830.

Li, F. & Fraumeni, J. (1969) Soft tissue sarcomas, breast cancer, and other neoplasms. A familial syndrome? *Annals of Internal Medicine*, **71**, 747–752.

Lipshultz, S. E., Lipsitz, S. R., Sallan, S. E. *et al.* (2002) Long term enalapril therapy for left ventricular dysfunction in doxorubicin-treated survivors of childhood cancer. *Journal of Clinical Oncology*, **20**, 4517–4522.

Lipshultz, S. E., Lipsitz, S. R., Sallan, S. E. *et al.* (2005) Chronic progressive cardiac dysfunction years after doxorubicin therapy for childhood acute lymphoblastic leukemia. *Journal of Clinical Oncology*, **23**, 2629–2636.

Lustig, R. H., Post, S. R., Srivannaboon, K. *et al.* (2003) Risk factors for the development of obesity in children surviving brain tumors. *Journal of Clinical Endocrinology & Metabolism*, **88**, 611–616.

Mackie, E. J., Radford, M., & Shalet, S. M. (1996) Gonadal function following chemotherapy for childhood Hodgkin's disease. *Medical & Pediatric Oncology*, **27**, 74–78.

Meadows, A., Baum, E., Fossati-Bellani, F. *et al.* (1985) Second malignant neoplasms in children: an update from the Late Effects Study Group. *Journal of Clinical Oncology*, **3**, 532–538.

Meeske, K. A., Slegel, S. E., Globe, D. R., Mack, W. J., & Bernstein, L. (2005) Prevalence and correlates of fatigue in long term survivors of childhood leukaemia. *Journal of Clinical Oncology*, **23**, 5501–5510.

Mertens, A. C., Yasui, Y., Neglia, J. P. *et al.* (2001) Late mortality experience in five-year survivors of childhood and adolescent cancer: the Childhood Cancer Survivor Study. *Journal of Clinical Oncology*, **19**, 3163–3172.

Moller, T. R., Garwicz, S., Barlow, L. *et al.*; Association of the Nordic Cancer Registries; Nordic Society for Pediatric Hematology and Oncology (2001) Decreasing late mortality among five-year survivors of cancer in childhood and adolescence: a population-based study in the Nordic countries. *Journal of Clinical Oncology*, **19**, 3173–3181.

Mora, S., Goodman, W. G., Loro, M. L., Roe, T. F., Sayre, J., & Gilsanz, V. (1994) Age-related changes in cortical and cancellous vertebral bone density in girls: assessment with quantitative CT. *AJR*, **162**, 405–409.

Mulhern, R. & Palmer, S. (2001) Neurocognitive late effects in pediatric cancer. Commissioned paper for the National Institutes of Health (www.iom.edu/ncpb).

Mulhern, R., Tyc, V., Phipps, S. *et al.* (1995) Health related behaviors of survivors of childhood cancer. *Medical & Pediatric Oncology*, **25**, 159–165.

Nagarajan, R., Neglia, J. P., Clohisy, D. R. *et al.* (2003) Education, employment, insurance, and marital status among 694 survivors of pediatric lower extremity bone tumors: a report from the Childhood Cancer Survivor Study. *Cancer*, **97**, 2554–2564.

National Comprehensive Cancer Network and the American Cancer Society (2005) *Cancer Related Fatigue and Anemia: Treatment Guidelines for Patients*, Version III, pp. 1–52 (www.cancer.org).

National Institute for Health and Clinical Excellence (2005) *Guidance on Cancer Services: Improving Outcomes in Children and Young People with Cancer*. National Institute for Health and Clinical Excellence, London.

Neglia, J., Friedman, D., Yasui, Y. *et al.* (2001) Second malignant neoplasms in five year survivors of childhood cancer: Childhood Cancer Survivor Study. *Journal of the National Cancer Institute*, **93**(8), 618–629.

Nysom, K., Holm, K., Michaelsen, K. F., Hertz, H., Muller, J., & Molgaard, C. (1998a) Bone mass after treatment for acute lymphoblastic leukemia in childhood. *Journal of Clinical Oncology*, **12**, 3752–3760.

Nysom, K., Colan, S. D., & Lipshultz, S. E. (1998b) Late cardiotoxicity following anthracycline therapy for childhood cancer. *Progress in Pediatric Cardiology*, **8**, 121–138.

Nysom, K., Holm, K., Lipsitz, S. R. *et al.* (1998c) Relationship between cumulative anthracycline dose and late cardiotoxicity in childhood acute lymphoblastic leukemia. *Journal of Clinical Oncology*, **16**, 545–550.

Oeffinger, K. C. & Wallace, W. H. (2006) Barriers to follow-up care of survivors in the United States and the United Kingdom. *Pediatric Blood & Cancer*, **46**, 135–142.

Oeffinger, K. C., Mertens, A. C., Sklar, C. A. *et al.* (2004) Obesity in adult survivors of childhood acute lymphoblastic leukemia: a report from the Childhood Cancer Survivor Study. *Journal of Clinical Oncology*, **21**, 1359–1365.

Ogilvy-Stuart, A. L., Clayton, P. E., & Shalet, S. M. (1994) Cranial irradiation and early puberty. *Journal of Clinical Endocrinology & Metabolism*, **78**, 1282–1286.

Olsen, J. H., Garwicz, S., Hertz, H. *et al.* (1993) Second malignant neoplasms after cancer in childhood or adolescence. Nordic Society of Paediatric Haematology and Oncology Association of the Nordic Cancer Registries. *BMJ*, **23**(307), 1030–1036.

Pein, F., Sakiroglu, O., Dahan, M. *et al.* (2004) Cardiac abnormalities 15 years and more after adriamycin therapy in 229 childhood survivors of a solid tumour at the Institut Gustave Roussy. *British Journal of Cancer*, **91**, 37–44.

Pemberger, S., Jagsch, R., Frey, E. *et al.* (2005) Quality of life in long term childhood cancer survivors and the relation of late effects and subjective well-being. *Supportive Care in Cancer*, **13**, 49–56.

Prince, R. L., Smith, M., Dick, I. M. *et al.* (1991) Prevention of postmenopausal osteoporosis. *New England Journal of Medicine*, **325**, 1189–1195.

Pui, C., Ribeiro, R., Hancock, M. *et al.* (1991) Acute myeloid leukemia in children treated with epipodophyllotoxins for acute lymphoblastic leukemia. *New England Journal of Medicine*, **325**, 1682–1687.

Puukko, L.-R. M., Hirvonen, E., Aalberg, V., Hovi, L., Rautonen, J., & Siimes, S. S. (1997) Sexuality of young women surviving leukaemia. *Archives of Disease in Childhood*, **76**, 197–202.

Relander, T., Cavallin-Stahl, E., Garwicz, S., Olssen, A. M., & Willen, M. (2000) Gonadal and sexual function in men treated for childhood cancer. *Medical & Pediatric Oncology*, **35**, 52–63.

Rimm, I., Li, F., Tarbell, N., Winston, K., & Sallen, S. (1987) Brain tumors after cranial irradiation for childhood acute lymphoblastic leukemia. A 13 year experience from the Dana Farber Cancer Institute and the Children's Hospital. *Cancer*, **59**, 1506–1508.

Ris, M. & Noll, R. (1994) Long term neurobehavioral outcome in pediatric brain tumor patients: review and methodological critique. *Journal of Clinical and Experimental Neurology*, **16**, 21–42.

Robertson, C. M., Hawkins, M. M., & Kingston, J. E. (1994) Late deaths and survival after childhood cancer: implications for cure. *BMJ*, **309**, 162–166.

Robison, L. L., Mertens, A. C., Boice, J. D. *et al.* (2002) Study design and cohort characteristics of the Childhood Cancer Survivor Study: a multi-institutional collaborative project. *Medical & Pediatric Oncology*, **38**, 229–239.

Rodgers, J., Horrocks, J., Britton, P. G., & Kernahan, J. (1999) Attentional ability among survivors of leukaemia. *Archives of Disease in Childhood*, **80**, 318–323.

Rogers, P. C., Meacham, L. R., Oeffinger, K. C., Henry, D. W., & Lange, B. J. (2005) Obesity in pediatric oncology. *Pediatric Blood & Cancer*, **45**, 881–891.

Ross, J. A., Oeffinger, K. C., Davies, S. M. *et al.* (2004) Genetic variation in the leptin receptor gene and obesity in survivors of childhood acute lymphoblastic leukaemia: a report from the Childhood Cancer Survivor Study. *Journal of Clinical Oncology*, **22**, 3558–3562.

Rueffer, U., Breuer, K., Josting, A. *et al.* (2001) Male gonadal dysfunction in patients with Hodgkin's disease prior to treatment. *Annals of Oncology*, **12**, 1307–1311.

Sanders, J. E., Buckner, C. D., Leonard, J. M. *et al.* (1983) Late effects on gonadal function of cyclophosphamide, total-body irradiation, and marrow transplantation. *Transplantation*, **36**, 252–255.

Sandler, E., Friedman, D., Mustafa, M., Winick, N., Bowman, W., & Buchanan, G. (1997) Treatment of children with epipodophyllotoxin-induced secondary acute myeloid leukemia. *Cancer*, **79**, 1049–1054.

Sentipal, J. M., Wardlaw, G. M., Mahan, J., & Matkovic, V. (1991) Influence of calcium intake and growth indexes on vertebral bone mineral density in young females. *American Journal of Clinical Nutrition*, **54**, 425–428.

Scottish Intercollegiate Guidelines Network (2004) *Long Term Follow up of Survivors of Childhood Cancer. A National Clinical Guideline.* Scottish Intercollegiate Guidelines Network, Edinburgh.

Silber, J. H., Cnaan, A., Clark, B. J. *et al.* (2001) Design and baseline characteristics for the ACE Inhibitor After Anthracycline (AAA) Study of cardiac dysfunction in long term pediatric cancer survivors. *American Heart Journal*, **142**, 577–585.

Skinner, R., Levitt, G., & Wallace, W. H. (2005) *Therapy Based LTFU Practice Statement.* UKCCSG (www.ukccsg.org.uk/public/followup/PracticeStatement/index.html).

Sklar, C. & La Quaglia, M. P. (1998) Rhabdomyosarcoma. In: *Paediatric Surgery and Urology: Long Term Outcomes* (eds M. D. Stringer, K. T. Oldham, D. E. Mouriquand, & E. R. Howard), pp. 688–701. W. B. Saunders, London.

Sorensen, K., Levitt, G. A., Bull, C., Dorup, I., & Sullivan, I. D. (2003) Late anthracycline cardiotoxicity after childhood cancer: a prospective longitudinal study. *Cancer*, **97**, 1991–1998.

Spunt, S. L., Sweeney, T. A., Hudson, M. M., Billups, C. A., Krasin, M. J., & Hester, A. L. (2005) Late effects of pelvic rhabdomyosarcoma and its treatment in female survivors. *Journal of Clinical Oncology*, **23**(1), 7143–7151.

Stamatakis, E., Primatesta, P., Chinn, S., Rona, R., & Falascheti, E. (2005) Overweight and obesity trends from 1974 to 2003 in English children: what is the role of socioeconomic factors? *Archives of Disease in Childhood*, **90**, 999–1004.

Stevens, M. C. G., Mahler, H., & Parkes, S. (1998) The health status of adult survivors of cancer in childhood. *European Journal of Cancer*, **34**, 694–698.

Stuber, M., Christakis, D. A., Houskamp, B., & Kazak, A. E. (1996) Posttrauma symptoms in childhood leukemia survivors and their parents. *Psychosomatics*, **37**, 254–261.

Talvensaari, K. K., Lanning, M., Tapanainen, P., & Knip, M. (1996) Long-term survivors of childhood cancer have an increased risk of manifesting the metabolic syndrome. *Journal of Clinical Endocrinology & Metabolism*, **81**, 3051–3055.

Tao, M., Guo, M., Weiss, R. *et al.* (1998) Smoking in adult survivors of childhood acute lymphoblastic leukemia. *Journal of the National Cancer Institute*, **90**, 219–225.

Taylor, A., Hawkins, M., Griffiths, A. *et al.* (2004) Long term follow-up of survivors of childhood cancer in the UK. *Pediatric Blood & Cancer*, **42**, 161–168.

Tillmann, V., Darlington, A. S., Eiser, C., Bishop, N. J., & Davies, H. A. (2002) Male sex and low physical activity are associated with reduced spine bone mineral density in survivors of childhood acute lymphoblastic leukemia. *Journal of Bone & Mineral Research*, **17**, 1073–1080.

Tokita, A., Matsumoto, H., Morrison, N. A. *et al.* (1996) Vitamin D receptor alleles, bone mineral density and turnover in premenopausal Japanese women. *Journal of Bone & Mineral Research*, **11**, 1003–1009.

Travis, L., Holowaty, E., Bergfeldt, K. *et al.* (1999) Risk of secondary leukemia after platinum-based chemotherapy for ovarian cancer. *New England Journal of Medicine*, **340**, 351–357.

Travis, L., Hill, D., Dores, G. *et al.* (2003) Breast cancer following radiotherapy and chemotherapy among young women with Hodgkin disease. *JAMA*, **290**(4), 465–475.

Tucker, M., D'Angio, G., Boice, J. *et al.* (1987) Bone sarcomas linked to radiotherapy and chemotherapy in children. *New England Journal of Medicine*, **317**, 588–593.

Tyc, V. L., Hadley, W., & Crockett, G. (2001) Prediction of health behaviors in pediatric cancer survivors. *Medical & Pediatric Oncology*, **37**, 42–46.

Van Dalen, E. C., Van der Pal, H. J., Van den Bos, C., Caron, H. N., & Kremer, L. C. (2003) Treatment for asymptomatic anthracycline-induced cardiac dysfunction in childhood cancer survivors: the need for evidence. *Journal of Clinical Oncology*, **21**, 3777.

Viner, R. (2003) Bridging the gaps: transition for young people with cancer. *European Journal of Cancer*, **39**, 2684–2687.

Wallace, H. & Green, D. (eds) (2004) *Late Effects of Childhood Cancer*. Arnold, London.

Wallace, W. H., Blacklay, A., Eiser, C. *et al.* (2001) Developing strategies for long term follow up of survivors of childhood cancer. *BMJ*, **323**, 271–274.

Wallace, W. H. B., Anderson, R. A., & Irvine, S. D. (2005) Fertility preservation for young patients with cancer: who is at risk and what can be offered. *Lancet Oncology*, **6**, 209–218.

Warner, J. T., Bell, W., Webb, D. K., & Gregory, J. W. (1998) Daily energy expenditure and physical activity in survivors of childhood malignancy. *Pediatric Research*, **43**, 607–613.

Williams, D., Levitt, G., & Crofton, D. (2005) Does ifosfamide affect male gonadal function? *Medical & Pediatric Oncology*, **45**, 419.

Winther, J. F., Boice, J. D., Mulvihill, J. J. *et al.* (2004) Chromosomal abnormalities among offspring of childhood cancer survivors in Denmark: a population-based study. *American Journal of Genetics*, **74**, 1282–1285.

Wong, F., Boice, J., Abramson, D. *et al.* (1997) Cancer incidence after retinoblastoma. Radiation dose and sarcoma risk. *JAMA*, **278**, 1262–1267.

Wyshak, G. (2000) Teenaged girls, carbonated beverage consumption, and bone fractures. *Archives of Pediatrics & Adolescent Medicine*, **154**, 610–613.

Zebrack, B. J. & Zeltzer, L. K. (2003) Quality of life issues and cancer survivorship. *Current Problems in Cancer*, **27**, 198–211.

Zebrack, B., Zeltzer, L., Whitton, J. *et al.* (2002) Psychological outcomes in long term survivors of childhood leukemia, Hodgkin's disease and non-Hodgkin's lymphoma: a report from the Childhood Cancer Survivor Study. *Pediatrics*, **110**, 42–52.

Zeltzer, L. K., Chen, E., Weiss, R. *et al.* (1997) Comparison of psychological outcome in adult survivors of childhood acute lymphoblastic leukemia versus sibling controls: a cooperative Children's Cancer Group and National Institutes of Health Study. *Journal of Clinical Psychology*, **15**, 547–556.

Chapter 9
Palliation and End of Life Care Issues

Maggie Bisset, Sue Hutton, and Daniel Kelly

Introduction

As a young person with cancer becomes aware that they are unlikely to recover, the emotional impact can be overwhelming. The reality of advancing disease means being asked to confront a situation of immense threat – a 'something' so powerful and mystical that it causes a 'frozen moment' where time is suspended, yet also, by its nature, limited and ticking away. It is in the turbulence of this situation that, without help, suffering can spiral out of control as the young person struggles to find meaning in repeated treatment attempts and failures, gradually advancing disease, and the prospect of their life being cut short.

Importantly, suffering not only impacts on the young person but also on those around them. At the outset of treatment the possibility of death in adolescence or young adulthood may represent a possibility that is best avoided. The focus of most interactions will be on the benefits of particular treatments in order to boost their resolve and morale. This avoidance of open disclosure about death is likely to include the person themselves, their carers, friends, and others in their wider social orbit. At this age cancer is so unusual that news of the initial diagnosis will already have spread rapidly – and even more rapidly will the news of the death of a young person from cancer.

This may be explained because society is 'affronted' at such a situation and cannot remain neutral in the face of a death from cancer in the young. We all struggle to make sense of death, even in those who have enjoyed a normal lifespan: in young people death is more difficult to comprehend. The aim of this chapter is to examine this phase of cancer care for adolescents and young adults.

The importance of experience

We begin by drawing on our own clinical experiences, which have suggested the journey towards death, even in the young, can be made easier. Contrary to what we may think, humans have an enormous capacity to understand and adapt to challenges that are beyond their experience. Age, we contend, does not necessarily need to affect this ability. In the face of death, new meanings can arise as the unfamiliar is confronted. As Saunders (2004) suggested:

> 'When a person is dying the family find themselves in a crisis situation, with the joys and regrets of the past, the demands of the present, and the fears of the future, all brought into stark focus. Help may be needed to deal with guilt, depression, and family discord, and in this time of crisis there is the possibility of resolving old problems and finding reconciliations that greatly strengthen the family' (p. xxiii).

Although highly relevant, Saunders (2004) was not writing here about young people specifically, where different dynamics may emerge in families at the dawning reality that time with the young person is limited. Added to the above is the context in which this realisation is taking place – acute hospitals, for example, are busy and impersonal places and do not always afford the privacy or open dialogue that can help facilitate this phase of care (Kelly *et al.*, 2005). This suggests the need for specialist help to be available to help those involved manage the symptoms of more advanced cancer and find some shared meaning in the time remaining (Dunlop and Hockley, 1998). We will return to the question of location of care later in this chapter.

Palliative care, if delivered well, can play a key role in helping young people to share their search for meaning and identify sources of physical or emotional suffering and how they can be helped to cope with these. A consistent message throughout this book has been the emphasis on age-appropriate care, and it remains true here. A more satisfying relationship between the professional and the young person facing the final phase of their life may be established through the adoption of a person-centred approach that incorporates awareness of the challenges of this life stage. This relationship, based on helping, may also assist the professional to make sense of what may also seem to them a 'senseless' death. Working with the belief that positive outcomes can emerge from such a situation can help deepen one's sense of professional integrity – essentially seeking ways to help the young person to 'die well'. This stance also links with the personal and professional ethics explored in the earlier chapter by Neale Hanvey and Alison Finch.

This chapter emphasises the importance of finding meaning within the sometimes-subtle transitions that characterise the phase of care towards the end of life. However, we do not intend to present a 'road map' of care where the route and destination are agreed in advance: rather, appropriate options are emphasised in order that the journey and direction of travel are dictated by individual as well as changing circumstances. We explore the main goals of palliation by supporting a philosophy of care that encourages accessibility and addresses the needs and expectations of young people and those close to them. It is not our intention to explore pharmacological interventions for addressing symptoms, as this information is already available for readers in specialist texts elsewhere (Doyle *et al.*, 2004). We have also chosen to use the terms adolescent and young person interchangeably throughout the chapter, knowing that each are relevant in describing this unique age group.

Constructions of palliative care

Defining palliative care

Questioning the meaning of palliative care for adolescents and young people is an appropriate starting point for understanding the nature of its delivery. Palliative care has been defined as:

'The active total care of patients whose disease is not responsive to curative treatment. Control of pain, of other symptoms and of psychological, social and spiritual problems is paramount. The goal of palliative care is achievement of the best quality of life for patients and their families. Many aspects of palliative care are also applicable earlier in the course of illness, in conjunction with anti-cancer treatment' (World Health Organization, 1990, p. 11).

The palliative approach to care therefore encourages clinicians to engage in a manner that is attentive to individual needs, fosters creative caring, and demands expertise to tackle the complexity of the needs that will emerge.

Palliative care for whom?

Expertise, however, may not always be available outside of major treatment centres, as life-limiting illness in young people is relatively rare. Extrapolating from existing figures, the annual mortality rate for young people aged 13–24 years with life-limiting conditions is said to be approximately 1.7 per 10 000, with the majority of deaths being due to cancer. In a review of death registrations in England between 1995 and 1999 Higginson and Thompson (2003) estimated that there had been 1472 cancer-related deaths in 16–24 year olds. The three most common diagnoses were acute lymphoid leukaemia, brain cancers, and diagnoses classified as 'other'. Importantly, some cancers have a higher associated mortality rate than others: for instance, some brain cancers may be less common in terms of incidence, but have a poorer prognosis and higher death rate. Despite the knowledge that a significant number of young people do eventually face death prematurely, the reality is that they may have been living with their cancer for some years. It has also been suggested that the need for palliative care services in this age group is likely to increase due to medical advancements that have extended the lifespan and survival rate for children diagnosed with illnesses that once would have been life limiting, but eventually become chronic – with survival now extending into teenage years and young adulthood (Robertson *et al.*, 1994).

What we mean by palliative care

Historically, palliative care has been synonymous only with the 'terminal' phase of care and considered relevant for people at the end of life and sometimes into the bereavement period. It was also usually confined to those with cancer.

However, a useful way of understanding current constructions of palliative care is to consider the life-limiting disease experience as part of a 'dying spectrum' (Addington Hall and Higginson, 2001).

At one extreme are those relatively predictable and relentless diseases – such as aggressive or widely disseminated cancers. At the other are those with more unpredictable and slowly progressing conditions that arise in childhood. In the centre are conditions that advance rapidly and may lead to unpredictable death (but these may also respond well to active treatment for a period of time). The term 'supportive care' has recently been adopted to suggest a more comprehensive range of interventions for all cancer patients, including those with advanced disease. Palliative care may be considered one element of this supportive care approach. There were a number of recommendations for healthcare providers to consider in the guidance published by the National Institute for Health and Clinical Excellence (2004), for example:

> Mechanisms need to be implemented within each locality to ensure medical and nursing services are available for patients with advanced cancer on a 24-hour, seven days a week basis, and that equipment can be provided without delay. Those providing generalist medical and nursing services should have access to specialist advice at all times (p. 10).

However, it is equally important to consider the needs of young people throughout the disease trajectory, especially in times of uncertainty and suffering when intensive support may be required. This approach was also recommended in the report of a joint working party of the Association for Children with Life-Threatening or Terminal Conditions and their Families (ACT); the National Council for Hospice and Specialist Palliative Care Services (NCHPCS) and the Scottish Partnership Agency for Palliative and Cancer Care (SPAPCC) (*Joint Report on Palliative Care for Adolescents and Young Adults*, 2001), who delineated four groups of young people for whom palliation is relevant. Box 9.1 shows that these groups include young people who may have had considerable experience of their illness or condition since birth or early childhood and who may be expected to die prematurely. However, it also includes those who will not be expected to survive cancer.

Therefore, an important feature of palliative care for young people is the need for it to be applied appropriately with an emphasis on flexibility and responsiveness to individual situations and needs. In practice, this is likely to rely on a team approach to care, where young people and those close to them work in partnership with skilled professionals including nurses, doctors, social workers, allied health professionals, psychologists, and educationalists across the hospital/home interface (Edwards, 2001).

In order to appreciate the nature of palliative support for adolescents and young people fully it is important to take account of the developmental issues that may impact on our practice when dealing with care during the advanced stages of cancer.

Box 9.1   Types of life-limiting conditions in young people

1.   Young people with life-threatening conditions for which curative treatment may be feasible but can fail. Palliative care may be necessary during periods of prognostic uncertainty and when treatment fails. Young people in long-term remission or following successful curative treatment are not included. Examples include cancer and irreversible organ failure of the heart, liver, or kidney.

2.   Young people with conditions where there may be long periods of intensive treatment aimed at prolonging life and allowing participation in normal activities, but premature death is still possible or inevitable. Examples include cystic fibrosis, Duchene muscular dystrophy, and human immunodeficiency virus/acquired immune deficiency syndrome.

3.   Young people with progressive conditions without curative treatment options, where treatment is exclusively palliative and may commonly extend over many years. Examples include Batten disease, mucopolysacharidosis, and Creutzfeldt–Jakob disease.

4.   Young people with a severe neurological disability that may cause weakness and susceptibility to heath complications. Deterioration may be unpredictable and not usually progressive. Examples include severe multiple disabilities following brain or spinal cord injuries and severe cerebral palsy.

From the Joint Report on *Palliative Care for Young People* (2001).

The search for meaning

As this book has emphasised throughout, the transition period between adolescence and young adulthood is characterised by physical growth, the development of personality and cognitive potential, the honing of intellectual abilities, and, inevitably, the challenging of social norms (Briggs, 2002). Great meaning is attached to 'belonging' and 'fitting in', behaviours that are usually reinforced through relationships with peer groups. Powerful friendships and group experiences are features of the adolescent world.

As Chapter 2 discussed, the rates of physical and cognitive development are individual and unpredictable, although there are central 'psychological tasks' that are considered important, no matter their actual sequencing. Abstract thinking and physical evidence of puberty may vary enormously in terms of when they occur. For this reason chronological age is not the most useful indicator of care needs, regardless of the stage of disease. In the case of a highly specialised surgery, for example, it may seem perfectly defensible and pragmatic to admit one 16 year old to an adult unit, whilst another would prefer to receive care in a children's oncology setting. This was the case for one young woman who recounted her experience earlier in this book. She was satisfied with her experiences of being cared for on a children's cancer unit and felt that it met her needs. Some of those who spoke to us about recommendations within the final chapter, however, emphasised the importance of having a choice in such situations.

The important point here is that age and the physical determinants of puberty do not, in themselves, always correspond to levels of maturity. Neither do they provide accurate indicators of the ability to absorb, reflect, and then deal with complex information about serious illness or treatment-related issues. Emotional or cognitive maturity can also seem to fluctuate rapidly, sometimes being demonstrated to a remarkable degree on one occasion and then dissolving (sometimes frustratingly) when the need arises for the next poignant conversation. Importantly, the transitory nature of insight or maturity may interrupt the natural flow of dialogue and the transfer of sensitive clinical information to young people. This apparent state of 'flux' is not uncommon in humans when confronted by the threat of loss. It is especially common in adolescents, however, and should be anticipated when planning care in advanced disease, especially if there is a likelihood that they will succumb to their disease (Flynn, 2000).

There is importance in considering the impact of this unpredictable but inherently natural way that young people may search for some meaning in their lives at this time. During adolescence two perspectives may coexist (i.e. child and adult), which will impact on all aspects of life. A clinical example of this would be the care of Lou (see the example below), where a childlike wish for the 'big bad thingy' of nightmares to go (death) is balanced by rage at its reality. This opposes the more adult recognition of death as an inevitable if unwelcome part of life. The impact of this balance between child and adult thinking in the face of existential threat is an important point of emphasis in relation to the focus of this chapter.

Encountering such reactions in young people facing the threat of death will present challenges when we attempt to deliver effective palliative care. A life-limiting disease process exists that is not responding to treatment and is now characterised by an unpredictable but inevitable decline. Obviously this will impact on all the life experiences (and related developmental tasks) necessary for maturation into adulthood. It is easy to see that, faced with this situation, young people will experience (and display) a range of powerful emotions. Not least is the frustration associated with becoming increasingly dependent on others and facing the reality of death, at the same time as the mind and body continue to develop (but may also be deteriorating) apace. From situations experienced in practice we now explore the importance of finding meaning in situations where effective care involved engaging with the reality of the imminent death of young people.

Working with the search for meaning

Palliation is concerned with issues of human suffering, and a biomedical perspective alone is unlikely to provide us with all the answers. Symptomatology is an inappropriate work ethic in such situations and one, in our view, that is likely to prove futile, as it will only partially address the needs of young people who are dying. In our experience many adolescents and young people actually have a greater capacity than some adults or even their adult carers to engage with the inherent meaning of their approaching death. This may be due to the fact that they have an increasing capacity to deal with abstract thinking – and usually without the cynicism of adults. This may be combined with finding a voice with which to negotiate care options and to discuss issues of meaning coherently, while still retaining some childlike capacity for playfulness. It is a unique constellation.

As a professional working with a palliative philosophy it is also important to engage in conversations with young people in ways that are relevant to the meanings they attach to death and loss. With time, narrative patterns may emerge that are recognisable, and it is within such interactions that many young people may reveal to us the extent of the emotional resources they have to draw upon to cope with the 'senselessness' of dying at such a young age. It is also during these interactions that professionals can intercede usefully to support patients when their search for a personal sense of meaning appears to get 'stuck'. This may happen when hopelessness overwhelms them or their parents or family, and may continue until some new understanding emerges, or at least until the situation is tolerable again.

Saunders (1988) talked about this situation and referred to Frankl's (1987) book *Man's Search for Meaning* (1987). In this he described his life in a Nazi labour and extermination camp and the hopelessness of the situation. However, as he said, 'The hopelessness of the situation did not detract from its meaning' (Saunders 1988, p.30). He argued that meaning can be found in the inner self, in relationships, and through moments of contemplation and spirituality. If there is no way out of suffering then we have an opportunity to shape the manner in which we suffer. However, no one can tell anyone else about the meaning of their life, according to Frankl (1987) and Saunders (1988), as this will be determined by our individual priorities. In young people, however, this is a difficult task due to the ever-present reality that a life is being cut short. Finding meaning in this situation, therefore, is challenging.

A key point of understanding may be reached when it is realised that, whilst the outcome cannot be changed, helping the young person to identify the meaning they attach to their life and the things they love can provide significant relief, especially during particularly distressing times. However, such fundamental issues require us to find ways of communicating with the young person and to do so in a way that is authentic and therapeutic.

Practice and challenges in palliative care

In order to explore the focus of meaning at the end of life we will now introduce some clinical examples to demonstrate its appropriate application.

'Why me man?'

Shanka was a smart 15 year old with a deep interest and talent for rap music. He was born and raised in poverty in south London, raised by his 20-year-old sister and his 'street' after his mum was put in the 'lunatic bin' (his dad did not interfere). He made a point of describing his ethnic origin on each admission as a 'Gangsta' – a clear provocation to one young nurse's sensibilities. Each time he thwarted her abilities to identify and record him on the computer system. He seemed to survive on his wits and rudeness and was always searching for 'total respect' . . . but invariably not finding it (and so thwarting himself too). He was frequently mean, moody, and disruptive. He had been diagnosed with a Ewing's sarcoma and endured complex neuropathic pain and an associated disfiguring disability as well as insomnia throughout his illness. The combination of his symptom burden and prescribed opioids caused sustained erectile dysfunction. He seemed to 'crash' on the admission when he was told no more chemotherapy would be offered and that his disease was overtaking him. 'Oh man . . . why me man?' he pleaded repeatedly for days, often crying himself into breathlessness, then panic.

At the moment we realise that a life-threatening illness has changed into a life-limiting situation, one's sense of meaning can disappear. Until this point Shanka had been able to function and find a role and purpose in his 'Gangsta' existence, despite the difficult manifestations of his disease. However, when told that his illness had progressed he became 'stuck in a moment' that lasted almost 2 weeks, as he struggled to make sense and to find some new meaning in his situation. Sometimes young people will spend inordinate amounts of energy trying to understand events like these – trying to make 'sense of the senseless', the sudden irrelevance of their previous persona (of a 'street kid' in this case) whilst their new identity remains unclear. The most vulnerable (perhaps the childlike parts) of the young person are suddenly exposed. There are no hiding places any longer and it can feel overwhelming and terrifying – both for them and for those witnessing what is happening. Helping can itself feel terrifying, as there is little to do apart from 'sticking with' the young person in their distress.

What are helpful palliative approaches here? Certainly being able to engage with a young man like Shanka is essential. Having the wisdom not to disenfranchise him whilst establishing some semblance of a clinical routine from the start of his illness was also useful. It also helped to have had some palliative input from the initial diagnosis that allowed relationships to be formed and negotiated before the most difficult point was reached. It was also helpful not to concentrate on the 'unfairness' of the disease, but instead to work with him to find out what was important to him and, more importantly, what was being lost. For Shanka this was his 'street cool', his independence, and being able to stay out of his home or hospital as long as possible (as home was full of overwhelming sadness about the loss of his mother). He was also preoccupied with the fact that he might die a virgin.

At this point it is also important to mention the bargaining that some young people may engage in to try to make sense of the senseless. For example, they may ask the question of whether 'if I had been a better person, this would not have happened'. If Shanka was encouraged to share such thoughts with someone he trusted they might be able help to explore and question his feelings of responsibility and to explore what was now important to him in the time left. Importantly, this requires a mixture of supportive interactions and the space to reflect free of symptoms, such as pain, which would simply add to his feelings of dependence and distress.

'Don't tell him he's dying'

We were called to see Dion, a 13 year old, to provide urgent advice about breathlessness secondary to heart failure following an aborted fourth attempt to control his acute myeloid leukaemia. He was a big lad being guarded on each side by his mother and aunt. As we walked into the room both stood to attention and, above his range of vision, gesticulated that, in no uncertain terms, were we to mention dying (or else!) With a mind to the nature of the situation we proceeded, with caution, to have a relatively safe discussion about breathlessness and treatment suggestions. Suddenly Dion said 'I think I'm dying' and looked straight at me with a knowing gaze. Hesitating, given the circumstances, I rather inarticulately managed to convey my hope he would get home, but I'm sure I looked embarrassed. Dion, of course, knew that this was not the case and he died that night.

Naming what is real and having faith in one's clinical judgement can help maintain professional integrity intact in this kind of work. The above case represents a common clinical dilemma: when is the right time to tell or confirm with a young person that death is likely? Transparency, we suggest, is a useful watchword, as adolescents can seem almost expert at seeking out the truth. It is our experience that most have an understanding of the outcome long before the adults around have allowed it to enter their minds as a reality. Therefore hesitancy, although natural, may prove unhelpful in aiding a young person to come to terms with events that serve to confirm rapidly advancing disease. However, some young people, such as Lou, will make it easy for us if given the chance:

MB: What's up?
Lou: I'm scared (talking like a 3 year old).
MB: What are you scared about, can you put your finger on it?
Lou: The big black thingy (tears flow).
MB: What is 'the big black thingy?' (Feeling careful, like a caring mum? I wonder inside in my mind, how will she react when I confirm her fears that the 'thingy' is her dying?)
Lou: Doh! . . . DEATH you DORK!! (Tears flow with laughter.)
MB: You knew, didn't you? (Relief is palpable.)

Note here that there is evidence of child and adult behaviours in Lou. This resulted in my hesitancy in terms of the best approach to take in confirming her fears. Given the space, however, she was able to make it easy for me.

One practical issue for palliative care clinicians is how to introduce oneself when first meeting a young person. This may be close to diagnosis, when their symptom burden can include pain, fatigue, and nausea. The difficulty arises because palliation has strong associations with death: hence, we fear letting 'the truth' out too soon. An easier process of communication may be established later if it was explicit from the start about the boundaries of engagement.

Parents and adult carers presented specific difficulties in the case of Dion. This is usually based on a conscious anxiety about expressing their emotions, especially in front of the adolescent affected, and their innate understanding of the capacity of their 'child' to cope compounds this. It is also understandable that inducing fear and uncertainty (common reactions to a poor prognosis) is a threat. However, most parents and adult carers may start to understand the necessity for open disclosure if given the space and time to explore their own emotions. Some may even prefer to be the bearer of bad news. For others, a more positive connotation is useful.

If more time had been available it might have been more useful to respond to Dion's mother and aunt by saying something like:

> It's really good that you are not answering Dion's questions about dying, otherwise you might be overwhelmed by feelings that you are finding hard to keep in . . .

Adopting a positive tone in this way can help address their unconscious wish that their imminent sense of sadness and loss could be avoided. His mother's response might then have been to realise that not allowing Dion to explore the possibility of death might thwart both of them from creating some meaning in the situation and, ultimately, the creation of a sense of calm before his death. If such situations do remain intractable, young people will often continue to 'play the game', but will then react by looking inwards to find a sense of calm. Despite our best intentions they can read the emotional tone by assessing the capabilities of the adults around them. In such a situation a professional may be best placed to initiate such conversations when a parent simply cannot. Bluebond-Langner (1978) confirmed this in a seminal ethnographic research work. This author described the way that a dying child with leukaemia willingly (apparently) entered into a display of mutual pretence:

> Ironically, these children came to see their own tasks as supporting others. They showed themselves to be responsive to the needs of their parents. Through the tactics they fashioned to follow rule 8 of mutual pretence, they gave their parents the opportunity to rehearse the ultimate separation.

Myra:	Jeffrey, why do you always yell at your mother?
Jeffrey:	Then she won't miss me when I'm gone.
Mrs Andrews:	Jeffrey yells at me because he knows I can't take it. He yells so I have an excuse for leaving.

'In essence, the children's ability to practice mutual pretence marked them as able to meet the most fundamental demand that society places on all its members – preservation of the social order . . . they contributed to society and its order in a fundamental and no less great sense by allowing the living their identities, their sense of self-worth, derived from their roles.' (Bluebond-Langner, 1978, pp. 232–233).

This suggests that, for these children, keeping their parents close was more important than overt discussions of their prognosis. These findings can help us appreciate the importance of the defences that families may use for coping with the almost unbearable situations they find themselves in. It is only with great care that we should breach these defences.

'My pain's no better . . . you're rubbish you are!'

We had been working with Lauren for months, mostly in the outpatient setting. She was 18 years old and, despite her illness (angiosarcoma), had maintained a university place and a clubbing schedule with friends. She lived between her boyfriend's flat and her grandmother's home and was considered a 'blithe spirit'. Over the course of a month, as her disease progressed, she developed complex pain, chest disfigurement, and profound weight loss. She also became sad and introverted and spoke of herself as a 'freak'. Neither pharmacological nor non-pharmacological interventions for the pain were reported as helpful by Lauren and she berated us constantly about how 'rubbish' we were. She started to alter her medication regime at will and did not adhere to the agreed plan, which may have been successful in easing her pain and other symptoms.

Suffering is inherently complex. Not least in the last few months of life, when it can manifest as overwhelming distress and agitation. It may be experienced as the struggle to find meaning in the physical deterioration and dependence. Psychological, spiritual, ontological, or existential crises can all come under the rubric of suffering. Despite our interventions Lauren's suffering seemed endless. In these circumstances it was impossible to make sense of an illness that caused such torment: however, the important message is that we had to keep trying.

Considerable effort is involved in engaging with a seemingly intractable problem. If the situation is considered almost impossible privately – meaning perhaps that this person is also 'impossible' – then unintentionally this message may be conveyed to the young person. Professional or personal frustration at 'being rubbish' may lead to feelings of anger and confusion.

When pain is particularly chronic or unrelenting the expectations of the young person or the professional may be unrealistic. Hence, when we repeatedly 'fail' to alleviate pain we are deemed failures. However, with hindsight a pattern emerged whereby, during an assessment, the pain was reported at about 10/10 on a visual analogue scale and her dialogue confirmed this. However, her gestures began to indicate small changes long before she reported them. Initially,

Lauren was reserved and did not gesture much. She would often hold her breath when talking about the nature of the pain experience. As time passed she would talk about her pain, but was also becoming more open in posture, gesturing freely to demonstrate anger (both at us and at the disease). Thus, body language can help meaning to be conveyed and is worth noticing as it can provide additional evidence that our interventions are not futile.

Suffering can also lead to a feeling of emptiness in the young person, especially when it is endured over a prolonged period of time. This feeling may be projected onto professionals, who may, in turn, share the dispiriting effect. Sometimes it can be useful to use conversational strategies to gain compliance and return a sense of control to the young person.

In Lauren's case we said that we recognised that changing medications sporadically was the best thing for her to do to deal with the terrible pain she undoubtedly endured (positive reinforcement) and on no account should she change her approach to managing her pain (paradoxical injunction). She rebelled and, in order to make us appear wrong (and so remain 'rubbish'), she started to adhere to the shared plan for the management of the pain. In this case relief of suffering in a life-limited situation required a somewhat unusual yet creative solution. Her suffering eventually lessened although it never ceased.

Near the end of life

Shanka, Dion, Lou, and Lauren all died requiring the support of palliative care services. Although each of their paths was unique, there were some common elements that can be extrapolated. These include (1) recognising when death is likely, (2) the place of death, (3) decision making, and (4) fundamental aspects of care.

Recognising when death is likely

Acknowledging that death is likely does not mean that we can predict when it will occur. Biological markers, although relevant, cannot always be relied upon either, as deaths from cancer can be very different, even in apparently similar cases. Some form of prediction about the possible timing of death may be important to the young person, those closest to them, and professionals, as it can help to frame the appropriateness of interventions. Recognising the closeness of death can also assist in achieving preparedness, in clarifying individual preferences, and in allowing time to complete tasks that are meaningful to an individual's personal biography. For example, Shanka wanted to know when death was likely to arise so he could go and say goodbye to his mother.

Death can be spoken about explicitly or through symbolic language if it is too distressing to acknowledge openly, as was the case with Dion. Even when predictions are made, however, events and coincidences take over. This was the case with Lou, who died more rapidly than we had prepared for and on a day that happened to be her birthday (which she shared with her mother).

Place of death

The place of death is often as meaningful to the adolescent themselves as to the people who love them. It is usually possible for the last year of life to be spent outside of hospital (especially with young people who have 'solid cancers') and young people themselves often clearly state their wish to be at home to die (Report of the Joint Working Party on Palliative Care for Adolescents and Young Adults, 2001). With responsive care provision and flexibility, this choice can often be achieved; and can do much to honour a persons' integrity, and may help improve the bereavement outcome. However, what is frequently not acknowledged is that people may change their minds, even at the last moment, and what is meant by 'home' can be a moot point.

For Lauren, going home meant being able to be independent: having a bath and having her friends round. However, it actually became too much for her to be at home without this happening as she became bed-bound. There was also her sister's unspoken terror (only given voice after her subsequent demise) at the prospect of Lauren dying in the same house, as she was then going to be living alone.

Often palliative care professionals can help to negotiate with the young person and others affected by their choices, especially where there is no agreement about the best way to proceed. It is time well spent, as those left can feel guilt that they failed, not only in halting the disease, but also at what they considered to be a hurdle (the choice of place of death). These discussions should not be seen as easy to engage in, and are often much more complicated in reality.

Some evidence exists about the place of death for young people in the UK. Higginson and Thompson (2003) reviewed death registrations for 16–24 year olds from 1995 to 1999 and found that a home death was less likely for those in lower social classes (according to parents' occupations) and for those with specific cancers (including leukaemia or lymphoma rather than solid cancers): 52% of children and adolescents and 30% of young adults died at home. These are higher figures than for the USA (20%) or for adults dying of cancer generally in the UK (26%). Brain tumours accounted for over half of those children who died in a hospice, perhaps reflecting the need for increased support as the condition worsens. These figures suggest that a home death, for those who prefer it, may be more problematic for some groups of patient than others.

Decision making

A fine balance also needs to be struck, particularly at the end of life, between making equally defensible decisions about distressing symptoms and medication choices. Often there will not be a completely 'right' or 'wrong' way to intervene. An adolescent may also fluctuate in their ability to cope with uncertainty, and may want us to make decisions on some occasions but not others. People commonly see an escalation of their symptom burden as a sign that death is approaching, and young adults are no different in this respect. However, their tolerability of a subcutaneous or rectal route of administration may differ from that of the average adult. This may be explained by a combination of body image and sensitivity, a situation that needs to be anticipated or avoided if at all possible. It is common in palliative practice to hone interventions towards individual needs, a situation that may be magnified in young adults. For example, in Dion's case we altered the level of sedation towards the end of his life according to his social schedule, as he had a differing threshold for attention span and general coping when his friends were present. He would also decide about his level of sedation at some times, whilst at others he became unable to negotiate (despite still being cognitively aware).

Fundamental aspects of care

What is common to all professionals involved in end of life care is our duty to attend to the fundamental aspects of care as death approaches – no matter what our clinical background. As dying is rare in young adults, people may have little experience in preparing them adequately for what can be a daunting challenge. A young person *in extremis* is not always easy to cope with when the physical effects of cancer become so visibly obvious. This is what Lawler (1991) talked about when she described the nursing work that goes on 'behind the screens'. Whilst this may be an aspect of cancer care that is less interventionist (from a treatment perspective), it is hugely important to the person who is dying and also helps ensure good memories of this time for those who will be left behind.

In our experience a care pathway approach can be useful in such instances, as it highlights the aspects of care that are required for most people. These can include monitoring symptoms and stopping unnecessary interventions. It will also necessitate dealing with unpleasant odours and toileting needs, and ensuring that comfort and cleanliness is maintained. Family can play a key role here (although some will find this easier than others) after coaching from professionals skilled in the care of the very ill (Kelly and Edwards, 2005).

There is no evidence available for the effectiveness of a care pathway approach in young adults: suffice it to say that its use is recommended for a wider dying population, where it has been shown to have great utility (Ellershaw and Wilkinson, 2003). Some worry that these approaches are too prescriptive. However, such criticism may be unfounded as the care pathway rarely represents the subtle nuances of care that invariably surround palliative practice.

In all of the above sections there is a heightened awareness of the emotional dimensions of care. This corresponds to an increasingly important theoretical and practical dimension of caring work known as emotional labour. This is defined as:

'The induction or suppression of feeling in order to sustain an outward appearance that produces in others a sense of being cared for in a convivial, safe place' (Hochschild, 1983, p. 7).

There is a need to acknowledge the significance of emotions, rather than ignoring their importance, in the care of adolescents and young adults at the end of life. To support young people and families means having to cope with a range of competing emotions. This has been demonstrated in studies exploring emotional labour in bone marrow transplant settings (Kelly *et al.*, 2000) and hospices (James, 1992). Clearly there is room for examining further how emotion management impacts on the perceptions and subsequent bereavement experiences of those left behind.

Is there meaning in bereavement?

To repeat an earlier point, society views the death of a young person as an abnormal event. The 'normal' trajectory of the life course is that parents and, indeed, grandparents are expected to die first. Death in the young is disruptive and, thus, it is more difficult to find any meaning in such a loss.

We now know that the death of a 'child', regardless of the age involved, increases the risk of complicated grief (Black, 1998). Following the death of a young person from a life-limiting illness, there is never just one bereaved person: there will be parents, siblings, grandparents, friends or peers, staff that have cared for the patient, and other adolescents and families they will have met along their cancer journey (Fig. 9.1). Although each will be thinking about the same person has died, their reflections, emotions, and experiences of them will be very different.

The feelings of grief experienced following the death of an adolescent or young adult can be very similar to those described at the time of diagnosis. Importantly, they can change from day to day, hour to hour, or even minute to minute. These emotions can include the following:

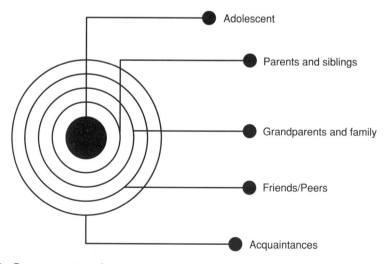

Fig. 9.1 Bereavement touches many people.

1. Shock: even though death from cancer is usually expected, the reality of the death is often accompanied by a sense of shock.
2. Relief: relief that the 'suffering' is over, relief that the person no longer has to endure further treatment/pain/immobility, or relief that the family can at last leave the hospital.
3. Guilt and self-reproach: guilt may follow feelings of relief or, as a parent, that you did not do more to save your 'child' (this can be particularly intense when there has been a late diagnosis of cancer) or guilt that your child/ sibling is dead and you are still alive.
4. Failure: that as a parent you could not protect your child from death, that as a sibling your bone marrow did not save your brother or sister, or that as a professional you could not cure the patient or control their pain completely.
5. Anger: that the death has occurred and that the professionals you trusted to have let you down – perhaps even God has let you down.
6. Helplessness: just not knowing what to do next.
7. Anxiety: arising from the emotional pain and sense of loss at the death, the practicalities of what to afterwards.
8. Numbness: feeling nothing at all, as if there are no emotions left.
9. Yearning: to see, touch, hold, or talk with the dead person once more, or wishing that life was back to 'normal'.
10. Loneliness: not necessarily due to being physically alone but due to a loss of connectedness to the person who has died. It should be remembered that some young adults will have been married or have had partners, and the sense of loneliness for the bereaved may be experienced through reminders, such as an empty space in the bed. Loneliness can therefore exist even when other people surround us.

As well as emotional reactions there can also be physical responses, which can include tightness in the chest or throat, an over-sensitivity to noise, feelings of breathlessness, a dry mouth, fatigue, or symptoms that mirror the disease itself. The mother of a 15 year old who had died of a brain tumour told us that:

> Of course any time one of us has a headache we always think it might be a brain tumour, we laugh about it of course but we do still wonder . . .

For parents and siblings, being able to share the experience of a life-limiting illness with others in similar situations is useful. Within our local Teenage Cancer Trust unit one of the specialist nurses runs a support group for parents. A theme that repeatedly emerges in the group is the importance of mutual support following the death of a young person. The issue is often raised at times when someone is dying on the unit or when someone has left hospital having exhausted all the treatment options or decided not to pursue further treatment and has instead chosen to go home to die (a choice that we will be involved in supporting). Parents will often ask 'Will there be groups like this for me after John has died?' This is asked out of a genuine need to know that there will be some supportive contact available if their child dies.

In a study carried out on a Teenage Cancer Trust unit (Kelly *et al.*, 2004) one mother spoke of endings with the unit being something she looked to with mixed feelings:

> 'Adjusting to normal life, yes, it will be a big gap in our lives when it's finished ... it's been our life and then it won't be ...'

Relationships with staff will have been built up over a long period of time and leaving the safety of this environment can be extremely traumatic, especially if death is the likely outcome. In these situations ongoing liaison services are essential. Subtle requests for support may also be put forward by young people on behalf of their parents through comments such as:

> 'Mum always goes to the parents' group when we are in (hospital). Sometimes I know she has been crying in there but she seems to find it helpful talking to the others about what it is like. There will be something for her after won't there, you know, when it's all over for me ...'

Not only do such statements offer us an opportunity to engage with the young person about the impact of their death on those closest to them, but they can also help support the need for a regular meeting or group for bereaved parents, as happened in our own setting.

Common occurrences in bereavement

Sometimes a group method is useful in helping facilitate the emergence of new insights or meaning after the death of a young person. Walter (1996) described such meetings as 'mutual help groups'. This means that help will be offered, as well as being received, by those who take part. Importantly, they will all have a similar shared experience to draw upon.

A clear message from the group that we established was how valuable it had been to have the chance to talk about the young person's decline towards death. As one bereaved parent told us:

> 'We all knew he was dying, we talked about it openly. We talked about what it might be like while it was happening and what life might be like for those of us left behind after he had died. It gave the rest of the family a chance to ask their questions too. Most of us don't see dying unless it's on TV. It was important for us to talk about what we might be frightened of so that his brother and sister could decide whether they might want to be with him at the end. It also gave us a chance to say the things we needed to say. If people had asked me a year ago how I would talk to my son about the fact that he was dying, I would have just said I wouldn't, but I am glad I did ...'

In contrast, another parent spoke about not talking about the inevitability of death in advance:

'You tried to give us the opportunity and we never took it, we chose not to hear what was being said, we know that now.'

We can infer from this that open acknowledgement that death is near may be helpful, not only at the time, but also subsequently when the bereaved person goes over the experience in order to find some meaning in it. We should therefore be aware of providing opportunities for honest communication, and not to be put off by the frustration or anger of relatives or friends (or sometimes even their raised voices, tempting as it might be). The sense of rage felt by those facing the loss of a young person may be directed towards the professionals involved: however, it is rarely about them in reality. Instead it is the situation that is provoking powerful emotions such as distress and helplessness that must be directed somewhere.

Having a hiding place

Following the death other issues arise for the bereaved, such as when to return to work. This was an issue for two fathers who attended a recent bereavement group. Even though both felt that their employers had been extremely understanding and helpful and no pressure was put on them to return to work, in reality there was little choice as bills still have to be paid. Both agreed that they had probably returned to work too soon (within a month in each case).

One father described how one of his colleagues had removed the photographs of his dead son, as she did not want him to be upset. Another talked about how often people are defined, in a social sense, by their offspring. When meeting new people, for example, an opening question may be about children or family life. When he talked about this situation one father's emotional pain was palpable:

'Do I say well I had three but one died of cancer so now I have two and then watch this person, who you might never have met before, wonder how the hell to respond? To say two would be to deny that he ever existed, so I just say three and leave it at that.'

Avoiding distress, both in themselves and others, is a common concern that was echoed by one mother who initially had gone to different shops to avoid encountering people who might (or might not) know that her child had died.

Very practical tasks that the bereaved must carry out include registering the young person's death. In the UK registry offices can often be places of celebration. The registering of the birth of a child is a happy occasion, for instance, and contrasts sharply with the registration of a young person's death. Witnessing the joy of others can feel like the final insult immediately after the death of a young adult. Requesting a private space for parents can be enormously helpful, and most registry offices are happy to oblige. As one mum told us:

'We had already been told by other parents to go as soon as it (the registry office) opened in the morning, that way you miss all the cooing and the balloons . . .'

Of course grief is not the exclusive preserve of parents. One sibling struggled to recount how she was feeling, as she was so ashamed of her negatives feelings:

'I felt I had been neglected for years, she had been ill for so long and mum was always with her. Then just when I got some time to be normal, I went on holiday with some friends, that's when she chose to die and I had to come back. I hate myself for feeling like this but that's how I feel. I need to talk about how I feel and I need to talk to her. You all have someone to talk to; there must be other brothers and sisters out there who feel the same.'

All this was said with her mother sitting at her side. They had stopped talking about her dead sister at home, despite the fact that her mother said she had wanted to. They both feared upsetting each other if they kept remembering the sister in shared conversations – perhaps if they did so they would never 'get over' the death. What was useful for them to hear from the group was that the expectation to 'get over it' is rather false. There is every likelihood, however, that the oscillation between the strong feelings that are present close to the time of death will eventually be balanced with concerns about a future life. This will eventually allow new meaning to emerge. It may be useful to consider bereavement as a process of adaptation and the emergence of a new sense of meaning, rather than being about forgetting or abandoning the dead person. This is a message that may be passed on more appropriately through group discussion with other parents who can draw on personal experience of grief.

Completing the construction of palliative care

Despite the advent of national policies and guidance on palliative and supportive care, palliative care for the needs of 13–24 year olds remains inadequate within the UK. Often there is limited choice in terms of service provision, despite choice being highlighted as a fundamental entitlement (Big Lottery Fund, 2006). Sometimes there is a lack of specialist palliative care available locally, combined with the fact that adult palliative care services may refuse to accept referrals for those under 18 years of age. Thus, adolescents and young adults face similar issues as they do during treatment – finding the most appropriate setting for end of life care, especially if home care is impossible. Specialist community paediatric teams or general practitioners, whilst willing to help, may also fear that they have inadequate knowledge or feel legally prohibited by providing end of life care with strong painkillers such as opioids.

This is a frustrating double bind for a young person and their family, whose only choice of care setting is to stay close to the original hospital care or to risk being at home without adequate help. This emphasises the need for appropriate advanced care planning when the prognostic indicators do change for the worse. Not all acute oncology units can offer beds for palliative care, and some hospices may feel alien to young people (although the care itself can be excellent, it does mean forming new relationships at a particularly vulnerable time). If the death is planned to occur at home there are also practical concerns that need to be considered. This includes the need for access to equipment and advice regarding symptoms when it is needed – such as overnight or at weekends – when there is often a dearth of professional support available (apart from over the telephone).

There are now more community palliative care support teams (both adult and paediatric) who are expanding their remit and addressing the end of life needs of the young adults in their communities. However, the evidence base for their interventions is currently weak and there is no service template that has yet been costed and commissioned. This means that different configurations of palliative care exist for young people dying of cancer. Despite this, for practitioners seeking to ensure the best death possible, it is important to consider the words of Saunders (1998): 'Palliative care may begin with symptom control, but in most cases it is only the beginning' (p. ix).

The practical challenge of a good death therefore extends beyond the walls of the hospital and into the communities where people live their lives (Freyer, 2004). If we want to encourage more people to die at home then the necessary services and infrastructure must be available to support them. What we deduce from practice at present is that palliation aimed at young people needs to be flexible and responsive to their needs. This supports the need to gather the necessary evidence from young people themselves, as the following chapter explores.

Summary

In this chapter we have emphasised that young people and their parents/siblings have clear ideas about what they need from our service. In summary these will include the following.

1. Involvement in decision making.
2. Attention to developmental needs.
3. An appropriate setting of care.
4. Ambivalence about taking on an adult role.
5. A desire for independent living.
6. The importance of school, college, and employment.
7. Opportunities to do things that other young people do.
8. Symptom relief and emotional support.
9. Planning of care to ensure the best end of life care possible.

Although each is important, awareness of young people being in a state of 'transition' is central to being able to provide effective palliation and end of life care for this population. Although adolescents and young people may have the same physical symptoms as adults, not all will be in a position to cope with them or to accept that death is unavoidable. Whilst this may also be true of adults, young people are especially vulnerable due to socialisation processes that reinforce, in the media and in everyday life, that they are simply 'dying at the wrong age'.

Good palliative care therefore means connecting with the physical, emotional, and existential aspects of death and dying. In this chapter we have suggested that finding some sense of meaning in advanced illness and death is a useful way of helping young people cope with their situation. This will involve them connecting with those closest to them and being helped to recognise the contribution that each life makes. With this route map in mind and applied wisely in practice, we believe outcomes can be achieved that are helpful, rather than leaving young people 'stuck in a moment' of fear and loneliness.

References

Addington Hall, J. M. & Higginson, I. (2001) *Palliative Care for Non-Cancer Patients*. Oxford University Press, Oxford.

Big Lottery Fund (2006) *Palliative Care. Year 3 Evaluation Findings*. Research issue 32, The National Lottery, London.

Black, D. (1998) Coping with loss: bereavement in childhood. *BMJ*, **316**, 931–933.

Bluebond-Langner, M. (1978) *The Private Worlds of Dying Children*. Princeton University Press, Chichester.

Briggs, S. (2002) *Working with Adolescents*. Palgrave, Basingstoke.

Doyle, D., Hanks, G., Cherny, N., & Calman, K. (2004) *Oxford Textbook of Palliative Medicine*. Oxford University Press, Oxford.

Dunlop, R. J. & Hockley, J. M. (1998) *Terminal Care Support Teams – The Hospital/Hospice Interface*. Oxford University Press, New York, NJ.

Edwards, J. (2001) A model of palliative care for the adolescent with cancer. *International Journal of Palliative Nursing*, **7**, 485–488.

Ellershaw, J. & Wilkinson, S. (2003) *Care of the Dying – A Pathway to Excellence*. Blackwell Publications, Oxford.

Flynn, D. (2000) Adolescence. In: *Adolescence* (ed. I. Wise), pp. 56–71. Institute of Psychoanalysis, London.

Frankl, V. E. (1987) *Man's Search for Meaning*, revised and enlarged edition. Hodder & Stoughton, London.

Freyer, D. (2004) Care of the dying adolescent: special considerations. *Pediatrics*, **113**, 381–388.

Higginson, I. & Thompson, M. (2003) Children and young people who die from cancer: epidemiology and place of death in England (1995–99). *BMJ*, **327**, 478–479.

Hochschild, A. (1983) *The Managed Heart. Commercialisation of Human Feeling*. University of California Press, Berkeley, CA.

James, N. (1992) Care = organisation + physical labour = emotional labour. *Sociology of Health & Illness*, **14**, 489–509.

Report of the Joint Working Party on Palliative Care for Adolescents and Young Adults (2001) *Palliative Care for Young People Aged 13–24*. Association for Children with Life threatening Conditions and their Families, Bristol.

Kelly, D. & Edwards, J. (2005) Palliative care for adolescents and young adults. In: *Handbook of Palliative Care*, 2nd edn (eds C. Faull, Y. Carter, & L. Daniels), pp. 317–331. Blackwell Publishing, Oxford.

Kelly, D., Ross, S., Gray, B., & Smith, P. (2000) Death, dying and emotional labour: problematic dimensions of the bone marrow transplant nursing role? *Journal of Advanced Nursing*, **32**, 952–961.

Kelly, D., Pearce, S., & Mullhall, A. (2004) 'Being in the same boat': ethnographic insights into an adolescent cancer unit. *International Journal of Nursing Studies*, **41**, 847–857.

Lawler, J. (1991) *Behind the Screens: Nursing, Somology and the Problem of the Body*. Churchill-Livingstone, London.

National Institute for Health and Clinical Excellence (2004) *Guidance on Cancer Services: Improving Supportive and Palliative Care for Adults with Cancer*. National Institute for Health and Clinical Excellence, London.

Robertson, C. M., Hawkins, M. M., & Kingston, J. E. (1994) Late deaths and survival after childhood cancer: implications for cure. *BMJ*, **309**, 162–166.

Saunders, C. (1988) Spiritual pain. *Journal of Palliative Care*, **4**, 29–32.

Saunders, C. (1998) Foreword. In: *Good Practices in Palliative Care: a Psychosocial Perspective* (eds D. Oliviere, R. Hargreaves, & B. Monroe), pp. ix–x, Ashgate, Aldershot.

Saunders, C. (2004) Foreword. In: *Oxford Textbook of Palliative Medicine* (eds D. Doyle, G. Hanks, N. Cherny, & K. Calman), pp. xvii–xviii, Oxford University Press, Oxford.

Walter, T. (1996) A new model of grief: bereavement and biography. *Mortality*, **1**, 7–25.

World Health Organization (1990) *Cancer Pain Relief and Palliative Care*. Technical Report Series 804, World Health Organization, Geneva.

Chapter 10

Building a Culture of Participation: Young People's Involvement in Research

Faith Gibson

Setting the scene

Respect for the views of young people is enshrined in the UN Convention on the Rights of the Child (adopted by the UK government in 1991) (Newell, 1993). Acceptance of this principle alone has led to an unprecedented swell in participation activity. In fact, participation has become a 'buzz word' in health care. Health care, however, is not the only arena to be influenced by the participation agenda, as the request for greater participative involvement of citizens and consumers has become an important feature of our society. We might go so far as to state that there is such an expectation of young people and families in our care that participation, in some form or another, will be a feature of their care pathway. In addition, as healthcare professionals working in adolescent cancer care we might well be championing the notion of participation at all levels in our respective organisations. However, can we be confident that participation is enshrined in the culture of our organisations and that we have in place strategies for meaningful participatory practice?

Patient participation is said to occur at three levels: practice, policy, and research (Beresford, 2005). In the UK this expectation of participation is reinforced by government policy directed at increasing consumer involvement in the National Health Service (NHS):

> 'Where the voices of patients, their carers and the public generally are heard and listened to through every level of the service, acting as a lever for change and improvement' (Department Health [DH], 2001, p. 2).

Patient participation in treatment decisions and decisions that affect their care is not new and we would anticipate that our agreed model of patient-centred care, supported by UK government policy such as the Children Act 1989, ensures that this level of participation is a feature of everyday clinical care. A further example of participation is in education and training, where already the views of young people as service users is evident through testimonials of their experience (see the database of personal experiences, www.youthhealthtalk.org/teenagecancer and the Teenage Cancer Trust, www.jimmyteenstv.com), as well through as presentations to health-related educational courses (McNamara *et al.*, 2007). What appears to be more of a challenge is the participation of young people in service evaluation and service developments (Sloper and Lightfoot, 2003). Likewise, the participation of young people in research, although beginning to be articulated on paper (McLaughlin, 2006), in practice would seem to be less than commonplace. There remains some uncertainty about how to involve young people, especially how we might do so in a way that is effective and brings about change, particularly change that is lasting (Sinclair, 2004).

Fundamentally, participation is about enabling young people to 'have their say' in all decisions that affect them: decisions that relate to them as an individual (for example, treatment and care) or those that relate to young people as a group (for example, research, monitoring, and service evaluation). The focus of this chapter is on how young people's participation can shape health services, specifically through their participation in research. All organisations providing health and social care services in the UK are expected to (1) seek the views and wishes of patients and service users, (2) act on these views, and (3) involve local people in decision making (DH, 2006; see also the National Youth Agency Hear by Right and Health, www.nya.org.uk/hearbyright).

Our success in achieving these expectations will depend on the development of strategies that both engage with and facilitate meaningful input from young people (Coad and Lewis, 2004). Cancer services can be improved through patient involvement. This chapter focuses primarily on two approaches that will enable young people to have their say:

1. Involving young service users as partners in research within a continuum of consultation, collaboration, and user-controlled research (Kirby, 2004).
2. The use of creative methodologies in consultation exercises and participatory research that allow young people to contribute their perspectives in a way that is most suited to their strengths and preferences (Veale, 2005).

This chapter begins with a brief description of the context of change: by this I mean, why participation now? What has influenced the way we view young people in our society, and what difference will participation mean to young people with cancer? The level of active participation will then be touched on. Remaining with the position of young people as active rather than passive in the research process, the range of partnerships that can be established when young people are involved in research will be described, highlighting some of the particular challenges we might face when seeking partnerships with young people. A description of some of the participatory approaches used in consultation and research will then be detailed. Key principles and obstacles to building a culture of participation will be threaded throughout the chapter. Evaluation and its crucial role in understanding the benefits of participation and measuring how effective methods are for involving young people will be highlighted. Finally, drawing on the National Youth Agency standards for the active involvement of children and young people, strategies to engage with young people meaningfully in cancer services research are then suggested.

Drivers towards increased participation of young people

The first driver is the 'consumer movement', which came to prominence in the 1970s and is now reflected in the much-used term in health care of 'user involvement'. One of the central tenets of 'consumerism' is that power shifts from those who provide services to those who consume them (Telford *et al.*, 2004). Increasingly, therefore, policies and practices in the NHS have acknowledged that patients are important and need to be 'heard' in order to make services more responsive to their needs as well as more acceptable, accountable, and equitable, and to improve quality and outcomes of care (DH, 2003a,b; Hubbard *et al.*, 2007). The involvement of consumers is central to NHS research and development policy (DH, 1999, 2000, 2004, Consumers in NHS Research Support Unit, 2000; Smith, 2005) and gradually the role of 'user' has been extended to include young people (Kirby, 2004).

Second, there has been a progressive shift towards the involvement of young people as informed and active participants in their treatment and care (DH, Department for Education and Skills, 2004). This increased commitment has become widely valued and respected as a right. The ratification of the United Nations Convention on the Rights of the Child (Newell, 1993) in the UK and many other countries signalled the growth of involving young people in public decision making. Article 12 in particular emphasises young people's right to have a say in decisions that affect their lives. In the UK, in both the NHS (DH, 2002, 2003a,b) and local government, legislation and policy development programmes are contributing to improving young people's participation. Thus, there is a solid policy infrastructure for supporting consulting with young people and encouraging decisions informed by this consultation (Roberts, 2004).

Finally, in tandem with policy and changes in the political scene, there has been a shifting position that children and young people are 'social actors' in their own right and 'agents of change' rather than passive recipients of others' intervention (James and Prout, 1997). As a result of this new emerging paradigm, methodological and theoretical support for listening to the voices of children and young people has grown (France, 2004). There is clear evidence, in health care and elsewhere, that adults are beginning to pay attention to what young people have to say and respect their competence to participate in health-related decisions (Mayall, 2006).

These developments are positive, and create opportunities to put the voice of young people at the centre of the research agenda. However, despite this commitment, there remain practical, ethical, and political problems, not just in listening to young people, but in taking the next step and ensuring their voices are heard and acted upon (Roberts, 2004).

Why participation is important

Translating these drivers towards participation of young people that mandates for involvement in the arena of global health care, it is anticipated that young people's participation will lead to improved and more appropriate services, improved decision making, better use of health services, and increased empowerment to manage their own health (www.nya.org.uk/hearbyright). Participation will also uphold young people's rights and fulfil legal responsibilities. Young people have the right to be heard and involved in shaping and evaluating services that affect them.

Specifically, in terms of cancer care, young people can anticipate to be part of the decision-making process about treatment and supportive care, discussions in which they should expect to be treated as an equal partner. Moreover, by developing a *listening* culture in adolescent cancer services professionals may have an increased understanding about what it is like to have cancer and receive treatment,which one young woman of 17 years described as making 'you feel like crap and you look like crap' (Gibson *et al.*, 2005, p. 16). Developing a listening culture is just the first step in participation, however: *hearing* and *responding* are two further and essential steps that, when absent, leave young people feeling disillusioned with a system that they feel 'asks but does not act' or remarking 'what's the point' (Sinclair, 2004, p. 115). Building a culture of participation will go some way towards showing young people that their contributions are important and providing reassurance that their concerns are being taken seriously.

In terms of cancer care research, young people's participation will help ensure that professionals have better knowledge of their views and priorities, and will help prioritise key issues and concerns amenable to future research studies. It might also mean that, with a contribution from young people, cancer care services can be designed, delivered, and evaluated based on actual rather than presumed needs. Measuring the effectiveness of a service will be more relevant in situations where young people have been involved in the process of deciding how to monitor it, what information to collect, how to interpret it, and how to make recommendations for change. By asking young people what is important, professionals will help to foster a more equal power relationship that acknowledges young people's experience as service users. But what level of participation might young people anticipate?

Levels of participation

In practice the involvement of young people may vary with the circumstances. User involvement has tended to be conceptualised in terms of hierarchical levels of user activities or roles illustrated in terms of inclusiveness: for example, 'the ladder of participation' (see Arnstein, 1969; Hart, 1992). The ladder has eight rungs, climbing from manipulation, through adult-led but sharing decisions, reaching towards young people initiating and sharing decisions with adults (Hart, 1992).

Sheir (2001) suggested that practitioners have found Hart's (1992) ladder to be most useful in exposing degrees of non-participation described as 'manipulation', 'decoration', and 'tokenism', levels that we might consider to be negative elements of participation.

Sheir (2001) offered an alternative model that emphasised the positive elements of participation and presented practitioners with a useable practical tool based on a pathway, guiding progression through an ordered sequence of 15 questions. Although describing the participation of children, its use in the context of young people is upheld, as their participation is also influenced by interactions between themselves and adults. The model has two functions: as a gauge to the nature of involvement and as a guide to how its quality might be improved. Using the ladder analogy, there are five levels of participation in Sheir's (2001) model, where the starting point on the pathway represents the statement 'young people are listened to', when they take it upon themselves to express a view, with the final level asking whether 'young people share power and responsibility for decision making' in situations where adults have chosen to relinquish some of their power. This shift in emphasis to more positive types of participation is an important one in clinical care, in recognition that young people have the right to participate.

Applying the ladder of participation to the research context is new, as, until recently, young people were viewed as 'objects of concern' and passive recipients in the research process (Alderson, 2005). Using the ladder in this context necessitates the terms of participation being applied to the research context, where participation is conceived as levels of control in the research process (Smith *et al.*, 2005). The range of participation is viewed from situations where adults initiate consultation and listen to young people through to projects directly initiated by young people themselves (Moules, 2005). Applying the ladder of participation to the research situation is a sound approach as the process remains at the fundamental level of decision making. In the research context practitioners could use the model of Sheir (2001), as the shift in emphasis and presentation from Hart's (1992) ladder achieves a number of important distinctions. Firstly, presenting a pathway to participation, rather than a ladder, removes any hierarchical conceptualisation that implies one type of involvement is better than another, and prioritises the purpose of involvement as fundamental to agreeing the level of participation. Secondly, removing types of non-participation, such as manipulation, decoration, and tokenism, reinforces the position of young people as social actors in their own right and asserts that the involvement of young people in the research process is meaningful. The aim for any research team would be to be open and honest about how far young people can be involved in the research process – and for young people to decide how far they want to be involved, recognising that this may fluctuate through the life of a project and may well depend on levels of 'wellness'.

Young people as partners in research

There are no absolute ways to approach the question, how far should I involve young people in research? The simple answer is that they can be involved at any stage, from identifying research questions, prioritising, and commissioning, through to planning, undertaking, evaluating, and dissemination (Kirby, 2004). The level of involvement will depend on a number of factors, such as the research question and the young person's abilities, experiences, and interests (Kirby, 2004). Careful planning and consideration is required at all stages, with early decisions also influenced by the skills of the research team, resources in terms of time and money, and the young person's choice and availability. Meaningful involvement is what we are aspiring to, where young people consent to participate in the knowledge of what is expected of them: the consequences, potential pitfalls, and benefits, as well as alternative options open to them (Steel, 2005). In terms of research, meaningful involvement will lie on a continuum from consultation to collaboration and user-controlled research.

Consulting with young people

In the majority of cases young people with cancer will be involved in research that has been adult initiated with *consultation* being an important feature of the research design. Consultation has been described as endemic within the UK and elsewhere (McLaughlin, 2006) and is in danger of instilling 'consultation fatigue' (Sinclair, 2004). Consultation means asking young people who use services about research, asking them for their views to inform decision making (Kirby, 2004) (see Box 10.1). For example, young people might be asked for their views on a research proposal, asked to identify and prioritise research questions, or asked what they want from a service. For example, in one study in the UK young people were consulted using a series of focus groups about their preference for single sex or mixed sex wards (S. Morgan, personal communication). This type of participation might involve a one-off face-to-face meeting, or more creative approaches may well include the use of online discussion groups that might be more appealing in terms of interest and the time required. For example, in the UK at the Teenage Cancer Trust 'Where's Your Sense of Tumour' annual conference for young people, interactive technology is used to consult with young people about their experiences and is one method of gaining views in 'real time' from young people (Smith *et al.*, 2007).

Care is needed in this process in order to ensure genuinely open communication rather than seeking confirmation of what professionals already think or want and dismissing young people's priority concerns (Stafford *et al.*, 2003). The need to build in a process of feedback and dissemination of findings to young people who have participated is also crucial in this type of participation: otherwise they may be left feeling that their contributions have been ignored.

Young people as collaborators in research

Collaboration implies a degree of ongoing service user involvement with the resultant power to affect decisions. There are a number of possibilities for participation, such as inviting young people to join a steering group for a research project, where they would play an important role in guiding a study and ensuring the

---

Box 10.1   Young people involved in consultations

These are usually one-off or short pieces of work that focus on a particular issue. For example, in the clinical studies group for teenagers and young adults from the UK National Cancer Research Institute two young people are taking an active role in the group. These young people are being supported by the chair of the group and its members to participate in meetings in order to develop research priorities for the clinical studies group in relation to health services research.

Strengths

1. Targeted and focused activity.
2. Time limited with clear expectations of involvement.
3. Cost-effective.
4. Immediate relevance to young people.
5. The results can be seen quickly.
6. A safe way to begin to work with young people in a research setting.

Limitations

1. Exclusive or unrepresentative.
2. Potential lack of follow-up once the period of consultation is over.
3. Lack of ownership.
4. Potential to be seen as a quick fix.
5. Limited time to prepare young people for their involvement.
6. Danger of 'consultation fatigue'.
7. Young people may be constrained by a professional agenda.

---

study remains focused on the needs of young people. In addition, assisting with research design, informing the development of recruitment materials and approaches to recruitment, acting as researchers, analysing and interpreting data, and contributing to the writing of the report and dissemination process are other possibilities. This is quite a commitment, particularly if there are frequent meetings or where the study is of a longitudinal nature, and hence it may be difficult for young people, other than those who have completed therapy, to participate. However, collaboration may occur at just one part of the research process or some or all of it and would constitute a decision about participation early on in a study. A further approach might be to tap into an established group or form a reference group to a study (see Box 10.2). Although input into a reference group may be less onerous, the ability to affect decisions may not be so obvious. Collaboration requires even more commitment than consultation: however, there might be an element of personal development for the young person that might appeal (Kirby, 1999), such as learning about the research process, increasing confidence in working with professionals, etc.

Box 10.2 Young people involved in reference groups

A group of young people (with or without adults) advise and inform those planning or reviewing a research study or who manage a project. There may be a series of face-to-face meetings over a period of time during the lifetime of a project. Other creative methods of engagement includes the use of webcams, email, and online discussion groups introduced to reduce the number of face-to-face meetings, which can be difficult to fit into a busy young person's life. For example, in our 'Listening to Children' project (Gibson *et al.*, 2005), we worked with a reference group of children and young people on active treatment using mail and telephone. These young people took on a number of roles, such as reviewing information sheets and recruitment material and advising on dissemination style and process. We involved the reference group throughout the study through the distribution of regular newsletters.

Strengths

1. Example of ownership.
2. Ensures researchers remain mindful of the needs of young people.
3. Representative.
4. Established and ongoing and can offer real support to young people.
5. Onus is not just on one or two people on an advisory group.
6. They can help interpret and understand data.

Limitations

1. Can be time-consuming.
2. Might be perceived as a rubber stamp exercise.
3. Irregular meetings and attendance due to other commitments.
4. Limited authority in the group to influence decision making.

User-controlled research

User-controlled research broadly refers to those research projects where power resides with service users who are responsible for the initiative and subsequent decision making (Turner and Beresford, 2005). This approach does not mean that young people undertake every stage of the research or that professionals are excluded from the process altogether. The key issue here is one of power (McLaughlin, 2006). Similar to consultation and collaboration, there is a range of potential options for user participation (see Box 10.3). User-controlled research might develop through membership of support groups, hospital-based user groups, patient forums, or the survivor network that exists through national and international organisations. At this level young people could establish a research agenda, commission research for others to undertake, or commission research in which they take on a researcher role (Moules, 2005). At present within the field of cancer care the involvement of young people in user-controlled research is not yet established, but it is beginning to happen in adult cancer care

---

Box 10.3   User-controlled research

Although I could find no examples of where young people are actively engaged in commissioning research and leading decision making at this level in cancer care, it is possible to suggest some potential strengths and limitations for this approach to participation.

Strengths

1. Maximises knowledge and experience of service users to improve practice.
2. Focuses research on what is important to young people.
3. Potential to ensure research is translated into clinical care.
4. Initiates collaboration with professionals.
5. Can empower young people.
6. Capacity to make change to a service more in line with what young people want.

Limitations

1. Time consuming.
2. Requires specific skills and training.
3. Requires support.

---

and in other fields, and its advocates have highlighted its validity (Beresford, 2005). There are, however, a number of examples where parents of young people with cancer are commissioning consumer-led research (for example, www. lauracranetrust.org). In addition, opportunities presented by young people participating in the role of a trustee of charities that support research, as has already happened at Cancer and Leukaemia in Childhood Sargent (www. clicsargent.org.uk), may well in the future present an opening for usercontrolled research. This is a complex area for participation, with some arguing that it can never be on an equal basis unless service users and their organisations are themselves fully and equally involved (Beresford, 2005). With respect to the continuum of participation, at this level it remains difficult to predict what this might mean in cancer care for young people.

At all levels of involvement young people will require support and guidance. There are a number of documents and publications available to guide research teams who seek to include the principles of user involvement in their research (Kirby, 1999, 2004; Combe, 2002; Lockey *et al.*, 2004; Beresford, 2005). Ensuring young people's health, safety, and wellbeing during their involvement in research must be an early consideration of any research team. In the UK the work of INVOLVE (Promoting Public Involvement in NHS, Public Health and Social Care Research, www.invo.org.uk) has been influential in enabling researchers to put the policy of user involvement into practice in a more structured and meaningful way (DH, 2004). The notion of a continuum, in terms of user involvement, remains a helpful term for practitioners wanting to engage with young people in research. Researchers need not think in terms of all or nothing (Beresford, 2005): a realistic appraisal of 'what is needed and what is possible' would seem to be a useful way forward (Children and Participation, www.savethechildren.org).

Methodologies used to facilitate participation in research

If our aim is building evidence for practice centres on the needs of young people through participation, more specifically consultation and collaboration, then these approaches must also feature in how we approach data collection. A number of research methods focusing on young people are available for consideration by researchers undertaking qualitative research. These are felt to hold the potential for success, especially when thought is given to the planning of the research with respect to specific ages, experiences, interests, and the ways in which young people feel most comfortable to communicate (Curtis *et al.*, 2004). The underlying philosophy of participatory research is that research participants are not simply regarded as 'subjects', but are empowered to participate truly and have their voices heard (Veale, 2005). Thus, participatory research is particularly relevant to individuals or groups who have in the past often been regarded as 'silent' or disempowered in research, such as young people (Cavet and Sloper, 2004). In participatory research there is a strong commitment to engaging with participants in a meaningful way and acknowledging that participants are the 'experts' on research topics (Coad and Lewis, 2004). When carrying out research that aims to enable young people to participate and give their views fully, the methods to be used must be considered very carefully.

A spectrum of data-gathering methods is available that can, depending on how it is used, fall within a category of participatory research. Chosen well, these methods can engage young people successfully. It is not the intention of this chapter to detail these approaches, as many authoritative publications exist that already do this, but simply to list some of the techniques of relevance. These include peer interviews, focus groups, mapping/drawing and posters, photographs and video, role play/drama and sculpting, and journals/scrapbooks and diaries, as well as information and communication technology that includes online questionnaires, discussion groups, webcams, etc. (see Coad and Lewis, 2004; Veale, 2005). More relevant to this chapter is to highlight the principles of participation embedded in some of these methods. These include the following.

1. Building a relationship: take time to get to know young people and find out something about them, not based on something someone else has told you but something they say themselves, and be willing to share something about yourself with them.
2. Providing choice: including a range of methods in a research study increases flexibility, maximises interest, reduces boredom, and may well fit more with young people's interests and preferences for engaging.

3. Taking into consideration developmental factors: adolescence spans a wide time period in which age might not be the most useful indicator of development. Here again, choice and appropriateness of data collection will facilitate engagement and value the experience and skills of young people.
4. Balancing differential power relationships: informality and sharing control, selecting a suitable environment in which the research takes place, understanding the need for reflexivity, be responsive, having fun, and allow young people greater participation and control.
5. Engaging with the process: be willing to have fun, show genuine interest in what young people have to say, value their knowledge and experience, and engage with young people at an active rather than passive level.

Evaluating participation

Knowing how best to involve young people in research, and what impact this can have, can only be realised if evaluation is a feature of the activity. The questions 'How are we doing?', 'Are young people meaningfully involved in research activities?', and 'What difference do you think your involvement has made?' can only be answered if evaluation, both informal and formal, is included in your overall participation strategy. Young people must be enabled to share their experience of the research process and their involvement in it openly and honestly. Patton's (1997) definition of evaluation has been applied to work that has involved young people in public decision making (Kirby and Bryson, 2002), and could easily be adapted to participation in research:

> 'Programme (i.e. participation of young people in research) is the systematic collection of information about the activities, characteristics, and outcomes of programs to make judgements about the program, improve the programme effectiveness, and/or inform decisions about future programming' (p. 23).

This definition is a useful guide, as it focuses on both the process of how evaluations are undertaken as well as their purpose.

A further useful potential evaluation tool that can be adapted for this purpose is that developed by the UK National Youth Agency, which presents a series of standards and statements for use in hospitals, primary care trusts, and health services in general (http://www.nya.org.uk/hearbyright).

Hear By Right is a standards framework used primarily for improving participation within health services. It consists of seven standards based on the 'seven S' model of organisational change: shared values, strategy, structures, systems, staff, skills and knowledge, and style of leadership. Each standard encompasses seven indicators, which provide a proven guide to the key elements of building in participation (www.nya.org.uk). It relies on self-assessment divided into three levels of 'emerging', 'established', and 'advanced', with each level building on the last: it is useful for organisations or research teams that are seeking to build, expand, and embed principles of participation into all their activities. It will allow organisations or research teams to gauge progress against each standard, indicating evidence, including that from young people themselves.

Evaluation of involvement must be planned from the outset. Doing so, it is possible to collect the information as you go along rather than thinking about evaluation at the end. Finding out what works in involvement is an underdeveloped area, and researchers need to perform this aspect of involvement much better (Royal College of Nursing, 2007).

Conclusion

Building a culture of participation is not straightforward, and relates to concepts of consumerism, partnership, and empowerment. Smith *et al.* (2005) described 'user involvement' as rather like apple pie: thought to be a good thing, but with limited evidence that explores the meaning and importance of involvement. For example, do we know when and in what context young people who are cancer service users should be involved in research? This question might be more easily answered if practitioners and researchers bear in mind the main reasons for involving service users before they make their decision: (1) to improve the relevance of research, (2) to improve the quality of the research process, and (3) to benefit the service users involved (Smith *et al.*, 2005).

Involving young people in health services research is about opening up opportunities to them for meaningful participation based on their own realities and enabling them to have a real impact on the way their care is managed and delivered (Moules, 2005). It is about building and sustaining a culture of participation in organisations and facilitating ongoing dialogue with young people rather than imposing fixed structures. Involving young people may mean taking risks and making mistakes is part of the process of getting it right (Combe, 2002): evaluation is our only way of understanding more about the process and the outcome.

There is an expectation across a range of health services of increased and more meaningful consumer participation, involvement, and attempts to see the world through the eyes of children and young people (Darbyshire *et al.*, 2005; Coyne, 2006). Although guidance on how to promote involvement has become more widely available, recent research suggests that currently, in reality, their involvement is often limited (Cavet and Sloper, 2004). However, the 'tide may well be turning': the final chapter of this book is just one example of involving users in informing future service developments through the use of focus groups. Engaging with the challenges of young people's involvement in research in order to promote their right to participate is demanded in the way forward. We have the policy: we must as practitioners and researchers now use this policy to influence and sustain the participation of young people at all levels in cancer care.

References

Alderson, P. (2005) Designing ethical research with children. In: *Ethical Research with Children* (ed. A. Farrell), pp. 27–36. Open University Press, Buckingham.

Arnstein, S. R. (1969) Eight rungs on the ladder of citizen participation. *Journal of the American Institute of Planners*, **35**(4), 216–224.

Beresford, P. (2005) Theory and practice of user involvement in research: making the connection with public policy and practice. In: *Involving Service Users in Health and Social Research* (eds L. Lowes & I. Hulatt), pp. 6–17. Routledge, London & New York.

Cavet, J. & Sloper, P. (2004) The participation of children and young people in decisions about UK service development. *Child: Care, Health and Development*, **30**(6), 613–621.

Coad, J. & Lewis, A. (2004) *Engaging Children and Young People in Research. Literature Review for The National Evaluation of the Children's Fund*. University of Birmingham, Birmingham.

Combe, V. (2002) *Up for it: Getting Young People Involved in Local Government*. National Youth Agency for the Joseph Rowntree Foundation, London.

Consumers in NHS Research Support Unit (2000) *Involving Consumers in Research & Development in the NHS: Briefing Notes for Researchers*. Consumers in NHS Research Support Unit, London.

Coyne, I. (2006) Consultation with children in hospital: children, parents' and nurses' perspectives. *Journal of Clinical Nursing*, **15**, 61–71.

Curtis, K., Roberts, H., Copperman, J., Downie, A., & Liabo, K. (2004) 'How come I don't get asked no questions?' Researching 'hard to reach' children and teenagers. *Child and Family Social Work*, **9**, 167–175.

Darbyshire, P., MacDougall, C., & Schiller, W. (2005) Multiple methods in qualitative research with children: more insight or just more? *Qualitative Research*, **5**, 417–436.

Department of Health (1999) *Patient and Public Involvement in the New NHS*. Department of Health, London.

Department of Health (2000) *Research and Development for a First Class Service*. Department of Health, London.

Department of Health (2001) *Involving Patients and the Public in Healthcare: Response to the Listening Exercise*. Department of Health, London.

Department of Health (2002) *Listening, Hearing and Responding: Department of Health Action Plan, Core Principles for the Involvement of Children and Young People*. Department of Health, London.

Department of Health (2003a) *Strengthening Accountability. Involving Patients and the Public*. Policy guidance section 11 of the Health and Social Care Act 2001, pp. 1–16. Department of Health, London.

Department of Health (2003b) *Listening, Hearing and Responding: Department of Health Action Plan*. Department of Health, London.

Department of Health (2004) *Patient and Public Involvement in Health: The Evidence for Policy Implementation*. Department of Health, London.

Department of Health (2006) *Our Health, Our Care, Our Say: a New Direction for Community Services: A Brief Guide*. Department of Health, London.

Department of Health and Department for Education and Skills (2004) *National Service Framework for Children, Young People and Maternity Services: Executive Summary*. Department of Health, London.

France, A. (2004) Young people. In: *Doing Research with Children and Young People* (eds S. Fraser, V. Lewis, S. Ding, M. Kellett & C. Robinson), pp. 173–190. Sage Publications, London.

Gibson, F., Richardson, A., Hey, S., Horstman, M., & O'Leary, C. (2005) Listening to children and young people with cancer. Final report submitted to Macmillan Cancer.

Hart, R. A. (1992) *Children's Participation: From Tokenism to Citizenship*. Innocenti essays no. 4, UNICEF, Florence.

Hubbard, G., Kidd, L., Donaghy, E., McDonald, C., & Kearney, N. (2007) A review of literature about involving people affected by cancer in research, policy and planning and practice. *Patient Education and Counselling*, **65**, 21–33.

James, A. & Prout, A. (1997) *Constructing and Reconstructing Childhood*, 2nd edn. RoutledgeFalmer, London.

Kirby, P. (1999) *Involving Young Researchers: How to Enable Young People to Design and Conduct Research*. Joseph Rowntree Foundation, London.

Kirby, P. (2004) *A Guide to Actively Involving Young People in Research: For Researchers, Research Commissioners, and Managers*. INVOLVE Support Unit, Eastleigh, Hampshire.

Kirby, P. & Bryson, S. (2002) *Measuring the Magic? Evaluating and Researching Young People's Participation in Public Decision Making*. Carnegie Young People Initiative, London.

Lockey, R., Sitzia, J., Gillingham, T. *et al.* (2004) *Training for Service User Involvement in Health and Social Care Research: a Study of Training Provision and Participants' Experiences (The TRUE Project)*. Worthing and Southlands Hospitals NHS Trust, Worthing.

McLaughlin, H. (2006) Involving young service users as co-researchers: possibilities, benefits and costs. *British Journal of Social Work*, **36**, 1395–1410.

McNamara, C., Sadler, C., & Kelly, D. (2007) Involving cancer patients in the education of healthcare professionals. *Cancer Nursing Practice*, **6**, 33–37.

Mayall, B. (2006) Values and assumptions underpinning policy for children and young people in England. *Children's Geographies*, **4**(1), 9–17.

Moules, C. (2005) Research with children who use NHS services: sharing the experience. In: *Involving Service Users in Health and Social Research* (eds L. Lowes & I. Hulatt), pp. 140–151. Routledge, London & New York.

Newell, P. (1993) *The UN Convention and Children's Rights in the UK*, 2nd edn. Calouste Gulbenkian Foundation, National Children's Bureau, London.

Patton, Q. (1997) *Utilisation-focused Evaluation*. Sage, London.

Roberts, H. (2004) Health and social care. In: *Doing Research with Children and Young People* (eds S. Fraser, V. Lewis, S. Ding, M. Kellett, & C. Robinson), pp. 239–254. Sage Publications, London.

Royal College of Nursing (2007) *RCN Guidance on User Involvement in Research by Nurses*. Royal College of Nursing, London.

Sheir, H. (2001) Pathways to participation: openings, opportunities and obligations. *Children & Society*, **15**, 107–117.

Sinclair, R. (2004) Participation in practice: making it meaningful, effective and sustainable. *Children & Society*, **18**(2), 106–118.

Sloper, P. & Lightfoot, J. (2003) Involving disabled and chronically ill children and young people in health service development. *Child: Care, Health & Development*, **29**(1), 15–20.

Smith, E., Ross, F., Donovan, S. *et al.* (2005) *User Involvement in the Design and Undertaking of Nursing, Midwifery and Health Visiting Research*. National Co-ordinating Centre for NHS Service Delivery and Organisation R&D, London.

Smith, G. (2005) The rise of the 'new consumerism' in health and medicine in Britain, c. 1948–1989. In: *Researching Health Care Consumers: Critical Approaches* (eds J. Burr & P. Nicolson), pp. 13–38. Palgrave Macmillan, New York, NY.

Smith, S., Davies, S., Wright, D., Chapman, C., & Whiteson, M. (2007) The experiences of teenagers and young adults with cancer – results of 2004 conference survey. *European Journal of Oncology Nursing*, **11**, 362–368.

Stafford, A., Laybourn, A., & Hill, M. (2003) 'Having a say': children and young people talk about consultation. *Children & Society*, **17**, 361–373.

Steel, R. (2005) Actively involving marginalised and vulnerable people in research. In: *Involving Service Users in Health and Social Research* (eds L. Lowes & I. Hulatt), pp. 18–29. Routledge, London & New York.

Telford, R., Boote, J. D., & Cooper, C. L. (2004) What does it mean to involve consumers successfully in NHS research? A consensus study. *Health Expectations*, **7**, 209–220.

Turner, M. & Beresford, P. (2005) *User Controlled Research: Its Meanings and Potential*. Final report, Centre for Citizen Participation, Brunel University.

Veale, A. (2005) Creative methodologies in participatory research with children. In: *Researching Children's Experience: Approaches and Methods* (eds S. Green & D. Hogan), pp. 253–272. Sage Publications, London.

Chapter 11

Developing an Integrated Approach to the Care of Adolescents and Young Adults with Cancer

Daniel Kelly and Faith Gibson

Introduction

The contributors to this book have emphasised the unique challenges facing teenagers and young adults (TYAs) who are confronted with a cancer diagnosis. Their professional and personal experiences confirm the need for individualised, appropriate models of care tailored to the specific life situation of young people, as well as to the stage of disease. This is a laudable aim and one that most would accept. However, changing practice for the better and delivering truly individualised care also raises a number of key challenges for those providing and commissioning TYA services in reality. Our aim in this final chapter is to summarise these challenges and suggest how they might best be approached. How, for example, can we prioritise developments and target finite resources in ways that will benefit young people effectively? How do we know that the care we are providing is responsive, effective, and appropriate? How can we adopt an 'evidence-based' approach to care when we need more evidence to draw upon? The recent launch of the policy document *Guidance on Cancer Services: Improving Outcomes in Children and Young People with Cancer* (National Institute for Health and Clinical Excellence [NICE], 2005) was viewed as a major step forward in this regard. It was intended to draw upon empirical evidence and expert opinion to produce a series of recommendations, which, in turn, should be used for informing service development and practice. Although discussed briefly in Chapter 1, with passing reference made in many of the other chapters, Boxes 11.1 and 11.2 provide a summary of the key recommendations. It remains to be seen, however, to what extent improvements to services flow from such policy initiatives – or how likely they are to be adopted when financial investment or reconfiguration of services will be required. Local champions being creative with local solutions, we suggest, might not be enough. Without a consensus on a range of approaches to care delivery, and supporting evidence about 'what works', TYA services may well remain patchy and vulnerable. Ongoing evaluations will be needed to

---

Box 11.1   Key Treatment-focused recommendations from *Guidance on Cancer Services: Improving Outcomes in Children and Young People with Cancer*

Planning, commissioning, and funding for all aspects of care for children and young people with cancer, across the whole healthcare system, should be coordinated to ensure that there is an appropriate balance of service provision and allocation of resources. The principle that underpins the guidance is age-appropriate, safe, and effective services as locally as possible, not local services as safely as possible.

Commissioners should ensure the following.

1. There is a clear organisational structure for these services, including a cancer network lead for children and young people with cancer.
2. Appropriately trained staff should undertake all aspects of care for children and young people with cancer.
3. Principal treatment centres for each cancer type are identified for children and young people, with associated referral pathways, including to centres outside the network of residence when necessary.
4. Principal treatment centres are able to provide a sustainable range of services, with defined minimum levels of staffing, as outlined in the guidance.
5. Shared care arrangements are established, which identify a lead clinician and lead nurse and have approved clinical protocols for treatment and care and defined areas of responsibility with principal treatment centres.
6. All sites delivering cancer therapy in this age group should be subject to peer review.
7. All relevant national guidance is followed.

*NICE (2005).

---

identify improvements and establish how best to ensure that best practice is built upon in the longer term.

Alongside the recent NICE (2005) recommendations are rising expectations alongside cost restraints facing all health systems, including the National Health Service in the UK (Kelly and Trevatt, 2006). In such a climate it will be even more important to emphasise the impact of cancer on young people's lives, and to understand their needs and how they change over the course of the cancer trajectory. As previous chapters have shown, those working with teenagers and young adults develop insight into their unique needs and wish to ensure that they are met by sharing their experiences more widely.

Decisions about service developments must be built on a sound evidence base, however, with young people's needs being central to service provision. In many cases the emphasis is usually placed on the acute phase of treatment. Whilst this may be understandable, less attention has been paid to the end phase of acute interventions – or to situations where the disease progresses despite treatment. These are more challenging aspects of cancer care for TYA populations that will also need to be addressed in the future. Similar challenges will undoubtedly confront colleagues in other countries, where considerable variation exists in the way that cancer services are funded and delivered. However, international collaborations are also now much more possible, with the Internet opening up

---

Box 11.2   Key recommendations from *Guidance on Cancer Services: Improving Outcomes in Children and Young People with Cancer*

Care should be delivered throughout the patient pathway by multidisciplinary teams, including all relevant specialist staff. Membership and governance of these teams should be explicit and include clearly defined responsibility for clinical and managerial leadership.

Appropriately skilled, professional key workers should be identified to support individual children and young people and their families by (1) coordinating their care across the whole system and at all stages of the patient pathway, (2) providing information, and (3) assessing and meeting the needs for support.

All care for children and young people under 19 years old must be provided in age-appropriate facilities. Young people of 19 years and older should also have unhindered access to age-appropriate facilities and support when needed. All children and young people must have access to tumour-specific or treatment-specific clinical expertise as required.

Theatre and anaesthetic sessional time should be adequately resourced for all surgical procedures, including diagnostic and supportive procedures, in addition to other definitive tumour surgery. Anaesthetic sessional time should be assured for radiotherapy and other painful procedures. The paediatric surgeon with a commitment to oncology should have access to emergency theatre sessions during working hours.

All children and young people with cancer should be offered entry to any clinical research trial for which they are eligible and adequate resources should be provided to support such trials. Participation in trials must be an informed choice.

Children and young people with cancer who are not participating in clinical trials should be treated according to agreed treatment and care protocols based on expert advice and resources provided to monitor and evaluate outcomes.

The issues related to the registration of cancers in 15–24 year olds and the potential value of a dedicated register within the structure of the National Cancer Registries should be addressed urgently.

The need for trained specialist staff across all disciplines able to work with children and young people with cancer should be included in workforce development plans by cancer networks in order to ensure the provision of a sustainable service.

Specific attention is required to address the shortage of allied health professional expertise in this area and the evaluation of the contribution of such services.

NICE (2005).

---

opportunities for larger scale studies in this field. Collaboration on service developments remains more of a challenge.

The milestones that mark the different phases of care are important to bear in mind as they can provide us with a framework against which to benchmark TYAs' needs. The time around diagnosis, the experience of treatment, and life beyond cancer provide a useful way of considering care issues across the cancer care trajectory. They also provide points of emphasis for educational programmes and awareness raising, as well as helping to identify future research questions. The context of cancer care requires some further consideration, however, before drawing the messages within this book towards a final conclusion.

Putting service developments into context

The last decade has witnessed significant progress in the development of care for TYAs with cancer in the UK. Clinical practice has been shaped, and approaches to care influenced, by cancer policy developments and lobbying organisations such as the Teenage Cancer Trust. Since the early 1990s the Teenage Cancer Trust has been championing the recognition of the medical and psychosocial needs of teenagers and young adults. Three consistent messages have been emphasised within much of the literature in the last decade and throughout the preceding chapters:

1. TYAs should receive care from experts and highly specialised teams of healthcare professionals.
2. TYAs should receive care in a specialist age-appropriate cancer unit.
3. TYA care should be evidence based whenever possible.

Importantly, failure to accomplish these principles may have implications for survival, as well as for the overall quality of care.

First, consider the unambiguous and easily measured influence on survival of treatment and care that is led by specialised teams of healthcare professionals. As Chapter 1 identified, there is evidence that the survival rates for TYAs are less acceptable than might be expected, particularly when compared to the results for children over the same period (Birch, 2005). There is also evidence that survival rates vary geographically across Europe and it is known that, in the UK and USA, the cancer incidence in 20–24 year olds is double that in children (Gatta *et al.*, 2003, Birch, 2005). In relation to treatment and survival there are two recurring arguments: the need for treatments tailored to disease biology rather than age, and the need to increase the uptake of clinical trials. Both, it is argued, would be resolved if TYAs were referred to dedicated units with a close interface between professionals from paediatric and adult practice (Stevens, 2006).

Second, the less obvious and the more difficult to measure influence on survival of care delivered in a dedicated TYA unit. Evidence suggests that the quality of the treatment experience is improved when TYAs are cared for in a dedicated unit providing age-appropriate management (Kelly *et al.*, 2002, 2004; Mullhall *et al.*, 2001). Although the treatment experience may not directly impact on survival, the quality of that survival may be influenced, with the TYAs having been guided confidently and sensitively in the short- and long-term management of their illness. As Chapter 1 also argued, however, the extent to which the care setting impacts upon adherence to therapy and follow-up, and on the willingness to enter clinical trials, factors that have all been linked to improved survival, is less clear. Despite the lack of research on the impact of the care environment, there is evidence focusing on the needs of TYAs that affirms the need to consider the physical, psychological, and social consequences of any disturbance to health in parallel with treatment (Lynam, 1995; Neville, 2005).

Third, the need for an evidence-based cancer policy. It has been argued elsewhere that tension exists between the twin aims of cure and care, suggesting that the current models of care may fail to facilitate integration (Lewis, 2005). Two

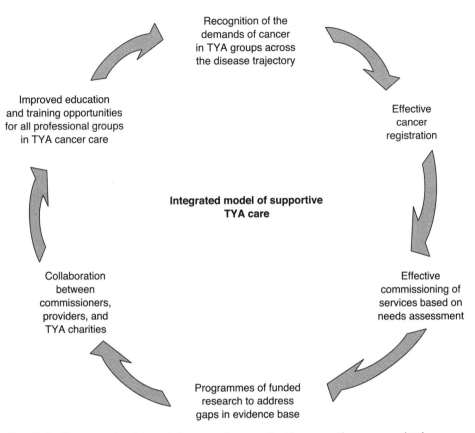

Fig. 11.1 Features of an integrated approach to meeting the supportive care needs of teenagers and young adults with cancer.

initiatives, however, herald hope for change: the recently published NICE (2005) document *Guidance on Cancer Services: Improving Outcomes in Children and Young People with Cancer* and the establishment of a clinical studies group for TYAs by the National Cancer Research Institute. The former policy document recommends that TYAs have access to age-appropriate facilities and the latter that TYAs have opportunities to enter disease-specific clinical trials and other research protocols. In addition to these two important initiatives, there is a growing range of policy and other professional and non-professional literature drawing on evidence and experience that clarifies both the purpose and outcome of dedicated TYA facilities, reference to which can be found in the preceding chapters. But how can we use the policy documents to effect change, and to continue to progress developments in the care of TYAs? How might we prioritise the steps to be taken? Clearly strong leadership and a desire to affect change in the delivery of services will be important if the current *status quo* is to be challenged (Kelly and Hooker, 2006).

Contributing to the evidence base

For the final chapter of this book we sought to draw on both professional and user views to examine how we might continue to shape developments in the care of TYAs: naturally this might also reveal current experiences that might illuminate both good and unhelpful aspects of current service provision. Our approach was to contact three established organisations in the UK: Teenagers and Young Adults with Cancer, the National Alliance of Childhood Cancer Parent Organisations, and the UK Survivors Group, inviting members to participate in a focused discussion. Three such discussion groups took place with six professionals, three mothers, and two young women. We note the female gender bias in the user group, however, this reflected the response to our invitations. The discussions were guided by one of the authors using a series of focused questions and were recorded on tape alongside brief notes taken by the second author. Each group lasted approximately 60–90 minutes. The tapes were not transcribed verbatim: instead a tape-based analysis was undertaken, noting recurring themes and areas of agreement. The discussions were integrated into the following discussion and shared with the participants prior to publication. In addition, research evidence and reflections on the content of the preceding chapters as well as the personal experience of the authors were combined to produce the conclusions in this final chapter. Cancer is never a welcome diagnosis, and its impact will always have ramifications beyond the physical effects. Its emotional and social impact will be felt far beyond the person before us in the clinic or hospital bed. For those of us who write about these issues there is the hope that sharing experiences can make a difference. By including some of the views of those with personal experience of cancer, however, we hope that this final chapter will have even more resonance.

Issues around diagnosis

Delay in diagnosis

Raising awareness of the risk of a cancer diagnosis was considered an important point of emphasis from everyone's perspective. The fact that many TYAs will experience delays and frustrations about their initial symptoms and being taken seriously might well present the first challenge. Within our discussions with young people and parents about this issue they had insight and realised that cancer may be a rare diagnosis for a general practitioner (GP) to consider. However, personal experience had suggested that delays added to the already considerable anxiety associated with the presenting symptoms. For instance, headaches or pain in one part of the body may have been reported several times before they were eventually referred for assessment. Whilst it is difficult to make concrete recommendations regarding a timely diagnosis for TYAs, this is an issue to be considered in any strategy to raise awareness of adolescent cancer, especially with primary care professionals and through health initiatives with young people. An analogy may be made with recent meningitis awareness campaigns with university students and parents in the UK – rather than raising unnecessary alarm it was intended to remind them (and health professionals) of the key signs of the disease and how important it is that they are detected early. A similar approach may be possible when awareness-raising strategies about cancer in TYAs are being developed. As cancer in this group may be considered rare and the presenting symptoms are diverse and non-specific, this may be a particularly difficult area of practice to influence: however, it remains important, given the experiences of many young people and parents who repeatedly visited their GP before their symptoms were taken seriously. Some experienced so much frustration and delay that they felt relieved when the diagnosis was eventually made, as they had begun to question their own sanity.

Impact of a cancer diagnosis

A diagnosis of cancer may be considered a traumatic and life-changing event at any age. In TYAs, however, it may have extra resonance, as it is so unexpected. Anxiety about treatment, side effects, and the longer-term prognosis are likely to be the most immediate concerns of most young people and those close to them. General negative associations with cancer are likely to compound the diagnostic experience significantly. The provision of effective, evidence-based care during the diagnostic phase of care is especially challenging due to the uncertainty and shock that many families experience at this time. The initial presenting symptoms of cancer, for instance, are problematic due to their often vague nature, a situation that is compounded by the fact that they can be experienced over a prolonged period of time with little insight of their eventual significance. Brain tumours, for instance, may be heralded by headaches of varying severity, mood changes, and associated physical or psychological symptoms. Previous research in this area is limited. However, those studies that are available suggest that, in childhood cancer, the diagnosis may often be delayed due to the symptoms being dismissed by professionals – despite parents' concerns that something is wrong (Dixon-Woods *et al.*, 2001). More recently, the significance of patient and professional delay has been examined, revealing that the older the young person the more likely that they will experience delay. The symptom interval was also longer in those presenting to a GP compared with an emergency department (Goyal *et al.*, 2004). These studies hypothesise reasons for patient delay in the older age group, suggesting that, in the absence of physician and parental awareness, including frequent observation, diagnosis relies on a process of self-reporting that may be unreliable. What is absent from this limited body of evidence is the voice of TYAs themselves, which might illuminate determinants for the lag time that may relate more to their behaviour or experiences of accessing healthcare.

Impact on the family

It must be remembered that cancer is a life-threatening disease and, as such, has implications for the whole of the TYA's life. As Chapter 2 discussed, besides the physical impact on the developing body, there are psychological effects due to the gravity of the illness: profound changes to everyday life and the impact on the young person's future. A diagnosis of cancer requires physical, social, and psychological effects of a life-threatening disease to be confronted. Among the psychological challenges is the profound uncertainty around the status and progression of the cancer: disruptions to everyday family and social life as well as fear about the long-term future. As previous chapters have highlighted, finding meaning in serious illness and dependence constitutes a challenge that all people with a cancer diagnosis will face. For the TYA, additonal burdens associated with this life stage may compound the distress experienced when a diagnosis of cancer is eventually made. This reinforces the need for adequate information and support being available around the diagnostic phase. The professionals recognised the importance of support that is necessary outside of the hospital and emphasised the role of parents, siblings, and friends in helping TYAs to cope with the ups and downs of cancer treatment.

Supporting young people at diagnosis

People who have been through a similar experience may be best placed to offer advice and support to others. The young people we spoke to about this issue concurred, but also felt that parents, siblings, and friends will need sources of support of their own. For some families there appeared to be considerable stress placed on marriages after the diagnosis. Gender differences were also discussed, with some fathers in particular being unable to communicate their fears to others. Some seemed to withdraw emotionally to protect themselves. Within friendships, some friends remained loyal and knew instinctively what to do, whilst others withdrew, probably indicating feelings of inadequacy added to a fear of the unknown. Clearly much more work is needed in this area of supportive care.

Websites or telephone helplines may be particularly useful to some when they are coming to terms with a cancer diagnosis. The availability of support and information when it is needed, rather than relying on a nine-to-five service, is also an important consideration. The ability to seek clarification and explanation of what has been said in clinical consultations is an important feature of any information resource, and the 24-hour nature of the Internet may be uniquely valuable in this regard. Caution, however, should also be advised when accessing unmonitored or non-sanctioned sites. Young people should be encouraged to seek expert guidance to interpret medical information in relation to their own circumstances. Nonetheless, the availablilty of Internet-based resources will mean they are likely to be important sources of information for young people from very early in their trajectory of care – despite variations in the accuracy of different sites.

Delivering appropriate care

An important point of note is that, once a cancer diagnosis has been made, the provision of appropriate care relies on support being on hand to help with the new 'destination map' that will now guide the TYA's life. A diagnosis of cancer may be constructed as something experienced 'internally' by the individual concerned or more 'externally' by other people (such as parents, friends, siblings, or health professionals). An internal perspective places value on the TYA's own perception of their situation. However, external (especially professionalised) perspectives may disregard – and may even devalue – subjective experience in favour of objective, measurable concerns (such as tumour volume reduction or response rates more generally) (Conrad, 1987). We would advocate the importance of recognising and seeking ways to understand the internal, subjective experience of a cancer diagnosis on the TYA. Without this there is a danger of failing to address the human costs of cancer and focusing instead on the more impersonal implications in this age group. Doing so may help to emphasise the balance between the need for supportive care/health services research and rigorous clinical trials for new drugs and other treatment advances.

The emotional impact of a cancer diagnosis may be difficult to appreciate in healthcare settings, which are often characterised by fixed routines, a rapid tempo of work, and a lack of privacy. Understanding events like a diagnosis of cancer, according to Ricouer (1985), will require time and the opportunity for explanation and interpretation as well as suggestions for how the experience may be improved for others in the future. Once diagnosed, the TYA will inevitably assume many different roles: that of a 'cancer patient', as well as, possibly, a 'family protector'. This will require them to learn the rules of these roles, as well as to manage the fluctuating demands of treatment and the associated side effects. Providing an integrated approach to TYA cancer care requires the diagnostic phase to be recognised as a crucial time that will change the life course for the whole family (Woodgate, 2005). By being supported at this time, the TYA may cope more effectively with the treatment phase. All of those we spoke to about the diagnostic phase emphasised the need for adequate support, explanation, and a person-centred approach to ensure that treatment can be faced with the belief that the best care available will be provided.

The treatment phase

The period spent as an inpatient will always be a defining feature of a cancer experience. Whether this is considered a good or less positive experience, young people and families do value being asked about their care and will take time to respond to such a question. Not surprisingly, therefore, the experience of hospital care featured prominently in the accounts of parents and young people.

Where should care be delivered?

The families we spoke with had experienced care from a cancer centre (paediatric), shared care, and a regional adult surgical unit: however, none had received care in a Teenage Cancer Trust unit, although one paediatric unit did have a 'teenage room'. The young women we spoke to about this issue had received cancer treatment on a paediatric oncology unit, with one receiving some care on a general adult surgical unit and the other spending some time on a general adolescent ward. Underpinning much of their discussions was the focus in the various care settings on meeting the needs of younger children: this included the types of information available, the way in which information was imparted, and, finally, the environment and facilities themselves.

Helpful and unhelpful ways of communicating

Information was considered essential throughout the treatment phase. Parents noted that this was often written for younger children or 'geared to little people', as were many of the resources they found when actively searching websites. Professionals who often used 'babyish' language when imparting information around the time of diagnosis compounded this by failing to provide appropriate explanations during treatment. The need for accurate and detailed information to be given directly was considered essential. One mother spoke about a doctor getting this right: 'he looked my son in the eye and told him exactly what was happening and spoke to him like a grown-up.' This response was from a doctor who normally cared for adults and was considered by the mother to have a 'better approach' than the professionals who cared for children, where the 'babyish' language was a 'turn-off'. There was a sense that young people were being 'spoken down to' and that some professionals were getting it wrong consistently. Sometimes it was felt that the appearance and perceived attitude of the young person may have hindered the process – with some professionals taking insufficient time to get to know the TYA and, hence, often being in danger of aiming information at the wrong level. In addition, parents spoke of professionals simply not 'being able to get through' TYA defence mechanisms because of an inappropriate approach – what one mother referred to as the 'Kevin attitude' (named after a particularly recalcitrant adolescent UK television character).

For the parents, 'knowing how to speak with young people' was considered an important skill through all the phases of care, and one that not everyone they had come into contact with had demonstrated. The young people echoed these concerns: they spoke of staff who seemed to find young people 'difficult' to care for as they lacked the necessary social skills or expertise to communicate with them. While this issue has been discussed at some length in recent years in the UK, it would appear that the setting of cancer care for young people who are on the cusp of adulthood remains relevant, especially from the perspective of those who have direct personal experience of cancer. The role of dedicated units, with specialist expertise, support structures, and age-appropriate environments that meet the individual needs of young people, seems to represent at least the core elements of a successful approach to TYA cancer care (Mulhall *et al.*, 2001; Kelly *et al.*, 2004; Smith, 2004; Arbuckle *et al.*, 2005; Gallini and Hooker, 2005; Lewis, 2005; Morgan, 2005).

It is arguable that knowing how to speak with young people has more to do with one's attitude and approach, and is a reflection of our personal values and confidence. However, there was a sense that much could be done about improving communication outside of TYA dedicated units. This may also be an issue for hospital, shared care, and social services to consider. All may be involved in the care of TYAs during cancer treatment, and all will need the appropriate skills and understanding of communication at this time.

Creating the right environment for care

The lack of education and training available to those choosing to work with TYAs was an issue noted by all the professionals we spoke to. Although there was mention of some well-developed local initiatives, national or multi-professional educational opportunities were not available. Some nursing courses, which were mentioned as being 'at risk' or diminishing in the present economic climate, were felt to provide only minimal content about the needs of TYAs. It was felt that specialist education and training did not receive sufficient endorsement from the medical, nursing, and allied health professional organisations. However, some educational initiatives appeared to be on the horizon, with web-based programmes being supported by organisations such as the Teenage Cancer Trust. All the professionals also highlighted clinical expertise as being crucial and this is supported by recent policy documents, with cancer treatment and supportive care needing to be considered in tandem. There was also mention of identifying and describing core competencies of TYA care in the future that might provide the focus for education and training.

All the mothers reflected on the positive and negative aspects of the environments in which they encountered TYA care. Choice was clearly a feature for some families and was usually offered because of the patient's age. However, when the question of whether they would like to be cared for in a children's ward or an adult ward was actually put to them, although considered an important and fundamental decision, the early treatment phase was actually a very difficult time to make such a decision. At the age of 16 years one of the young women we spoke to had opted for a children's ward and had no regrets. When reflecting on place of care our discussions also revealed mothers weighing up the advantages and disadvantages in terms of 'family care' issues and the benefits to their child's ongoing social and supportive needs, rather than the cancer treatment itself. It was almost assumed, however, that treatment expertise would exist in either setting. The mothers spoke about the Teenage Cancer Trust developments and the availability of specialist units, and about distance from home being important. The closeness of friends who could visit, as well as having the opportunity to go home during the day when TYAs were admitted, for example, with febrile neutropenic episodes, was an important element in the location of care decision. Similarly, a parent being able to stay with the TYA when necessary, yet still being able to keep home life going, was considered a beneficial option. There was a strong and negative feeling of isolation from the family unit when the distance to home from the treatment centre was considered to be too great. Families were clearly faced with making very difficult decisions about the place of care early in their relationship with healthcare professionals. Ensuring that this is an informed decision that families make, balancing what they know is available alongside the needs of all members, is an important information message for healthcare professionals.

Mothers spoke about receiving excellent care, but felt that the 'children's' environment, although not a major issue, had impacted negatively on their child's experience and, hence, their response to a hospital admission. For example, cartoon character duvet covers, inappropriate pictures on the walls, and small children making lots of noise were memorable features of the children's unit. Other support services, such as the need for appropriate play specialists/activity workers that could focus on the specific needs of TYAs, were also mentioned. One young woman spoke with some anger about being approached by a play specialist to play with children's clay during cancer treatment when she was 14 years old.

The contentious question of location of care, although a significant feature at diagnosis, may recur when access to other treatment options, such as surgery, plays a part in the treatment trajectory. Paediatric units may be deemed preferable for younger teenagers (or for those with what may be considered a cancer of childhood, such as a Wilms' tumour). However, the young women and parents we talked with did not always remember this in a positive light. One young woman spoke about being cared for in a mixed sex bay when she considered herself an 'almost fully developed woman' at 14 years old. The primary problems with this situation included a lack of privacy, embarrassment, and feeling awkward (issues not likely to be confined to this age group). She spoke with some mortification about having to use a commode in a mixed sex bay. There may be a view that, in contrast with older adults, TYAs are happy to be cared for in mixed sex bays – however, this clearly may not be the case. Respecting individual choice regarding privacy and dignity is paramount in such situations. Few criticisms were directed at the medical or nursing care, however, the long-term nature of admissions for radiotherapy or surgery meant that the setting of care does assume greater importance for some. Examples were also given of too much emphasis being placed on education in hospital, when all they needed was the space 'to be ill'.

Supporting young people during treatment

Psychosocial care that included the young person and other family members featured highly in our discussions. This was important during as well as after treatment when 'less allowance is made and you're treated as more normal'. The need to get on with life and focus on survival and attaining life goals were also issues reflected upon. Activities that could be maintained, such as keeping up with friends, going back to school, playing sport, and having 'treats' when feeling well, had an important part to play in keeping spirits up and making treatment feel worthwhile. Internet access, keeping in touch with friends, and life outside of hospital, such as school or college, were important, but rarely available at the time these families received treatment. There was also tension around the issue of making friends with other young people with cancer or choosing to remain more isolated as an inpatient. Wanting to talk to others in the same boat, whilst also feeling afraid to get close to the few other young people they encountered, was described as 'worrying'. Yet the need to talk about the experience, for some young people and mothers, was an important coping strategy and has been supported by research on a specialist TYA unit (Kelly *et al.*, 2004). Talking to other young people on such a unit might be an option for some, but the anxieties of getting close to someone who then dies was implicit in some of our discussions. The double worry that 'I could lose a mate' and 'that could be me next' might well be ongoing unspoken fears that some might find difficult to express. Counselling services had been found to be sparse yet useful if they focused on the needs of young people. Counselling and being able to talk about the challenges of cancer treatment are clearly not a universal expectation: however, they do highlight once again the importance of individual approaches to the planning and delivery of care and social support for TYAs. A telephone help line was also mentioned as a possible alternative to face-to-face services. There is new evidence emerging on the benefits of care being delivered on a specialist unit from surveys with young people themselves. Smith *et al*, (2007) questioned 350 young people in the UK at a Find Your Sense of Tumour Conference and found that the majority who have had cancer preferred to be treated on a specialist unit. This finding supports the need for more research to be undertaken to understand young people's reasons more fully. There is also a need to compare the setting of care with other outcome variables, such as survival, as well as patient and family satisfaction.

Role and significance of family members

There was an overwhelming sense of feeling 'on your own', with mothers speaking about needing to take the lead in finding resources and being proactive in advocating for the young person's needs. At the same time they wanted to be recognised as having a role and their own individual needs as a person, not simply seen as 'mum' whose only role was to look after their child. Similarly, they wanted to be referred to by name and not simply as 'mum', thereby being seen as people with specific supportive care needs separate from their child. Once again these findings are supported by recent empirical work on the needs of parents at this time (Grinyer, 2002; Young *et al.*, 2002). The availability of facilities for parents, such as a quiet room and access to a kitchen, was variable and constituted some of the 'little things' necessary to provide the space and opportunity to look after oneself or to allow all the parents on the unit to share experiences. These are examples of the more nuanced features of supportive care that service providers should consider when establishing integrated facilities or approaches to care.

There were central concerns shared about the impact of cancer on the whole family. The young people emphasised the multiple needs that parents have to be informed and supported about what is happening to their child. In some sense this seems to be a prerequisite if they themselves are to cope with the demands of the illness (Woodgate, 2006). There may be some gendered aspects to this situation, with mothers expressing different needs to fathers (Grinyer, 2002; Hovey,

2003). It may also be common for mothers to be present when the child is undergoing treatment, with fathers having to work and, thus, connecting with the everyday reality of treatment less often. This may be implicated in extra stress being placed on the marriage at such a difficult time, and an extra source of worry for TYAs, who may pick up on signs of relationship discord. This situation suggests the need for more awareness of the strain imposed on relationships (as well as other family members) when cancer is diagnosed in this age group. Whilst services may be unlikely to offer dedicated relationship support, it may be necessary to examine this aspect of supportive care in less formal ways, as well as in dedicated research studies, to ensure that enough is being done. The evidence base could certainly be strengthened in the future in this regard.

As Chapters 5 and 6 show, there are multiple issues to consider when supporting TYAs through the treatment experience. Many revolve around recognition of the individual within a system that is usually based on routines and predetermined schedules. Integrated approaches to treatment-related support emphasise individual and family needs alongside the challenges (such as boredom, depression, or other side effects) that will be encountered during arduous treatments. Importantly, however, they also recognise that life will continue beyond treatment and place importance on considering how best to see beyond immediate concerns to the future and all that it will bring.

Beyond treatment

As survival rates improve there are concerns about those TYAs who may need to be transferred to adult services for ongoing care (such as fertility assessment or reconstructive surgery). Once again, this raises practical as well as philosophical questions about age-appropriate care and the need for it to be available to as many young people as possible. Fertility is only one of the physical and emotional sequelae of cancer and its treatment. However, it is a good example of how 'the future' will always impact on the cancer experience. Importantly, it may serve as a reminder of all that is being lost in order to effect a cure. Young women may experience concerns about their fertility that will require intensive investigations over a long period of time. Those TYAs who survive cancer then face new challenges when confronted with the need to engage partners in discussions about fertility and their life together. This may bring them into contact with endocrinology services – a further reminder of the profound change that their body has undergone as a result of cancer. For young men sperm banking may have been completed without much thought being given to the existential message associated with this procedure (Quinn and Kelly, 2000).

The need for continuing care

More awareness of the lasting impact of cancer seems to be the recurring theme here, and it emphasises the need for appropriate models of rehabilitation, in its broadest sense, for this patient group. Once again, there is a weak evidence base at present upon which policy or services may be planned (Doyle and Kelly, 2006). Whilst life continues after treatment the quality of this life should be a concern for service providers (Hokkanen *et al.*, 2004). For those who do survive there may be a need for late effects services, as Chapter 8 has argued. Seamless care will remain an important feature for follow-up services. The young women spoke passionately about the need for continuing care from those professionals with whom they had already formed a crucial and supportive relationship, a finding supported through ongoing research (Gibson *et al.*, 2005). One worry about follow-up was the requirement of accessing multiple professionals as health needs became more complex. This was influenced both by the complex nature of cancer and its treatment and by normal developmental changes. Integrated models of service provision should include consideration of this requirement – an inevitable consequence of improved survival rates.

Sexual and relationship concerns are inevitable within the TYA population. Both young women in our discussions, for instance, spoke about being kept 'in the dark' and 'uninformed' about their own fertility. Given this fact, it is important to recognise the value placed on those who have the necessary time and expertise to support this aspect of care. Social workers, counsellors, voluntary groups, and websites can each offer different means of support – and at a time when it is actually needed (and not necessarily determined by chronological age). Once again it is important to emphasise that support needs do not always emerge during the working day, an issue which those commissioning TYA services need to consider when putting programmes of support into place. From our discussions and from the literature available, there is a sense of limited resources being available when treatment is completed. In addition, there appear to be variable levels of support available from schools or colleges when TYAs return to them. Tension may exist between being recognised and supported as a young person who has survived cancer and being treated as 'normal' (Kyngäs *et al.*, 2001). The support gained from others who have had cancer, received through the UK Survivors Group and other groups, was of definite benefit to some (although less so to others). However, knowing about the support available, as well as being informed and aware of where to access help, are key requirements when coping with the long-term uncertainty associated with cancer (e.g. the Birmingham Study Centre Survivors Help Line).

Supporting young people after treatment

Self-help or lobbying groups, such as the UK Survivors Group (www.clicsargent.org.uk/Aboutchildhoodcancer/OnlineCommunity) and the International Survivors Group (www.icccpo.org/articles/general/survivors_group_2003.html), clearly have a role to play in informing young people about adapting to life after treatment as well as coping with late effects. However, information will also have to be gained from expert professionals, as well as other young people, families and siblings, and friends who have also survived cancer. Each can provide helpful insights that help to shape an integrated approach to TYA cancer care. The danger is that we adopt a 'fight or flight' approach to cancer and focus on treatment and survival rates alone, without considering the long-term needs of all of those who have to live with the reality of survival.

As Chapter 9 has also shown, we must be mindful of those TYAs who, despite treatment, will succumb to their cancer. End of life care must always be a necessary feature of any integrated approach. Inevitably, this relies on expert symptom control, access to the services necessary as required, and a flexible and person-centred philosophy that allows the dying process to be the best that can be achieved (Kelly and Edwards, 2005). A model of care that encompasses a programme for the bereaved would also be welcome. In reality, however, there is remarkably little research about the end of life experiences of TYAs and, hence, a poor research base of evidence upon which to base palliative care (Hinds *et al.*, 2004). This, we suggest, should be addressed in empirical studies drawing on a range of research methods and sponsors (such as cancer charities and statutory funding bodies).

Towards an integrated approach to TYA cancer care

This chapter has drawn the key messages of the preceding chapters together to consider the diagnostic, treatment, and longer-term dimensions of TYA cancer care. Figure 11.1 captures the key elements of an integrated approach in a diagrammatic form. Undoubtedly there is a need for further research and development in this area, and debates will continue about the most appropriate setting for TYAs to receive cancer care. More positively, however, we can see a groundswell of awareness generally, with the publication of policy documents and the work of charities such as the Teenage Cancer Trust and professional interest groups such as Teenagers and Young Adults with Cancer (www.tyac.org.uk) and the National Cancer Research Institute TYA Clinical Study Group in the UK, in addition to the UK Survivors Group and the International Survivors Group. The need for accurate registration systems as well as more appropriate clinical trials in order to improve survival is now increasingly acknowledged. To this extent the times do seem to be changing. The expertise gathered in this book is testament to how far we have come in advancing the care needs of this unique cancer population. The young people, mothers, and professionals we spoke to emphasised the need to recognise the age-related 'differences' that shape the cancer experience. These focus primarily on the additional demands of facing cancer during the time of life normally associated with growing up, leaving home, and finding a place in the world.

The psychological, social, and educational impacts of cancer in TYAs are important factors to be considered alongside survival statistics: importantly, each may be influenced by the current approach to care (which all agreed was open to improvement). Although concerns regarding the failure of the current service to meet the needs of this patient group have been well described and soundly articulated, the reality remains that care is inconsistent and gaps do remain in service provision (Whiteson, 2005). The recent NICE (2005) guidance places specific emphasis on the role of cancer networks and charges them with some responsibility, through commissioners, for the implementation of a clear organisational structure that provides 'age-appropriate, safe and effective services as locally as possible, not local services as safely as possible' (p. 7). Some of this may require investment in new facilities and a new workforce, for example, or the development of care pathways, improved models of multi-professional follow-up, or end of life support. The existence of policy recommendations, however, does not automatically deliver improved services: prioritising investment in TYA services over other patient groups remains a significant and fundamental barrier to be overcome. However, this situation simply makes the messages within this book even more, rather than less, relevant.

The real challenge of achieving an integrated approach to TYA cancer care rests on ensuring that service providers both recognise that what exists may no longer be appropriate and are able to deliver change. Local champions and political lobbying are two approaches mentioned that can influence the direction and rate of change. Expert opinion leaders were also felt to be necessary, particularly where evidence is lacking. Users of the service have a role in calling for tangible improvements where they are needed and professionals have an opportunity to advance the registration, clinical trial recruitment, and health services research agenda to ensure that the present weaknesses are recognised and addressed, with the corresponding positive impact upon both treatment success and patient outcomes. Voluntary and professional groups need to develop more effective forms of dialogue (at a local and international level) and commissioners of services should be encouraged to engage with the challenge of providing equitable, effective, and sustainable systems of TYA care provision throughout the patient pathway. This will, in the end, help to ensure that the individual young person behind the cancer statistic remains the focus of our attention.

Acknowledgements

We would like to thank the following individuals who took part in discussions about the focus of this chapter: Di Braithwaite, Lorraine Case, Simon Davies, Bryony Carr, Caroline Field, Anna Jones, Louise Hooker, Rebecca Lofts, Ginny Macintyre, Maria Michelagnoli, and Jeremy Whelan.

References

Arbuckle, J., Cotton, R., Eden, T. O. B., Jones, R., & Leonard, R. (2005) Who should care for young people with cancer. In: *Cancer and the Adolescent*, 2nd edn (eds T. Eden, R. Barr, A. Bleyer, & M. Whiteson), pp. 231–240. Blackwell, Oxford.

Birch, J. M. (2005) Patterns of incidence of cancer in teenagers and young adults: implications for aetiology. In: *Cancer and the Adolescent*, 2nd edn (eds T. Eden, R. Barr, A. Bleyer, & M. Whiteson), pp. 13–32. Blackwell, Oxford.

Conrad, P. (1987) The experience of illness: recent and new directions. *Research in Sociological Health Care*, **6**, 1–31.

Dixon-Woods, M., Findlay, M., Young, B., Cox, H., & Heney, D. (2001) Parents' accounts of obtaining a diagnosis of childhood cancer. *Lancet*, **357**, 670–674.

Doyle, N. & Kelly, D. (2006) So what happens now? Issues in cancer survival and rehabilitation. *Clinical Effectiveness in Nursing*, **9**, 147–153.

Gallini, A. & Hooker, L. (2005) Young people's and carer's views on the cancer services they receive. *Cancer Nursing Practice*, **4**, 27–32.

Gatta, G., Capocaccia, R., De Angelis, R., Stiller, C., & Coeberg, J. W.; The EUROCARE Working Group (2003) Cancer survival in European adolescents and young adults. *European Journal of Cancer*, **39**(18), 2571–2786.

Gibson, F., Aslett, H., Levitt, G., & Richardson, A. (2005) Follow up after childhood cancer: a typology of young people's health care needs. *Clinical Effectiveness in Nursing*, **9**, 133–146.

Goyal, S., Roscoe, J., Ryder, W. D. J., Gattamaneni, H. R., & Eden, T. O. B. (2004) Symptom interval in young people with bone cancer. *European Journal of Cancer*, **40**(15), 2280–2286.

Grinyer, A. (2002) *Cancer in Young Adults. Through Parents' Eyes.* Open University Press, Buckingham.

Hinds, P. S., Pritchard, M., & Harper, J. (2004) End-of-life research as a priority for pediatric oncology. *Journal of Pediatric Oncology Nursing*, **21**(3), 175–179.

Hokkanen, H., Eriksson, E., Ahonen, O., & Salantera, S. (2004) Adolescents with cancer: experience of life and how it could be made easier. *Cancer Nursing*, **27**(4), 325–335.

Hovey, J. K. (2003) The needs of fathers parenting children with chronic conditions. *Journal of Pediatric Oncology Nursing*, **20**(5), 245–251.

Kelly, D. & Edwards, J. (2005) Palliative care for adolescents and young adults. In: *Handbook of Palliative Care*, 2nd edn (eds C. Faull, Y. Carter, & L. Daniels), pp. 317–331. Blackwell, Oxford.

Kelly, D. & Hooker, L. (2006) Evidence based cancer policy: the needs of teenagers and young adults. Editorial. *European Journal of Oncology Nursing*, **11**, 4–5.

Kelly, D. & Trevatt, P. (2006) NHS Finances. *Cancer Nursing Practice*, **5**(8), 14–17.

Kelly, D., Pearce, S., & Mulhall, A. (2002) Adolescent cancer – the need to evaluate current service provision in the UK. *European Journal of Oncology Nursing*, **7**, 53–58.

Kelly, D., Pearce, S., & Mullhall, A. (2004) 'Being in the same boat': ethnographic insights into an adolescent cancer unit. *International Journal of Nursing Studies*, **41**, 847–857.

Kyngäs, H., Mikkonen, R., Nousiainen, E. M. *et al.* (2001) Coping with the onset of cancer: coping strategies and resources of young people with cancer. *European Journal of Cancer Care*, **10**, 6–11.

Lewis, I. (2005) Patterns of care for young people with cancer: is there a single blueprint of care? In: *Cancer and the Adolescent*, 2nd edn (eds T. Eden, R. Barr, A. Bleyer, & M. Whiteson), pp. 241–259. Blackwell, Oxford.

Lynam, J. (1995) Supporting one another: the nature of family work when a young adult has cancer. *Journal of Advanced Nursing*, **2**, 116–125.

Morgan, S. (2005) Managing professional relationships across the services. In: *Cancer and the Adolescent*, 2nd edn (eds T. Eden, R. Barr, A. Bleyer, & M. Whiteson), pp. 259–269. Blackwell, Oxford.

Mullhall, A., Kelly, D., & Pearce, S. (2001) Naturalistic approaches to health care evaluation: the case of a teenage cancer unit. *Journal of Clinical Excellence*, **3**, 167–174.

National Institute for Health and Clinical Excellence (2005) *Guidance on Cancer Services: Improving Outcomes in Children and Young People with Cancer*. National Institute for Health and Clinical Excellence, London.

Neville, K. (2005) The impact of cancer on adolescents and their families. In: *Cancer and the Adolescent*, 2nd edn (eds T. Eden, R. Barr, A. Bleyer, & M. Whiteson), pp. 165–179. Blackwell, Oxford.

Quinn, B, & Kelly, D. (2000) Sperm banking and fertility concerns: enhancing the support available to men with cancer. *European Journal of Oncology Nursing*, **4**, 55–58.

Ricouer, P. (1985) *Time & Narrative*. University of Chicago Press, Chicago.

Smith, S. (2004) Adolescent units – an evidence-based approach to quality nursing in adolescent care. *European Journal of Oncology Nursing*, **8**, 20–29.

Smith, S., Davies, S., Wright, D., Chapman, C. and Whiteson, M. (2007) The experience of teenagers and young adults with cancer – results of 2004 conference survey. *European Journal of Oncology Nursing*, **11**: 362–368.

Stevens, M. (2006) The 'lost tribe' and the need for a promised land: the challenge of cancer in teenagers and young adults. *European Journal of Cancer*, **42**, 280–281.

Whiteson, M. (2005) A right. Not a privilege! In: *Cancer and the Adolescent*, 2nd edn (eds T. Eden, R. Barr, A. Bleyer, & M. Whiteson), pp. 1–10. Blackwell, Oxford.

Woodgate, R. L. (2005) Life is never the same: childhood cancer narratives. *European Journal of Cancer Care*, **15**, 8–18.

Woodgate, R. (2006) The importance of being there: perspectives of social support by adolescents with cancer. *Journal of Pediatric Oncology Nursing*, **23**(3), 122–134.

Young, B., Dixon-Woods, M., Findlay, M., & Heney, D. (2002) Parenting in a crisis: conceptualising mothers of children with cancer. *Social Science & Medicine*, **55**, 1835–1847.

Useful Contacts

Aftercure: information and support on long-term survival issues (www.aftercure.org).

Befrienders worldwide: (www.befrienders.org).

British Association of Counselling and Psychotherapy: advises on sources of individual and family therapy in the UK (www.counselling.co.uk; tel. 0870 443 5252).

Cancerbacup: general cancer information and support (www.cancesbacup.org.ok; tel. 0808 800 1234).

CLIC Sargent: childhood cancer information and support (www.clicsargent.org.uk; email: helpline@clicsargent.org.uk; free child cancer help line (09.00–17.00 Monday to Friday) tel. 0800 197 0068).

Cruse Bereavement Care: offers support and telephone help to young people (aged 12–18 years) (www.crusebereavementcare.org.uk; youthline tel. 0808 808 1677; general line tel. 0208 939 9530).

The Compassionate Friends: support for bereaved parents and families (www.tcf.org.uk; tel. 08451 23 23 04).

George Easton Memorial Trust (www.cancerinyoungadults-throughparentseyes.org).

Group Loop: online support for teenagers with cancer (www.grouploop.org).

Fertility Friends: online support and information on infertility issues (www.fertilityfriends.co.uk).

Leukaemia Care: support and information on blood cancers (www.leukaemiacare.org.uk; 24-hour care line 0800 169 6680).

Macmillan Cancer Support (www.macmillan.org.uk; Macmillan YouthLine 0808 808 0800 (09.00–22.00 Monday to Friday)).

Maggie's Centres: supportive spaces for patients, families, and friends (www.maggiescentres.org).

Mattdotcom: UK organisation dedicated to providing ill adolescents access to computer technology by funding for laptops and computers (www.mattdotcom.org.uk).

Samaritans: 24-hour emotional support (www.samaritans.org.uk; tel. 08457 90 90 90).

Further contacts

Teenage Cancer Trust: a UK charity devoted to improving the lives of teenagers and young adults with cancer (www.teenagecancertrust.org).

Teenagers and Young Adults with Cancer: national UK group for professionals (www.tyac.org.uk).

tic: information for teenagers about cancer (www.click4tic.org.uk/).

United Kingdom Childhood Cancer Study Group: clinical trial information about childhood cancers (www.ukccsg.org/; Email: info@ccsg.org.uk; Tel.: + 44 (0)116 249 4460).

The Willow Foundation: special days for seriously ill young adults age 16–40 years (www.willowfoundation.org.uk; Email: info@willowfoundation.org.uk; Tel.: 01707 259777).

Index